Traumatic Brain Injury Rehabilitation

Editors

AMY HAO
BLESSEN C. EAPEN

PHYSICAL MEDICINE AND REHABILITATION CLINICS OF NORTH AMERICA

www.pmr.theclinics.com

Consulting Editor
BLESSEN C. EAPEN

August 2024 • Volume 35 • Number 3

ELSEVIER

1600 John F. Kennedy Boulevard • Suite 1800 • Philadelphia, Pennsylvania, 19103-2899

http://www.theclinics.com

PHYSICAL MEDICINE AND REHABILITATION CLINICS OF NORTH AMERICA Volume 35, Number 3
August 2024 ISSN 1047-9651, 978-0-443-12897-4

Editor: Megan Ashdown
Developmental Editor: Nitesh Barthwal

Reprints. For copies of 100 or more of articles in this publication, please contact the Commercial Reprints Department, Elsevier Inc., 360 Park Avenue South, New York, NY 10010-1710. Tel.: 212-633-3874; Fax: 212-633-3820; E-mail: reprints@elsevier.com.

Physical Medicine and Rehabilitation Clinics of North America (ISSN 1047-9651) is published quarterly by Elsevier Inc., 360 Park Avenue South, New York, NY 10010-1710. Months of issue are February, May, August, and November. Business and Editorial Offices: 1600 John F. Kennedy Blvd., Suite 1800, Philadelphia, PA 19103-2899. Customer Service Office: 3251 Riverport Lane, Maryland Heights, MO 63043. Periodicals postage paid at New York, NY and additional mailing offices. Subscription price per year is $352.00 (US individuals), $100.00 (US students), $400.00 (Canadian individuals), $100.00 (Canadian students), $506.00 (foreign individuals), and $210.00 (foreign students). For institutional access pricing please contact Customer Service via the contact information below. Foreign air speed delivery is included in all *Clinics* subscription prices. All prices are subject to change without notice. **POSTMASTER:** Send address changes to *Physical Medicine and Rehabilitation Clinics of North America*, Customer Service Office: Elsevier Health Sciences Division, Subscription Customer Service, 3251 Riverport Lane, Maryland Heights, MO 63043. **Customer Service: 1-800-654-2452 (US). From outside of the United States, call 314-447-8871. Fax: 314-447-8029. E-mail: JournalsCustomerService-usa@elsevier.com (for print support); JournalsOnlineSupport-usa@elsevier.com (for online support).**

Physical Medicine and Rehabilitation Clinics of North America is indexed in *Excerpta Medica, MEDLINE/ PubMed (Index Medicus), Cinahl, and Cumulative Index to Nursing and Allied Health Literature.*

Contributors

CONSULTING EDITOR

BLESSEN C. EAPEN, MD
Chief, VA Greater Los Angeles Health Care System, Associate Clinical Professor, Division of Physical Medicine and Rehabilitation, Department of Medicine, David Geffen School of Medicine at UCLA, Los Angeles, California

EDITORS

AMY HAO, MD
Medical Director, Division of Physical Medicine and Rehabilitation, Evernorth Health Services, Los Angeles, California

BLESSEN C. EAPEN, MD
Chief, VA Greater Los Angeles Health Care System, Associate Clinical Professor, Division of Physical Medicine and Rehabilitation, Department of Medicine, David Geffen School of Medicine at UCLA, Los Angeles, California

AUTHORS

NICHOLAS ABRAMSON, MD
PGY-4, Department of Physical Medicine and Rehabilitation, Vanderbilt University Medical Center, Nashville, Tennessee

DERRICK ALLRED, MD
Associate Professor, Director of Brain Injury Rehabilitation, Department of Physical Medicine and Rehabilitation, University of Utah Health, Salt Lake City, Utah

PATRICK ARMISTEAD-JEHLE, PhD
Chief, Department of Veterans Affairs, Concussion Clinic, Munson Army Health Center, Fort Leavenworth, Kansas

HARSHA AYYALA, MD
Assistant Professor, Specialist, Department of Physical Medicine and Rehabilitation, Hackensack Meridian School of Medicine, JFK Johnson Rehabilitation Institute, Edison, New Jersey

SHEITAL BAVISHI, DO
Associate Professor – Clinical, Department of Physical Medicine and Rehabilitation, Medical Director, Brain Injury Program, Dodd Inpatient Rehabilitation Hospital, Ohio State University Wexner Medical Center, Columbus, Ohio

MERIDETH BYL, DO, MBA
Resident Physician, Physical Medicine and Rehabilitation Residency Program, Greater Los Angeles VA Healthcare System, Los Angeles, California

ZEKE CLEMMENS, DO
Physiatrist, Department of Physical Medicine and Rehabilitation, HonorHealth John C. Lincoln Medical Center, Scottsdale, Arizona

DOUGLAS B. COOPER, PhD
Adjunct Associate Professor, Departments of Psychiatry and Rehabilitation Medicine, University of Texas Health Science Center (UT-Health), South Texas VA Healthcare System, San Antonio Polytrauma Rehabilitation Center, San Antonio, Texas

BLESSEN C. EAPEN, MD
Chief, VA Greater Los Angeles Health Care System, Associate Clinical Professor, Division of Physical Medicine and Rehabilitation, Department of Medicine, David Geffen School of Medicine at UCLA, Los Angeles, California

STUART J. GLASSMAN, MD, MBA
Chief, Department of Physical Medicine and Rehabilitation, VA Northern California Healthcare System, Associate Professor, Department of Medicine, David Geffen School of Medicine at UCLA, Los Angeles, California

DUSTIN J. GORDON, PhD
Director, Neuropsychologic and Clinical Services, Rehabilitation Specialists, Fair Lawn, New Jersey

BRIAN D. GREENWALD, MD
Department of Physical Medicine and Rehabilitation, Professor, Medical Director of Center for Brain Injuries, Hackensack Meridian School of Medicine, Associate Medical Director, JFK Johnson Rehabilitation Institute, Edison, New Jersey

KRISTEN A. HARRIS, MD
Assistant Professor, Department of Physical Medicine and Rehabilitation, JFK Johnson Rehabilitation Institute, Edison, New Jersey

ZAYD HAYANI, MD
HonorHealth John C. Lincoln Medical Center, Scottsdale, Arizona

ANNE HUDAK, MD
Associate Professor, Department of Physical Medicine and Rehabilitation, Virginia Commonwealth University, Central Virginia Veterans Affairs Medical Center, Richmond, Virginia

CHERRY JUNN, MD
Assistant Professor, Department of Rehabilitation Medicine, University of Washington, Seattle, Washington

SCOTT R. LAKER, MD
Professor, Department of Physical Medicine and Rehabilitation, University of Colorado School of Medicine, Aurora, Colorado

KATHERINE LIN, MD
Physiatrist, Department of Physical Medicine and Rehabilitation, Palo Alto VAMC, Palo Alto, California

ASHLEY LUJAN, DO
Adjunct, Assistant Professor, Department of Rehabilitation Medicine, South Texas VAHCS, San Antonio, Texas

MAKINNA MOEN, MD
Resident Physician, Department of Physical Medicine and Rehabilitation, Virginia Commonwealth University, Richmond, Virginia

DIANE SCHRETZMAN MORTIMER, MD, MSN, FAAPMR
Medical Director, Department of Physical Medicine and Rehabilitation, Inpatient Brain Injury, Polytrauma Rehabilitation Center, Minneapolis VA Health Care System, Site Director, Brain Injury Medicine Fellowship, Department of Rehabilitation Medicine, University of Minnesota, Minneapolis, Minnesota

UDAI NANDA, DO
Chief, Pain Management Section, Director, Headache Center of Excellence, Department of Physical Medicine and Rehabilitation, Pain Management, VA Greater Los Angeles Healthcare System, Associate Program Director, Pain Medicine Fellowship Program, Division of Physical Medicine and Rehabilitation, Department of Medicine, UCLA David Geffen School of Medicine, Los Angeles, California

CHRISTIAN NICOLOSI, MD
Resident, Department of Physical Medicine and Rehabilitation, University of Colorado School of Medicine, Aurora, Colorado

VICTORIA O'CONNOR, PhD
Post Doctoral Researcher, Department of Veterans Affairs, W. G. (Bill) Hefner VA Healthcare System, Salisbury, North Carolina; Veterans Integrated Service Networks (VISN)-6 Mid-Atlantic Mental Illness, Research Education and Clinical Center, Durham, North Carolina; Wake Forest School of Medicine, Winston-Salem, North Carolina

SANJOG PANGARKAR, MD
Professor, Division of Physical Medicine and Rehabilitation, Department of Medicine, UCLA David Geffen School of Medicine, Department of Physical Medicine and Rehabilitation, Pain Management, VA Greater Los Angeles Healthcare System, Los Angeles, California

QUYNH GIAO PHAM, MD
Clinical Professor, Division of Physical Medicine and Rehabilitation, Department of Medicine, David Geffen School of Medicine at UCLA, Los Angeles, California; Physical Medicine and Rehabilitation Residency Program, Greater Los Angeles VA Healthcare System, David Geffen School of Medicine at UCLA, Palos Verdes Estates, California

CLAUSYL J. PLUMMER II, MD
Assistant Professor, Department of Physical Medicine and Rehabilitation, Vanderbilt University Medical Center, Nashville, Tennessee

DAVID ROTHMAN, PhD
Psychologist, Department of Physical Medicine and Rehabilitation, Virginia Commonwealth University, Richmond, Virginia

ROSANNA SABINI, DO
Physiatrists, Department of Physical Medicine and Rehabilitation, Donald and Barbara Zucker School of Medicine at Hofstra/Northwell Health, South Shore University Hospital, Bay Shore, New York

GABRIEL SANCHEZ, DO
Internal Medicine Specialist, Physical Medicine and Rehabilitation Residency Program, Greater Los Angeles VA Healthcare System, Los Angeles, California

ROBERT SHURA, PhD
Neuropsychologist, Department of Veterans Affairs, W. G. (Bill) Hefner VA Healthcare System, Salisbury, North Carolina; Veterans Integrated Service Networks (VISN)-6 Mid-Atlantic Mental Illness, Research Education and Clinical Center (MIRECC), Durham, North Carolina; Wake Forest School of Medicine, Winston-Salem, North Carolina; Via College of Osteopathic Medicine, Blacksburg, Virginia

BRUNO SUBBARAO, DO
Physician, Director of Whole Health, Wellness and Administrative Medicine, Phoenix Veterans Healthcare System, Phoenix, Arizona

DAVID UNDERHILL, MD
Resident Physician, Division of Physical Medicine and Rehabilitation, Department of Medicine, UCLA David Geffen School of Medicine, Los Angeles, California

ALLISON WALLINGFORD, MD
Physiatrist, Department of Rehabilitation Medicine, University of Washington, Seattle, Washington

LEVI WEITZEL, BS
Medical Student, Department of Physical Medicine and Rehabilitation, Ohio State University College of Medicine, Columbus, Ohio

GRACE ZHANG, MD
Chief Resident Physician, Division of Physical Medicine and Rehabilitation, Department of Medicine, UCLA David Geffen School of Medicine, Los Angeles, California

Contents

The focus of this article is on the acute management of traumatic brain injury. The article focuses on the classification of traumatic brain injury, general acute management of traumatic brain injury, the role of the physiatrist on this team, and lastly, behavioral and family considerations in the acute care setting. The article includes a focus on physiologic systems, strategies for the management of various aspects of brain injury, and consideration of factors associated with the continuum of care. Overall, the article reviews this critical period of brain injury recovery and provides a primer for the physiatrist.

This article reviews the definition, assessment, neuroimaging, treatment, and rehabilitation for disorders of consciousness after an acquired brain injury. It also explores special considerations and new neuromodulation treatment options.

According to the Centers for Disease Control, in 2019, there were approximately 223,135 hospitalizations in the United States related to traumatic brain injury (TBI). If not managed properly, these patients can suffer complications with significant negative implications with respect to morbidity, mortality, and long-term functional prognosis. It is imperative that medical providers who care for patients with TBI across the entire spectrum of care readily diagnose and treat the sequela associated with moderate–severe brain trauma. This article will focus on some of the key medical issues that providers may encounter during acute inpatient rehabilitation.

Concussions are the most common type of traumatic brain injury. They result from external force to the head that causes a neuro-metabolic cascade to unfold. This can then lead to a variety of symptoms in the domains of physical, cognition, mood, and sleep. Concussions are a clinical diagnosis but it is important to rule out acute intracranial pathology through a detailed history and physical examination in addition to possible head imaging. Treatment should include an individualized approach that focuses on what domains are affected after concussion.

Persistent symptoms following a mild traumatic brain injury are challenging to treat and pose a significant threat to community reintegration. Early recognition and intervention play a pivotal role in preventing the development of persistent symptoms by providing education that emphasizes clear recovery expectations and the high likelihood of full symptom resolution. We recommend early development of a personalized treatment plan, offering guidance on gradual return to activity and specific symptom-targeted treatments that may incorporate both pharmacologic and nonpharmacologic interventions.

Sports-related concussions (SRC) have been a topic of interest for decades and are a prevalent risk of sports participation. The definition of SRC continues to evolve but includes a plausible mechanism and associated symptoms of injury. Rates of concussion vary among sports, and many sports have adopted rule changes to limit this risk for its athletes. There has been a considerable effort to prevent the occurrence of SRC, as well as a focus on safe return to learn and sport alike. There is growing concern about the ramifications of concussions, which will continue to warrant further investigation.

Traumatic brain injury (TBI) in the military can involve distinct injury mechanisms, diagnostic challenges, treatments, and course of recovery. TBI has played a prominent role in recent conflicts, causing significant morbidity and mortality. Blast-related TBI in combat settings is often accompanied by other physical injuries. Military TBIs of all severities can lead to prolonged recoveries and persistent sequelae. The complex interplay between TBI, pain, and mental health conditions can significantly complicate diagnosis and recovery. Military and veteran health settings and programs provide comprehensive care along the continuum of TBI recovery rehabilitation with the goal of optimizing recovery and function.

This article will identify common causes of pain following traumatic brain injury (TBI), discuss current treatment strategies for these complaints, and help tailor treatments for both acute and chronic settings. We will also briefly discuss primary and secondary headache disorders, followed by common secondary pain disorders that may be related to trauma.

Neuropsychological evaluations can be helpful in the aftermath of traumatic brain injury. Cognitive functioning is assessed using standardized assessment tools and by comparing an individual's scores on testing to normative data. These evaluations examine objective cognitive functioning as well as other factors that have been shown to influence performance on cognitive tests (eg, psychiatric conditions, sleep) in an attempt to answer a specific question from referring providers. Referral questions may focus on the extent of impairment, the trajectory of recovery, or ability to return to work, sport, or the other previous activity.

This article focuses on neuropathologic diagnostic criteria for chronic traumatic encephalopathy (CTE) and consensus research diagnostic criteria for traumatic encephalopathy syndrome (TES). CTE as a tauopathy has a unique pattern for diagnosis and differs from other neurodegenerative diseases. We discuss the history, neuropathology, and mechanism of CTE as well as the preliminary reasearch diagnostic criteria for TES, which is the proposed clinical presentation of suspected CTE.

One of the primary goals in traumatic brain injury (TBI) treatment is to minimize secondary brain damage and promote neuroprotection. In TBI rehabilitation, we seek to facilitate neurologic recovery and restore what independence is possible given a patient's physical and cognitive impairments. These goals must be balanced with treatment of the various symptoms that may occur following TBI. This is challenging given the fact that many of the typical treatments for certain symptoms also come with side effects which could be problematic in the TBI population.

Achieving effective community reintegration is important to maximize recovery in patients with traumatic brain injury, simultaneously limiting caregiver burden and improving satisfaction with quality of life. Certain medical complications that are common after brain injury may impact community reintegration, and should be addressed by the physician in a systematic approach. Additionally certain social and environmental factors such as mobility or return to work or school may arise, and should be addressed proactively by the physician. Inpatient/residential or outpatient programs with case management and a multi-disciplinary team can facilitate community reentry for patients, and should be considered when available.

Bruno Subbarao, Zayd Hayani, and Zeke Clemmens

Traumatic brain injury (TBI) is a complex condition associated with a range of persistent symptoms including headaches, cognitive dysfunction, mental fatigue, insomnia, and mood disorders. Conventional treatments for TBI-related symptoms can be insufficient, leading to interest in complementary and integrative medicine (CIM) approaches. This comprehensive article examines the existing literature on CIM modalities, including mind-body interventions, acupuncture/acupressure, herbal remedies, nutritional supplements, biofeedback, yoga, and tai chi in the context of managing secondary complications following TBI. The article highlights potential benefits and limitations of CIM modalities, while acknowledging the need for further research to better establish efficacy and safety in this specific population.

Stuart J. Glassman

Traumatic Brain Injury (TBI) cases often involve both medical and legal issues, litigation and prolonged recovery timelines. As TBI cases are often complex, and can have a significant impact on the lives of the patients and their families/caregivers, having a comprehensive understanding of the causes, diagnoses, treatments and long term outcomes will be valuable in understanding the medical and legal aspects of this type of injury. Patients, families, and health care professionals will all benefit from a deeper understanding of the medical and legal aspects of TBI, which should help improve rehabilitation and recovery outcomes.

PHYSICAL MEDICINE AND REHABILITATION CLINICS OF NORTH AMERICA

VISIT THE CLINICS ONLINE!
Access your subscription at:
www.theclinics.com

PHYSICAL MEDICINE AND REHABILITATION CLINICS OF NORTH AMERICA

RECENT ISSUES

May 2024

November 2023

Foreword

Assessment, Management, and Rehabilitation of Traumatic Brain Injury

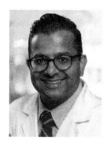

Blessen C. Eapen, MD
Consulting Editor

Traumatic Brain Injury (TBI) is defined as a violent jolt or blow to the head or body, by an external force, causing a physiologic disruption in brain function. TBI is often considered a significant cause of morbidity and mortality worldwide. In the United States, the annual incidence of TBI is estimated to be over 1.7 million, while the worldwide incidence ranges from 20 million to 79 million individuals sustaining TBI.

While there are varying classification schemaa for the grading of TBI severity (mild, moderate, or severe), it typically involves one of the following criteria for diagnosis: loss of consciousness, loss of memory before or after the injury (posttraumatic amnesia), alteration of mental status (eg, dazed or confused), Glasgow Coma Scale (after 30 minutes), structural imaging changes, and/or focal neurologic deficits. TBI can be present with a variety of symptoms depending on the severity of injury. For example, mild TBI (concussions) can present as physical (eg, headache, nausea, dizziness), sensory (eg, blurry vision, tinnitus, photosensitivity), or cognitive/behavioral/mental health (eg, insomnia, mood changes, concentration) symptoms. Moderate to severe TBI symptoms can present with a variety of complications, such as spasticity, endocrine abnormalities, behavioral conditions, cranial nerve injuries, autonomic instability, posttraumatic epilepsy, posttraumatic agitation, and so forth. The management of brain injuries is a complex process, often ongoing, individualized, and best managed by an interdisciplinary team.

We hope this timely special issue provides a comprehensive overview of the evaluation, management, and rehabilitation of all severities of TBI. In addition, we provide a succinct review of special populations (military TBI, sports concussions, disorders of consciousness) and discuss the evolution of Chronic Traumatic Encephalopathy. We

Phys Med Rehabil Clin N Am 35 (2024) xiii–xiv
https://doi.org/10.1016/j.pmr.2024.05.002
1047-9651/24/© 2024 Published by Elsevier Inc.

especially want to thank our esteemed colleagues for sharing their valuable experience and expertise with the physical medicine and rehabilitation community!

Blessen C. Eapen, MD
Division of Physical Medicine and Rehabilitation
David Geffen School of Medicine at UCLA
VA Greater Los Angeles Health Care System
11301 Wilshire Boulevard
Los Angeles, CA 90073, USA

E-mail addresses:
beapen@ucla.mednet.edu; blessen.eapen2@va.gov

Preface

Traumatic Brain Injury Rehabilitation

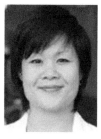
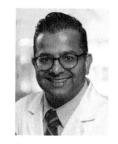

Amy Hao, MD   Blessen C. Eapen, MD

Editors

Traumatic brain injury (TBI) is a major cause of death and disability worldwide. The field of TBI rehabilitation is constantly evolving with advances in research, technology, and clinical practice guidelines. Since the previous issue of TBI Rehabilitation, there has been increased attention to the management of sports concussions and disorders of consciousness, clinical criteria and diagnosis of Chronic Traumatic Encephalopathy (CTE), and continued expansion of TBI treatment options both pharmacologic and nonpharmacologic.

Rehabilitation specialists manage a spectrum of TBI from mild to severe injuries from presentation to the chronic phase of disease, with the goal of minimizing impairments and promoting functional independence and quality of life after TBI. This issue of *Physical Medicine and Rehabilitation Clinics of North America* seeks to provide a comprehensive and current review of TBI rehabilitation by experts in the field. Articles cover the continuum of care starting with initial management in the acute hospital and inpatient rehabilitation settings. This includes the approach to those with disorders of consciousness, a particularly complex clinical condition. There is a focus on common persistent symptoms and pain syndromes, such as headache. We delve into the role of neuropsychological testing on evaluation and ongoing assessment of TBI. Of great interest for research and media in recent years is the relationship between TBI, especially sports-related concussions, and the development of CTE. We cover the subject of military TBI, as TBI is the signature injury of the post-9/11 conflicts, and service members with combat injuries are distinctive in that many injuries are the result of blast exposures, and they have trauma-related comorbidities. Pharmacologic options are detailed for treatment of TBI symptoms of all severities, as well as integrative medicine treatments that can enhance and supplement the treatment plan. Finally, we review

Phys Med Rehabil Clin N Am 35 (2024) xv–xvi
https://doi.org/10.1016/j.pmr.2024.05.001
1047-9651/24/© 2024 Published by Elsevier Inc.

complications that impact community reintegration as well as the intricacies of medicolegal issues with TBI.

The goal of this issue is to give clinicians the tools needed to provide up-to-date, evidence-based care to the TBI population. We hope readers find it to be a valuable resource.

DISCLOSURES

The authors have nothing to disclose.

Amy Hao, MD
Division of Physical Medicine
and Rehabilitation
Evernorth Health Services
Los Angeles, CA, USA

Blessen C. Eapen, MD
Physical Medicine and Rehabilitation Service
VA Greater Los Angeles Health Care System
Division of Physical Medicine
and Rehabilitation
David Geffen School of Medicine at UCLA
Los Angeles, CA, USA

E-mail addresses:
amyhao@gmail.com (A. Hao)
Blessen.Eapen2@va.gov (B.C. Eapen)

Acute Management of Moderate to Severe Traumatic Brain Injury

Anne Hudak, MD[a,b], Rosanna Sabini, DO[c], Makinna Moen, MD[a], David Rothman, PhD[a],*

KEYWORDS

- Acute traumatic brain injury • Assessment and management • Continuum of care
- Behavioral intervention

KEY POINTS

- Moderate to severe brain injury effect multiple systems that require consistent assessment and management in acute care settings.
- Physiatrists have a unique and vital role in consultation due to their unique set of skills.
- Behavior management and family intervention are important in acute settings to promote long term wellbeing.

INTRODUCTION

The goals of this article are to provide background and highlights of acute moderate-severe traumatic brain injury (TBI) care for the physiatrist. TBI which occurs in all age groups and populations, results from the application of force to the brain, causing a disturbance or disruption of brain function with heterogeneous macroscopic and microscopic injury.[1] There are varied mechanisms of injury, including motor vehicle-related, falls, violent trauma, sports, and being struck by an object. While there are a reported 27 million injuries per year globally,[2] this number is an underestimation as many who sustain a mild TBI or concussion do not present for medical care. The CDC estimates there are approximately 60,500 TBI-related deaths in the United States.[3]

[a] Department of Physical Medicine and Rehabilitation, Virginia Commonwealth University, 223 E. Marshall Street Box 980677, Richmond, VA 23284-0667, USA; [b] Central Virginia Veterans Affairs Medical Center, 1201 Broad Rock Boulevard, Richmond, VA 23249-4915, USA; [c] Department of Physical Medicine & Rehabilitation, Donald and Barbara Zucker School of Medicine at Hofstra/Northwell Health, South Shore University Hospital, Bay Shore, NY 11706, USA
* Corresponding author.
E-mail address: david.rothman@vcuhealth.org

Phys Med Rehabil Clin N Am 35 (2024) 479–492
https://doi.org/10.1016/j.pmr.2024.02.002
1047-9651/24/© 2024 Elsevier Inc. All rights reserved.
pmr.theclinics.com

TBI can be classified in several ways, with the most traditional of these by using the Glasgow Coma Scale (GCS)[4] which separates injury severity utilizing clinical responses to stimuli (ie, verbal response, motor response, eye response); scores of 3 to 8 are categorized as severe, 9 to 12 as moderate, 13 to 15 as mild. While common clinical interventions, such as intubation and neuromuscular blockade, and the concurrent use of alcohol or illicit drugs may limit the application of this scale, it does not require specialized equipment or movement of the injured individual, so it is easily applied. The Marshall[5] and Rotterdam[6] CT Classification systems use imaging findings, such as basal cistern compression, midline shift, and mass lesions for stratification; however, imaging represents only one time point and reevaluation requires further imaging, making these systems less user-friendly. Mechanism of injury, such as blast, closed, or penetrating injuries, is another way to classify TBI.[7]

Advancements in medical knowledge and technology have led to improved understanding and care for TBI. Care for individuals with an acute TBI starts in the prehospital setting by applying the ABC's of resuscitation.[1] Lack of attention to these critical elements can lead to further disease burden. Primary injury results from the initial direct force to the brain tissue or cranium; examples of primary injuries include intracranial hemorrhage, skull fractures, and diffuse axonal injury.[7] Activated by primary injury, secondary injury are the elaborate biochemical and cellular interactions leading to oxidative stress, free radical formation, cell membrane failure, mitochondrial dysfunction, and apoptosis.[1,7,8] Disruption of the blood brain barrier can lead to inflammatory processes and disruption of cerebral autoregulation.[8] While there are a number of efforts in prevention for primary brain injury (ie, seat belt usage, air bags, helmet wearing), second injury has the most potential for intervention.

SYSTEMIC EFFECTS
Cardiovascular

The impact of moderate-severe TBI is felt not just in the central nervous system. Numerous bodily systems are affected by the flooding of catecholamines and inflammatory responses. Sympathetic overload leads to cardiovascular system changes that include elevated blood pressure and heart rate. The resultant increased cardiac oxygen demands can lead to cardiac ischemia. Just as easily, a stunned myocardium without ischemia can manifest from a neurologic injury. This can lead to cardiogenic pulmonary edema and systemic hypotension.[8] Given its association with cerebral edema and poorer outcomes, hypotension should be addressed immediately.[8] Raith and colleagues recommend targets of SBP greater than 100 mm Hg in ages less than or equal to 60 years of age and SBP greater than 120 mm Hg in those greater than 60 years, citing limitations in the recommendations of Brain Trauma Foundation Guidelines.[8] Hypotension is typically corrected through fluid administration, and the use of vasopressors and inotropes. Normotonic crystalloids are preferred for resuscitation; albumin and hypotonic fluids are not recommended.[2] Hypotonic fluids may lead to fluid shifts across the blood brain barrier, leading to or exacerbating cerebral edema and elevation of the ICP.[9] To date, no definitive recommendations are available regarding when to transfuse red blood cells.[2,8] Norepinephrine is the most commonly used first line vasopressor, but there are no high quality studies directly comparing vasopressors in TBI management.[2,8]

Pulmonary

Intubation for individuals with moderate-severe TBI is used for airway protection and maintenance of oxygenation, but there is the possibility of aspiration or other lung injury from the time of the injury.[8] Protective ventilation techniques include the avoidance of high tidal volumes. Positive end expiratory pressure (PEEP) up to 15 cm H20 may be used without an increase in ICP. Besides maintaining oxygenation within normal physiologic parameters ($Pa_{O_2} > 60$ mm Hg), a main goal of ventilation is the maintenance of normocapnia (35–45 mm Hg) due to the direct relationship between cerebral blood flow and levels of CO_2. Both hypercapnia and hypocapnia exacerbate secondary injury. Hypercapnia causes cerebral vasodilatation resulting in increased intracranial pressure (ICP) and hypocapnia causes cerebral vasoconstriction leading to decreased ICP and possible ischemia.[7] Hypoventilation should be considered as a temporary emergency measure to manage cerebral herniation.[7,8,10]

Coagulopathy

Moderate-severe TBI can lead to hyper- and hypo-coagulable states occurring in a range from 7% to 63% of individuals.[7,11] While not fully understood, trauma is associated with the release of procoagulant molecules and platelet activating molecules,[11] endothelial dysfunction and hyperfibrinolysis.[2] In addition, prolonged immobility is associated with hypercoagulable states.[11] Treatment should prioritize stopping hemorrhage and targeting the underlying mechanism.

Hypothalamic-pituitary-adrenal Axis

Endocrine dysfunction after TBI results from direct damage to the hypothalamus, pituitary stalk, and pituitary gland. It is estimated that more than 25% of individuals with TBI develop hypopituitarism.[8] The anatomy of this system, with its location at the base of the skull and long hypophyseal vessels, makes it vulnerable to direct trauma, ischemic injury, and elevated ICP.[12] Risk factors for pituitary dysfunction include TBI severity, hypotension, hypoxia, older age, and prolonged ICU stay.[8] Twenty-two to 26% of individuals with severe TBI develop diabetes insipidus (DI), and 12.7% develop the syndrome of inappropriate ADH secretion (SIADH) during the acute period.[12] Screening is recommended when there are signs of pituitary insufficiency: refractory hypotension, hypoglycemia, hyponatremia, or electrolyte abnormalities.[8,12] The management of DI can include fluid replacement to maintain euvolemia and DDAVP when high urine output is present.[8] The management of SIADH involves free-water restriction, hypertonic saline, urea, and potentially vaptans.[13] The majority of individuals with TBI recover endocrine function over time.

MANAGEMENT
Sedation

The use of sedation is appropriate in the critical care setting to decrease metabolic demand. Typical sedative agents are midazolam, and propofol,[9] with propofol having the added benefit of ICP reduction.[8] Ketamine is emerging as an alternative sedative agent.[14] It has been associated with the lowest occurrence of spreading depolarizations[15] and provides a potential target to reduce secondary brain injury. Daily breaks in sedation are recommended except in the face of uncontrolled ICP.[8,9] Barbiturate coma is used to improve control of refractory ICP when maximal medical management has failed[8] and should use continuous EEG monitoring for burst suppression. Opioids are appropriate for pain management. Neuromuscular blockade helps to further reduce metabolic demand.

Sympathetic Hyperactivity

Sympathetic hyperactivity is characterized as excessive sympathetic nervous system activity manifesting as cycles of agitation, tachycardia, diaphoresis, temperature elevation, hypertension, and posturing.[7,8] Resulting from the loss of inhibition of excitation, sympathetic hyperactivity is present in 8% to 10% of individuals.[7] It typically manifests about 1 to 2 weeks postinjury and can be triggered by noxious stimuli.[7] Sympathetic hyperactivity is associated with longer ICU stays, longer ventilation times, and lower Glasgow Outcome Scores.[11] Treatment should be individualized and often consists of adrenergic blockers, typically propranolol.[11] Other agents such as centrally acting alpha-2 agonists and opioids are other commonly used medications.[8]

Posttraumatic Seizures

This topic is covered in depth elsewhere in this). Seizure activity after brain injury is delineated by time of occurrence as early (within 7 days) or late (after 7 days).[7] Early PTS is found in 16.9% to greater than 20% of individuals, and can lead to neurologic deterioration through increased cerebral metabolic demands and excitotoxicity.[8,11] Subclinical seizures occur in up to 30% of individuals with moderate and severe TBI, therefore supporting the use of continuous EEG monitoring to ensure detection.[7] The presence of early seizures increases the risk of posttraumatic epilepsy.[7] According to the Brain Trauma Foundation Guidelines, there is sufficient evidence to recommend phenytoin to decrease the incidence of early posttraumatic seizures if the benefit is determined to outweigh the risks.[10] The report indicates there was insufficient data to support the use of levetiracetam,[10] despite its more advantageous drug profile and its frequent use.[9] Research does not substantiate the use of seizure prophylaxis beyond 7 days.[7]

GENERAL SUPPORTIVE MEASURES
Nutrition

TBI results in a catabolic situation with caloric demand up to 50% to 100% of baseline.[9] The Brain Trauma Foundation Guidelines recommend the replacement of basal caloric needs at least by the fifth day but no more than the seventh day post injury.[10] Whenever possible enteric feeding is recommended.[10] Delayed gastric emptying must be taken into account when planning enteral nutrition.[2] Previous guidelines have recommended post-pyloric over gastric feeding in severe TBI to reduce the risk of ventilator-associated pneumonia.[10,16] However, other meta-analyses[17] have not demonstrated clinical benefit in postpyloric versus gastric feeding in the intensive care setting.

Thromboprophylaxis

Trauma is a hypercoagulable state due to the release of platelet activating molecules, immobility, and release of procoagulant molecules.[11] The obvious risk of utilizing pharmacologic agents for deep vein thrombosis (DVT) prevention in moderate and severe TBI is increased intracranial hemorrhage. The Brain Trauma Foundation guidelines note that pharmacologic agents as well as pneumatic compression devices may be used for DVT prophylaxis as long as the brain injury is stable.[10] There is insufficient evidence to recommend the exact timing to initiate DVT prophylaxis, but delaying prophylaxis beyond 72 hours increases the risk of thromboembolism.[11] The modified Berne-Norwood Criteria are available to assist in decision making.[11]

Glycemic Control

Recommendations for glucose management after TBI have varied over time. Studies using tight glucose control had a higher incidence of hypoglycemia with varied outcomes, from improved neurologic outcomes to no difference.[2] It is prudent to aim for intermediate glucose levels of between 60 and 180 mg/dL.[7,8]

Gastrointestinal Ulcer Prophylaxis

Gastrointestinal bleeding is a serious complication for individuals in neurocritical care, but the frequency is low.[9] Risk factors include ventilator dependence, coma, coagulopathy, and previous GI bleeds. Preferred medications are proton pump inhibitors and H2 receptor blockers, with an enteral over IV route preferred.[9] Early enteral feeding is appropriate.[8]

Bowel Care

The avoidance of constipation and straining for bowel movements is important due to the associated elevation of ICP. The use of laxatives is appropriate to avoid this scenario.[8]

MANAGEMENT OF INTRACRANIAL PRESSURE

The classic Monro-Kellie Doctrine describes the cranium as a closed space filled with 3 components: CSF, brain tissues, and blood. Due to the closed space, an increase in one of these will result in a decrease in the others. Of those listed, fluid is the most difficult to compress, therefore, it is more likely that the brain tissue will bear the brunt of the space limitations. Intracranial pressure (ICP) is the force exerted by the contents of the cranium (CSF, brain tissue, and blood). Measured via external or internal monitors,[2] the target is less than 22 to 25 mm Hg.[8] Increased ICP commonly occurs after severe TBI and is can present as a set of signs known as Cushing's Triad: tachycardia, hypertension, and irregular or depressed respiration. In severe TBI, 4 patterns of ICP elevation have been observed: (1) Early less than 72 hrs, (2) Late greater than 72 hrs, (3) Bimodal less than 72 hrs and greater than 72 hrs, and (4) Continuous elevation.[7]

As the intracranial pressure rises, not only is brain tissue compressed, but there is also compression of the vasculature, limiting the delivery of oxygen and vital components. The measurement of cerebral perfusion pressure (CPP) is critical and is defined as the difference between the mean arterial pressure (MAP) and intracranial pressure (ICP). The preferred CPP target varies between 60 and 70 mm Hg, with age and cerebral autoregulation taken into account.[2] To achieve the target CPP, either ICP or MAP can be altered based on the situation.[2] MAP can be adjusted through the changes in volume status or vasoactive medications.[2] Decrease of ICP is accomplished via sedation, removal of CSF, and/or hypoventilation.

Identified as a key to the management of severe TBI,[1] a stepwise approach is recommended for the management of ICP. Based on intracranial pressure and brain oxygenation, recommendations are divided into tiers. Tiers range from 0 to 3, with Tier 0 covering basic strategies for individuals with ICP monitoring, up to Tier 3, which includes barbiturate coma, mild hypothermia, and secondary decompressive craniotomy.[18] Failure to manage elevated ICP can lead to the herniation of the brain which can present with pupillary change (fixed, dilated), motor posturing (decorticate or decerebrate) and the presence of Cushing's Triad: tachycardia, hypertension and irregular or depressed respiration.[7] Herniation of the brain often leads to death.

SURGICAL INTERVENTIONS

When refractory intracranial hypertension is present, surgical decompressive craniotomy is considered with a goal to improve brain tissue oxygenation and reduce

ICP. The Brain Trauma Foundation recommended larger flaps over smaller flaps for improved neurologic outcomes with severe TBI.[9] The RESCUEicp trial indicated the use of secondary decompressive craniotomy resulted in shorter ICU length-of-stays and decreased mortality compared with medical management.[19] The mortality rates at 6 months for the surgical and medical groups were 26.9% and 48.9%, respectively.[2] However, the rates of good recovery with higher levels of functional outcomes were similar between groups.

ACUTE CARE SETTING AND ROLE OF PHYSIATRY CONSULTATION
Initial Assessment

As a consult service in Physical Medicine & Rehabilitation (PM&R), physiatrists are well equipped to meet the comprehensive needs of individuals with moderate and severe traumatic brain injuries. Physiatrists have the expertise in functional assessment, coordination of multidisciplinary care, and conceptualization of goals, which ultimately provides the foresight into the challenges that lay in the short- and long-term care of these individuals. In the acute care management of TBI, the primary and immediate focus is to stabilize the individuals and prevent secondary injuries and complications. The initial Physiatry assessment includes a history of the traumatic event, including the mechanism of injury (eg, motor vehicle accident, fall, sports-related injury), timing, and associated factors (eg, alcohol use) associated with the injury. Any assessments and interventions performed at the scene, during transportation, and acute care hospitalizations should be summarized, as they can have an influence on outcomes. Specifically, the duration and details of loss of consciousness and post-traumatic amnesia, as well as the Glasgow Coma Scale (GCS), can impact recovery trajectories.[20–23] Additional relevant documentation in a consultation of moderate to severe traumatic brain injuries includes.

- Imaging results (extent, location, progression of brain injury, additional injuries sustained)
- Diagnostic test results (eg, EEG)
- Medical interventions (eg, intubation, cardiac arrest)
- Surgical procedures (eg, craniotomies, fracture repairs)
- Complications (eg, hypoxia, intracranial hypertension, hydrocephalus, difficulties in wakefulness, aphasias, weakness, deep venous thrombosis, infections, aspirations, seizures, sleep difficulties, pain, headaches, and so forth)
- Restrictions in range of motion (ROM) or weight-bearing
- Pending or planned interventions

The PM&R consultation should also contain relevant medical history of pre-existing conditions, previous head injuries, psychiatric disorders, substance abuse, and medications to identify potential risk factors that can impact recovery.[24,25] A social history and the community support available need to be explored to provide insight into the individual's past functional abilities, living environment, and available resources, as this can influence rehabilitation recommendations.

Physical and Functional Assessment

When performing the physical xamination, the neurologic, musculoskeletal, cognitive, and behavioral aspects should be documented while noting vital signs, as they may offer insight into response to stressors including pain or autonomic stability. Pertinent positives noted in the examination of pupillary response, cranial nerves, motor and sensory, including weakness, paralysis, posturing, involuntary movements (tremors or spasticity), vision or hearing impairments, fine motor control, abnormal reflexive responses, dysmetria, or impaired balance/sense of position or neglect should be sought out. Memory, attention, executive function, as well as language impairments are essential to note. Formal assessment using specific tools such as the MOCA,[26] can be confounded by distractions and pain. Instead, one can perform and acquire such relative cognitive findings indirectly. Although seemingly simplistic, a question such as "Can you show me how to turn on the TV?" or "Can you sit at the edge of the bed?" can provide significant information about the individual's functional status, coordination, language comprehension, attention, working memory, executive function, verbal and visual memory, problem-solving skills, sensory and perceptual abilities as well as behavior in response to the request.

For individuals with Disorders of Consciousness (DOC), the Coma Recovery Scale-Revised (CRS-R)[27] can be a valuable tool for objectively measuring the level of consciousness, monitoring recovery, as well as providing discussion points on potential outcomes.[27,28] If possible, the CRS-R should be administered by several trained clinicians at multiple time points to the emergence of patterns or trends across the spectrum of DOC.[29–31]

When a formal assessment can be obtained by Physical and Occupational Therapists and is combined with the Physiatrists' assessment of the individual, it guides short term functional goals. A speech and language pathologist can perform a more formal cognitive assessment in addition to the evaluation of language and swallowing dysfunctions.

Ongoing Assessments and Interventions

During the acute care stay, from the initial visit to discharge planning, implementing early rehabilitation interventions plays a significant role in the recovery of individuals with moderate to severe TBI. Initially, physical intervention may need to be passive such as providing range of motion and using appropriate positioning aides to ensure the ongoing prevention of complications related to immobility. For those with DOC, interventions may include sensory stimulation interventions (eg, tactile, thermal stimulation, and/or visual). If individuals improve physically and cognitively, as they are being medically optimized, individuals should be transitioned to performing more active and functional exercises (eg, grasping, fine hand motor exercise).

Subsequent physiatry encounters should continue to document and track ongoing physical examination findings, specifically the neuromusculoskeletal and cognitive status, to guide treatment decisions and alter goals on progress for improving ongoing outcomes and recovery. Rehabilitation interventions should be monitored and tailored to the individual's specific impairments for optimizing progress through the acute hospital stay, which will ultimately derive the rehabilitation discharge recommendations. Limitations in neurocognitive, musculoskeletal, and function will also determine the need for pharmacologic and nonpharmacological interventions used by the physiatrist to manage the complications that may arise from the indirect and direct effects of moderate to severe brain injuries. Goals for medications are to improve wakefulness while monitoring for impulsivity and limiting the need for constant supervision or restraints, which ultimately are barriers to achieving discharge. Hence, sleep should be prioritized to occur at night to ensure a routine daytime/nighttime routine with maximal daytime participation with staff.[32]

Challenges with behavior can arise if one is not already anticipating the psychocognitive pathophysiology of traumatic brain injuries.

Discharge Planning

Discharge planning can begin early into to the acute care setting to ensure a smooth transition. Achieving medical optimization, individual and/or family education, and postacute care rehabilitation decisions also highlights the Physiatrist's important role in the coordination of care. Factors involved in deciding rehabilitation discharge planning should include.

- Admission Diagnosis
- Prior level of function
- Current level of function
- Expected time for recovery and transition into community living
- Need for active medical comorbidity management
- Need for multidisciplinary care (ie, neuropsychology, occupational therapy, physical therapy, speech and language pathology, recreational therapy)
- Health insurance coverage

Typically, most of the above factors are required for admission into inpatient rehabilitation facilities. Unfortunately, for some individuals who are either considered significantly impaired or unable to return to community living, the alternate discharge plan is to subacute rehabilitation programs or long-term acute care hospitals (L-TACHs). Home discharges are usually reserved for higher functioning individuals who can mobilize without significant assist and have adequate support or supervision from their families. Some individuals may have significant challenges if limited by financial resources and may require extensive family training in providing rehabilitative and medical care. Community resources and services should be identified to support the individual's long-term integration into the community.

Continuum of Care

Physiatrists should be part of the acute care hospital discharge plans to ensure individuals with moderate to severe brain injuries are maintained in the rehabilitative continuity of care. Whether discharge to a postacute care facility of home, follow-up will ensure that any emerging needs or challenges are addressed, and adjustments are made to the rehabilitation plan accordingly. This will ensure a relatively smoother transition to gaps that may develop in active medical management or appropriate therapy interventions, as well as establish a monitor on progress toward achieving optimal functional outcomes and quality of life, including cognitive, physical, and emotional readiness for reentering the workforce or pursuing educational goals. Therefore, Physiatrists play a vital role in optimizing outcomes and improving the quality of life for individuals with individuals in all aspects of traumatic brain injured individuals. Collaborative efforts among health care professionals, individuals, and families are crucial throughout the acute care phase into the discharge to facilitate successful recovery and rehabilitation outcomes.

Mental Health Management

Within the context of moderate to severe TBI, there is an increasing focus on mental health, especially as we consider TBI as a chronic condition.[33] For the purposes of this article, we will focus on the acute period of moderate/severe TBI, which in this context will typically include individuals in the ICU and acute care. In the context of mental health, while the setting is important, the most important factors are considered under the lens of the biopsychosocial model.[34] For our mental health section in this article, our focus will be on assessment and intervention depending on these biopsychosocial factors in an effort to promote longer-term wellbeing for individuals as they move though the chronic condition of TBI.

When an individual first arrives in the ICU following an incident, the primary focus as noted earlier in this article is on life-saving measures. Thus, it is common that upon initial arrival to the ICU, mental health is not a primary element. From a physiatrist's (and if available, mental health provider's) standpoint, the management of behavior in the ICU/acute care setting soon becomes one of the most important aspects of recovery. As noted above, assessment in a consultation focuses on comprehensive factors, including posttraumatic amnesia (PTA). Currently, guidelines highlight the use of various measures, with strong support for the use the Orientation Log.[35,36] PTA represents one of the most important constructs in recovery prediction from TBI.[37] As individuals are removed from sedation and orientation can be assessed, often agitation becomes a major factor and is implicated in long term outcomes.[38] To determine cognitive and behavioral status, individuals are assessed based on the Rancho Los Amigos Scale, see **Table 1** later in discussion.

For individuals who are at a stage between Rancho IV to Rancho VI behavioral concerns become a primary focus due to confusion. This phase may occur across the care continuum including in the acute and chronic phase of recovery. These individuals are typically alert and awake but due to their confusional state often attempt to get out of bed, can be angry/violent, and may be considered a danger to themselves. Thus, there is typically a focus on pharmacologic and non-pharmacologic management.[40] As noted earlier in our chapter, pharmacologic management often plays a major role. Providers though may be asked to provide recommendations/treatment plans for behavior management due to concerns around sedation.[14] Typically, behavior management focus on the principles associated with delirium treatment including the regulation of the sleep/wake cycle via environmental cues. There is a focus on creating a structured schedule, cues for day/night awakening (eg, opening blinds in the morning/closing at night), and reorientation to time. Additionally, there is a focus on low stimulation environments including: limiting visitors, identifying, and removing any noxious stimulus, and helping family members learn how to talk with their affected loved one to decrease distress. Finally, the creation of consistency becomes important to increase predictability for those with TBI as a factor that decreases distress.[36] The primary directive at this point of treatment is to find factors that promote agitation. Later in discussion is a clinical care point with recommendations for behavior management.

Table 1 Rancho Los Amigos scale[39]	
Level of Functioning	**Response**
Level I	None
Level II	Generalized
Level III	Localized
Level IV	Confused and Agitated
Level V	Confused and Inappropriate
Level VI	Confused and Appropriate
Level VII	Automatic and Appropriate
Level VIII	Purposeful and Appropriate

Clinics Care Point Recommendations to manage behavioral agitation in the ICU for patients with TBI (adapted from Ponsford and colleagues (2023) INCOG guidelines[36]),

Use low stimulation environments which focus on limiting noise, light, and discomfort (for example, sheets/blanket textures
Consider the impact of visitors, time of meds/assessment, and therapy on agitation and limit those which cause fatigue/behavior change
Allow and facilitate rest and sleep as needed with a focus on sleep occurring mostly at night to reduce daytime sleepiness
Minimize the use of restraints as possible. These can act as an agitating factor
Allow for safe movement when able
Focus on consistency of providers/faces for the patient. Limit changing of staffing
Encourage family to visit patient at specific times to create consistency and predictability
Provide and model frequent reassurance – including both family/caregivers and providers
Provide limited and consistent reassuring information
Provide education to family about agitation
Use low stimulation environments which focus on limiting noise, light, and discomfort (for example, sheets/blanket textures

As agitation begins to decrease, individuals often begin to progress toward improving insight and cognition. This often leads to a set of new challenges as an individual is developing the ability to make new memories each day. Depending on the individual, there may continue to be impaired self-awareness[41] impacting behaviors, cognitions, and emotional functioning. Yet, there is often an increase in awareness of what has happened, the impact of their injury, and distress associated with their injury. During the acute phase of recovery, there is a focus initially on providing individuals with education. Moreover, frequently, when individuals are seen in acute care or ICU settings, the focus from a mental health perspective is on engagement in in rehabilitation therapies. During this stage, the focus is on engagement as this has been shown to be the primary factor in the promotion of outcomes for individuals with TBI.[42] Moreover, there may begin to be evidence of depressed mood, anxiety, or post-traumatic stress symptoms associated with their hospitalization. Treatment at this point often focuses on cognitive behavioral, motivational interviewing, and mindfulness-based therapies to decrease the distress associated with these symptoms, often with a focus on helping patients engage in care. This may fall outside of physiatry and require a consult to psychology/psychiatry, though the assessment of these factors is important in the acute phase.[43]

Family Interventions

While there is a focus on the treatment of agitation in the acute setting when focused on the patient, there is also an important role in the treatment of family members when an individual remains in PTA. For families of individuals who are currently in acute care there is often a high degree of distress due to the uncertainly of their family member's condition. In a qualitative study of family members in critical and acute care, their experiences occurred across the timeline from learning the news to moving on/forward.[44] There was an identification of themes for family members that include being involved in care, looking for progress, managing life while in the hospital, and hoping for hope.[44] Within this context, families are often provided with education by staff including nursing, medical, and psychology staff about brain injury. Moreover, they often benefit from feelings of being involved in care and information on how best to do this, based on the above recommendations. This information can often be provided by bedside staff. At this time, helping family members be appropriately involved and provision of information to decrease uncertainty can be the most important way to promote wellbeing for the family and the individuals themselves. Inventions for family across acute and outpatient settings focuses on 5 major topics.[45] These include the effects of brain injury on the survivor and family, understanding recovery, solving problems and goal setting, managing stress and intense emotions, and promotion of strategies for recovery. There is often a shifting between caregiver role demands and the emotions associated with the changes in the person with TBI.[46] It is noteworthy that family members of individuals with TBI endorse higher levels of depressed mood and posttraumatic stress symptoms than non-TBI counterparts.[47,48] Thus, interventions with individuals and family focus on behavior and emotion management following TBI. Initially, the focus is on behavior management while an individual remains in posttraumatic amnesia and support of family. As they progress out of posttraumatic amnesia the focus shifts to emotional needs for both individuals and families following traumatic brain injury. While these needs begin in inpatient acute settings, they continue over time, consistent with TBI as a chronic disease and early intervention is an important part of this recovery.

SUMMARY

After acute stabilization and management, individuals with acute moderate-severe TBI have a wide range of needs that are optimally managed by PM&R professionals and teams. Physiatry care should focus on reducing common medical morbidities, stabilizing overall health, and optimizing recovery using basic medical and rehabilitation principles.

DISCLOSURE

None.

REFERENCES

1. Khellaf A, Khan DZ, Helmy A. Recent advances in traumatic brain injury. J Neurol 2019;266(11):2878–89.
2. Meyfroidt G, Bouzat P, Casaer MP, et al. Management of moderate to severe traumatic brain injury: an update for the intensivist. Intensive Care Med 2022;48(6):649–66.
3. Centers for Disease Control and Prevention. Surveillance Report of Traumatic Brain Injury-Related Deaths by Age Group, Sex, and Mechanism of Injury—United States, 2018 and 2019.; 2022.
4. Teasdale G, Jennett B. Assessment of coma and impaired consciousness: A practical scale. Lancet 1974;304(7872):81–4.
5. Marshall LF, Marshall SB, Klauber MR, et al. The diagnosis of head-injury requires a classification based on computed axial-tomography. J Neurotrauma 1992;9:S287–92.
6. Maas AIR, Hukkelhoven CWPM, Marshall LF, et al. Prediction of outcome in traumatic brain injury with computed tomographic characteristics: a comparison between the computed tomographic classification and combinations of computed tomographic predictors. Neurosurgery 2005;57(6):1173–81.

7. Robinson CP. Moderate and Severe Traumatic Brain Injury. Continuum 2021; 27(5):1278–300.

8. Raith EP, Reddy U. Critical care management of adult traumatic brain injury. Anaesth Intensive Care Med 2023;24(6):333–9.

9. Al-Mufti F, Mayer SA. Neurocritical Care of Acute Subdural Hemorrhage. Neurosurg Clin N Am 2017;28(2):267–78.

10. Carney N, Totten AM, O'Reilly C, et al. Guidelines for the Management of Severe Traumatic Brain Injury, Fourth Edition. Neurosurgery 2017;80(1):6–15.

11. El-Swaify ST, Kamel M, Ali SH, et al. Initial neurocritical care of severe traumatic brain injury: New paradigms and old challenges. Surg Neurol Int 2022;13(431). https://doi.org/10.25259/SNI_609_2022.

12. Mahajan C, Prabhakar H, Bilotta F. Endocrine Dysfunction After Traumatic Brain Injury: An Ignored Clinical Syndrome? Neurocrit Care 2023;1–10. https://doi.org/10.1007/S12028-022-01672-3/FIGURES/2.

13. Gross P. Clinical management of SIADH. Ther Adv Endocrinol Metab 2012;3(2): 61–73.

14. Oddo M, Crippa IA, Mehta S, et al. Optimizing sedation in patients with acute brain injury. Crit Care 2016;20(1).

15. Hertle DN, Dreier JP, Woitzik J, et al. Effect of analgesics and sedatives on the occurrence of spreading depolarizations accompanying acute brain injury. Brain 2012;135(Pt 8):2390–8.

16. Acosta-Escribano J, Fernández-Vivas M, Grau Carmona T, et al. Gastric versus transpyloric feeding in severe traumatic brain injury: a prospective, randomized trial. Intensive Care Med 2010;36(9):1532–9.

17. Marik PE, Zaloga GP. Gastric versus post-pyloric feeding: a systematic review. Crit Care 2003;7(3):R46.

18. Hawryluk GWJ, Aguilera S, Buki A, et al. A management algorithm for patients with intracranial pressure monitoring: the Seattle International Severe Traumatic Brain Injury Consensus Conference (SIBICC). Intensive Care Med 2019;45(12): 1783–94.

19. Hutchinson PJ, Kolias AG, Timofeev IS, et al. Trial of Decompressive Craniectomy for Traumatic Intracranial Hypertension. N Engl J Med 2016;375(12):1119–30.

20. Zafonte RD, Mann NR, Millis SR, et al. Posttraumatic amnesia: Its relation to functional outcome. Arch Phys Med Rehabil 1997;78(10):1103–6.

21. Frey KL, Rojas DC, Anderson CA, et al. Comparison of the O-Log and GOAT as measures of posttraumatic amnesia. Brain Inj 2009;21(5):513–20.

22. Bishara SN, Partridge FM, Godfrey HPD, et al. Post-traumatic amnesia and Glasgow Coma Scale related to outcome in survivors in a consecutive series of patients with severe closed-head injury. Brain Inj 2009;6(4):373–80.

23. Ellenberg JH, Levin HS, Saydjari C. Posttraumatic Amnesia as a Predictor of Outcome After Severe Closed Head Injury: Prospective Assessment. Arch Neurol 1996;53(8):782–91.

24. Xie E, Pellegrini M, Chen Z, et al. The Influence of Substance Use on Traumatic Brain Injury Recovery and Rehabilitation Outcomes: The Outcome-ABI Study. Arch Phys Med Rehabil 2023;104(7):1115–23.

25. Roy SJ, Livernoche Leduc C, Paradis V, et al. The negative influence of chronic alcohol abuse on acute cognitive recovery after a traumatic brain injury. Brain Inj 2022;36(12–14):1340–8.

26. De Guise E, Alturki AY, LeBlanc J, et al. The Montreal Cognitive Assessment in persons with traumatic brain injury. Appl Neuropsychol Adult 2014;21(2):128–35.

27. Giacino JT, Kalmar K, Whyte J. The JFK Coma Recovery Scale-Revised: Measurement characteristics and diagnostic utility. Arch Phys Med Rehabil 2004; 85(12):2020–9.

28. Kalmar K, Giacino JT. The JFK Coma Recovery Scale - Revised. Neuropsychol Rehabil 2005;15(3–4):454–60.

29. Seel RT, Sherer M, Whyte J, et al. Assessment Scales for Disorders of Consciousness: Evidence-Based Recommendations for Clinical Practice and Research. Arch Phys Med Rehabil 2010;91(12):1795–813.

30. La Porta F, Caselli S, Ianes AB, et al. Can we scientifically and reliably measure the level of consciousness in vegetative and minimally conscious states? Rasch analysis of the coma recovery scale-revised. Arch Phys Med Rehabil 2013;94(3): 527–35.e1.

31. Nakase-Richardson R, McNamee S, Howe LL, et al. Descriptive Characteristics and Rehabilitation Outcomes in Active Duty Military Personnel and Veterans With Disorders of Consciousness With Combat- and Noncombat-Related Brain Injury. Arch Phys Med Rehabil 2013;94(10):1861–9.

32. Aubanel S, Bruiset F, Chapuis C, et al. Therapeutic options for agitation in the intensive care unit. Anaesthesia, Crit care pain Med. 2020;39(5):639–46.

33. Corrigan JD, Hammond FM. Traumatic brain injury as a chronic health condition. Arch Phys Med Rehabil 2013;94(6):1199–201.

34. Williams WH, Evans JJ. Biopsychosocial Approaches in Neurorehabilitation: Assessment and Management of Neuropsychiatric, Mood and Behavioural Disorders : A Special Issue of Neuropsychological Rehabilitation. Biopsychosoc Approaches Neurorehabilitation Assess Manag Neuropsychiatr Mood Behav Disord 2003. https://doi.org/10.4324/9780203009017.

35. Novack TA, Dowler RN, Bush BA, et al. Validity of the Orientation Log, relative to the Galveston Orientation and Amnesia Test. J Head Trauma Rehabil 2000;15(3): 957–61.

36. Ponsford J, Trevena-Peters J, Janzen S, et al. INCOG 2.0 Guidelines for Cognitive Rehabilitation Following Traumatic Brain Injury, Part I: Posttraumatic Amnesia. J Head Trauma Rehabil 2023;38(1):24–37.

37. Walker WC, Ketchum JM, Marwitz JH, et al. A multicentre study on the clinical utility of post-traumatic amnesia duration in predicting global outcome after moderate-severe traumatic brain injury. J Neurol Neurosurg Psychiatry 2010; 81(1):87–9.

38. Prendergast NT, Onyemekwu CA, Potter KM, et al. Agitation is a Common Barrier to Recovery of ICU Patients. J Intensive Care Med 2023;38(2):208–14.

39. Rancho Los Amigos Hospital. Professional Staff Association. Rehabilitation of the head injured adult : comprehensive physical management. 1979:89.

40. Wiles MD, Braganza M, Edwards H, et al. Management of traumatic brain injury in the non-neurosurgical intensive care unit: a narrative review of current evidence. Anaesthesia 2023;78(4):510–20.

41. Richardson C, McKay A, Ponsford JL. Does feedback influence awareness following traumatic brain injury? Neuropsychol Rehabil 2015;25(2):233–53.

42. Seel RT, Corrigan JD, Dijkers MP, et al. Patient Effort in Traumatic Brain Injury Inpatient Rehabilitation: Course and Associations With Age, Brain Injury Severity, and Time Postinjury. Arch Phys Med Rehabil 2015;96(8 Suppl):S235–44.

43. Hart T, Benn EKT, Bagiella E, et al. Early trajectory of psychiatric symptoms after traumatic brain injury: relationship to patient and injury characteristics. J Neurotrauma 2014;31(7):610–7.

44. Keenan A, Joseph L. The needs of family members of severe traumatic brain injured patients during critical and acute care: a qualitative study. Can J Neurosci Nurs 2010;32(3):25–35.

45. Kreutzer JS, Rapport LJ, Marwitz JH, et al. Caregivers' well-being after traumatic brain injury: a multicenter prospective investigation. Arch Phys Med Rehabil 2009;90(6):939–46.

46. Kratz AL, Sander AM, Brickell TA, et al. Traumatic brain injury caregivers: A qualitative analysis of spouse and parent perspectives on quality of life. Neuropsychol Rehabil 2017;27(1):16–37.

47. Warren AM, Rainey EE, Weddle RJ, et al. The intensive care unit experience: Psychological impact on family members of patients with and without traumatic brain injury. Rehabil Psychol 2016;61(2):179–85.

48. Jackson JC, Jutte JE. Rehabilitating a missed opportunity: Integration of rehabilitation psychology into the care of critically ill patients, survivors, and caregivers. Rehabil Psychol 2016;61(2):115–9.

Disorders of Consciousness

Levi Weitzel, BS[a],*, Sheital Bavishi, DO[b]

KEYWORDS

- Disorder of consciousness • Rehabilitation • Coma
- Unresponsive wakefulness state • Minimally conscious state • Traumatic brain injury
- Acquired brain injury

KEY POINTS

- Disorders of consciousness (DOCs) are altered states of pathologic consciousness, sub-divided into coma, unresponsive wakefulness state (UWS), and minimally conscious state (MCS) based on neurobehavioral function.
- Emergence from MCS is defined as reliable and consistent functional object use and functional communication.
- The Coma Recovery Scale-Revised assessment scale is recommended in DOC for clinical practice and research.
- Neuroimaging and electrophysiology are an essential component of the diagnostic/prognostic assessment of patients but should be used in conjunction with appropriate behavioral assessments.
- Amantadine is recommended by the 2018 AAN/ACRM/NIDILRR DOC guidelines for patients in UWS or MCS 4 to 16 weeks after injury.

INTRODUCTION

There are approximately 50 to 60 million new traumatic brain injury (TBI) cases worldwide each year, with approximately 3.5 million of those occurring in the United States alone.[1] TBIs exact a profound economic toll, illustrated by the estimated lifetime cost per TBI being $555,000 in the United States.[2] Not only are severe TBIs the most economically detrimental, but approximately 0.3% of these cases can result in a disorder of consciousness (DOC).[3] DOC is a state of prolonged, altered arousal and/or awareness, which is categorized into coma, unresponsive wakeful state (UWS), formally vegetative state (VS), minimally conscious state without language (MCS–), and MCS with language (MCS+).[4] Despite continual progress in objective diagnostic

[a] Department of Physical Medicine and Rehabilitation, Ohio State University College of Medicine, 370 W 9th Avenue, Columbus, OH 43210, USA; [b] Department of Physical Medicine and Rehabilitation, Brain Injury Program, Dodd Inpatient Rehabilitation Hospital, Ohio State University Wexner Medical Center, 480 Medical Center Drive, Room 1036, Columbus, OH 43210, USA
* Corresponding author.
E-mail address: levi.weitzel@osumc.edu

Phys Med Rehabil Clin N Am 35 (2024) 493–506
https://doi.org/10.1016/j.pmr.2024.02.003
pmr.theclinics.com

assessments, misdiagnosis in DOC remains as high as 40%.[5] Due to the difficult nature of diagnosis, prognosis, and treatment, DOCs present a unique challenge that negatively impacts the quality of life and well-being of the individuals affected and their loved ones.[6] In this article, the authors review the latest definitions, diagnoses, imaging techniques, and treatment intervention.

CONSCIOUSNESS

Continued insights into the neural correlates of consciousness have proven valuable clinically as the 2 components that separate consciousness from unconsciousness are arousal and awareness.[7] On a neuroanatomic level, arousal is mediated by the ascending reticular activating system of the upper brainstem. Consciousness in a clinical sense is mediated by activation of heterogeneous neuronal populations within the brainstem, hypothalamus, and basal forebrain that diffusely promote the depolarization of thalamic and cortical neurons, providing the conditions necessary for effective interactions among cortical area.[8] From neurobiologic perspective, the conscious awake state is associated with a high-energy demand and electrical activity within the corticothalamic system, and this is further supported by electroencephalogram (EEG) recordings and functional MRI (fMRI) studies.[9,10] Conversely, a decline in arousal is associated with reduction in excitatory neuromodulator influences. Awareness is the ability of an individual to respond to both external and internal stimuli in an integrated manner. In healthy individuals, an increase in arousal is associated with an increase in awareness in a linear manner along the continuum of conscious state.[11] A dissociation of these 2 components of consciousness is seen in pathologic states, like UWS and MCS.

CLINICAL DEFINITION
Coma

Coma is a state of unconsciousness characterized by lack of arousal and awareness. The defining clinical feature is complete loss of spontaneous or stimulus-induced arousal.[12] There is no eye opening, and EEG testing reveals the absence of sleep–wake cycles. The usual pathophysiological mechanism is broad withdrawal of excitatory synaptic activity across the cerebral cortex.[4] Those who survive this stage will begin to awaken and transition to a UWS or MCS within 2 to 4 weeks.[12,13]

Unresponsive Wakefulness State

The UWS is an unconscious, dissociative state of wakefulness without awareness. The individual's eyes open spontaneously, and they demonstrate preserved behavioral sleep. However, sleep–wake patterns are not detected on electroencephalography.[14] Individuals demonstrate reflexive movement and arousal but show no signs of conscious perception. These individuals may also smile, cry, or grimace, though they appear unrelated to context.[15] The presence of wakefulness suggests preserved brainstem functioning, but the lack of awareness suggests underlying cortical dysfunction. Likewise, functional neuroimaging has shown sensory stimuli will activate primary cortical areas, but not higher order cortical areas thought necessary for awareness.[9] With proper medical care, an individual in UWS can survive for many years.

Minimally Conscious State

The MCS is characterized by a severe impairment of consciousness, with evidence of wakefulness and partial preservation of awareness. Unlike the UWS, there are discernible, purposeful behaviors that can be differentiated from reflexive behavior.

The hallmark of MCS is inconsistent but reproducible, command following. The preservation of corticothalamic connections might explain why individuals in MCS retain the capacity for cognitive processing. The patient may exhibit visual pursuit, emotional responses, and gestures to appropriate environmental stimuli, but are unable to functionally communicate their thoughts or feelings. Based on the presence or absence of receptive and expressive language, MCS can be further subcategorized into MCS+ and MCS–.[15]

Post-Traumatic Confusional State

Once emerged from MCS, individuals continue to exhibit signs that they are not fully recovered either cognitively or behavioral. The full array of symptoms associated with the post-traumatic confusional state (PTCS) can also include attention deficits, anterograde amnesia, restlessness, emotional lability, perceptual disturbances, and a disrupted sleep–wake cycle.[16] While the level of functional ability indicative of resolution is not widely agreed upon, global improvements in attention, memory retrieval, and executive function resulting in greater independence are features.[16]

Locked in Syndrome

Locked in syndrome (LIS) is a rare condition characterized by intact consciousness and cognition with anarthria and quadriplegia. This state is caused by damage to the ventral pons and is often due to basilar thrombosis.[15] Individuals with classic LIS have intact sensation and spared vertical eye movement, enabling gaze-based communication. Over time, individuals may recover some control of the fingers, toes, or head. This atypical presentation, with lost speech and motor control, places these individuals at risk for misdiagnosis as a DOC, explaining why the average time of diagnosis is 2.5 months post-onset.[15]

CLINICAL EXAMINATION AND QUANTITATIVE ASSESSMENT

A focused clinical examination is essential to diagnose DOCs. Specifically, 7 domains should be tested and include sleep–wake cycles, awareness, motor skills, auditory function, visual function, communication, and emotional integrity.[17] Behavioral sleep–wake cycles alone, detected through observation of intermittent eye-opening, helps differentiate someone in a UWS from someone in a coma. The presence of awareness will further distinguish someone in an MCS from those in UWS. When testing the remainder of the domains, certain caveats exist. First, yes/no responses can be given through direct verbal communication or through gestures, like a thumbs-up. These responses can be incorrect contextually, but they must be reproducible. Second, behavioral responses should demonstrate a definite relationship with their stimuli, such that reflexive activity cannot explain the response. It is important to test a wide array of behavioral responses within the patient's abilities and perform serial examinations to ensure accuracy. Last, it is imperative that comprehensive physical examination be done to provide insight for any findings that may obscure appropriate diagnosis, including effects of sedative medications, aphasia, apraxia, motor impairments, or sensory deficit.[17] As the patient continues along the spectrum of recovery, emergence from an MCS would be evidenced by 2 distinct behaviors. The first is functional, interactive communication, which would have to be demonstrated through means of correct yes/no responses to 6 situational questions on 3 consecutive examinations. Responses can be gestural, written, or verbal. The second behavior is the functional use of 2 different objects that can be validated on 3 consecutive examinations.[17]

BEHAVIORAL ASSESSMENT SCALES

Standardized neurobehavioral assessments and clinical observation are the basis of DOC diagnosis. These assessment scales require fixed administration, standardized scoring procedures, and the ability to assess a broad range of neurobehavioral function.[15] Several scales are described later and outlined in **Table 1**. Of these scales, the Coma Recovery Scale-Revised (CRS-R) is the clinical standard of care. The current recommendation for serial evaluation of patients with neurobehavioral assessment scales is based on clinical judgment as there are insufficient data regarding interval between assessments.[5]

Coma Recovery Scale-Revised

The CRS-R is a 23 item scale comprising 6 subscales, whose items are arranged hierarchically from reflexive to cognitively mediated processes. Subscales address visual, auditory, motor, oromotor, communication, and arousal categories. Emergence criteria are assessed by the communication (yes/no accuracy) and motor subscales (functional object use).[18,19] Training consists of establishing interdisciplinary and particularly trained teams, using instructional videos, multicenter residency agreements, workshops, and video conferences.[20] The Coma Recovery Scale Pediatrics (CRS-P) is a modified version of the CRS-R that accounts for functional and behavioral differences in a developing child, while maintaining sensitivity to underlying neurologic function.[21]

Sensory Modality and Rehabilitation Techniques

Sensory modality and rehabilitation techniques (SMART) was developed as both an assessment and treatment tool for patients in UWS or MCS.[22] SMART comprises 2 components. The formal component, conducted by the SMART assessors, includes the SMART Sensory Assessment and the SMART Behavioral Observation Assessment. The informal component consists of exploring family, friend, and team

Table 1
Summary of psychometric and clinical characteristics reported for commonly utilized behavioral assessment scales

Scales	Psychometric Properties					Clinical Use			
Name	IRR	TRR	CV	Sensitivity	Specificity	TTA	Dx	Px	Tx
CRS-R[18]	✔	✔	✔			15–30 min	✔	✔	✔
SMART[22]	✔	✔	✔			~60 min	✔	✔	✔
GCS[24]	✔	✔	✔			~5 min	✔		
C-NC[25]	✔		✔			~15 min	✔	✔	
WHIM[27]	✔	✔	✔			30–120 min	✔		
WNSSP[28,29]	✔	✔				20–40 min	✔	✔	
DOCS[30]	✔		✔	✔	✔	~45 min		✔	✔
MATADOC[31]	✔	✔	✔	✔		15–30 min	✔	✔	

Abbreviations: C-NC, coma-near coma scale; CRS-R, coma recovery scale-revised; CV, construct validity; DOCS, disorders of consciousness scale; Dx, diagnosis; GCS, Glasgow Coma Scale; IRR, inter-rater reliability; MATADOC, music therapy assessment tool for awareness in disorders of consciousness; Px, prognosis; SMART, sensory modality assessment and rehabilitation technique; TRR, test-retest reliability; TTA, time to administer; Tx, treatment; WHIM, Wessex Head Injury Matrix; WNSSP, Western Neurosensory Stimulation Profile.
✔ = $P<.05$.

interpretations of observed behaviors.[23] The SMART requires a 5 day training course to become an assessor and prior submission of a portfolio to gain access to the assessment tool.

Glasgow Coma Scale

Glasgow Coma Scale (GCS) independently measures motor responsiveness, eye opening, and verbal performance to assess depth and duration of DOCs.[24] This scale is useful in longitudinally assessing DOC patients for different levels of responsiveness; thus, the GCS is primarily used as a prognostic tool.

Coma Near Coma Scale

Coma Near Coma Scale was designed to measure small clinical changes for DOC patients in UWS or coma. This scale consists of an 11 item test with specific and structured sensory stimulation for auditory, visual, olfactory, and tactile modalities. Vocalization and command response are also tested. Training consists of 2 or more raters observing items independently and repeating this process on 5 to 10 patients until raters can place patients in the same category range.[25]

Wessex Head Injury Matrix

Wessex Head Injury Matrix (WHIM) is a 62 item scale, ordered in hierarchy, that assesses communication ability, cognitive skills, and social interaction by observing tasks used in everyday life. The WHIM was created to follow a patient from emergence from coma to emergence from PTCS as a prognostic tool, but recent studies have explored the scale's diagnostic utility.[26] There is a fee to obtain the rating scale and training manual. Training is required because interrater reliability and test–retest reliability relies on experience.[27]

Western Neurosensory Stimulation Profile

Western neurosensory stimulation profile (WNSSP) consists of 32 items, which assess patients' arousal/attention, expressive communication, and response to auditory, visual, tactile, and olfactory stimulation. The WNSSP has shown internal consistency, as well as standardized scoring and administration. It relies on visual comprehension and tracking.[28,29]

Disorders of Consciousness Scale

Disorders of Consciousness Scale consists of 23 items with 8 subscales including social knowledge, taste and swallowing, olfactory, proprioceptive and vestibular, auditory, visual, tactile, and testing-readiness. It is a free test requiring training with a 2 h DVD and observation by a trained practitioner.[30]

Music Therapy Assessment Tool for Awareness in Disorders of Consciousness

The Music Therapy Assessment Tool for Awareness in DOC (MATADOC) is a 14 item measure assessing auditory responsiveness and functional ability. A patient's level of awareness is determined by measuring whether he or she responds differently and purposefully to contrasting musical stimuli. A 3 day specialized training is required and must be administered by trained music therapists.[31]

Individualized Quantitative Behavioral Assessment

Individualized Quantitative Behavioral Assessment employs the principles of single-subject experimental design enabling the creation of a unique protocol suited to a patient's injury and constellation of impairments.[32] The first step is identifying 2 potential voluntary movements (eg, command following, visual tracking). Second, this selected behavior is recorded following either appropriate or incompatible commands. These data are then used to determine whether the selected behavior occurs significantly more often in relation to the command.[15] While the individualization of this assessment controls for examiner and response bias, there remains a lack of psychometric property data.

Nociception Coma Scale

The Nociception Coma Scale-Revised (NCS-R) is composed of motor, verbal, and facial expression response subscales to a nociceptive pain stimulus.[15] Noxious stimuli are introduced in the form of pressure applied to the patient's fingernail bed while they exhibit spontaneous eye opening to ensure sufficient level of arousal. The NCS-R provides clinicians with a tool to specifically tailor pain management plans to individuals with DOC.[33]

IMAGING AND COMPLEMENTARY STUDIES

With a lack of individualized prognostic tools and the misdiagnosis of DOC consistently hovering around 40%, there remains a need for objective measures through neuroimaging.[5] Debate persists regarding the utility of structural neuroimaging by means of computed tomography and MRI apart from initial evaluation or in the event of an acute neurologic deterioration, but use of functional neuroimaging to assess brain processes has been useful in characterizing DOC at acute and chronic stages.[34]

PET Scan

Prior studies using PET scans demonstrated that auditory stimuli activated secondary brain regions thought to be associated with awareness in MCS patients but remained inactive in patients categorized in UWS.[13] An additional study concluded that different levels of neuronal activity in response to pain could be detected in UWS patients compared to MCS patients.[35] While additional studies are necessary to substantiate the correlation between brain activity on PET and corresponding behavior, PET can be utilized to reveal disruptions of functional networks and provide evidence of neuronal response in patients who seem to be unresponsive.[4]

MRI

MRI's role in treating individuals with DOC has grown as imaging techniques have evolved. The combination of structural MRI, fMRI, and diffusion tensor imaging (DTI) allow clinicians to obtain a more accurate diagnosis and prognosis for individuals, without exposure to radiation. However, accessibility, repeatability, and sensitivity remain major limitations.[34]

Structural MRI

Structural MRI enables 3 dimensional high-resolution characterization of both gray and white matter injury following TBI.[34] The ability to localize and assess the extent of damage makes structural MRI the method of choice beyond the acute phase of DOC.[36]

Functional MRI

In a study by Monti and colleagues,[37] fMRI was able to detect neuronal activity associated with creating volitional mental imagery in individuals thought to be in a UWS. Several other studies have also shown that stimulus-based fMRI paradigms can detect signatures of awareness in individuals without behavioral signs.[10] fMRI's capability to measure neural activity at rest or in response to a passive or active paradigm makes it a promising diagnostic tool if accessible.

Diffusion Tensor Imaging

DTI has shown the ability to reveal disruption of white matter connections within subcortical and cortical networks in acute and chronic DOC patients.[38] This ability to generate a quantitative measurement of differential connectivity between brain regions or networks correlated to areas responsible for perceived consciousness makes DTI a potentially powerful prognostic modality.[10]

Electroencephalograms

EEGs are a cheaper alternative to fMRI, yet they still retain diagnostic utility.[34] One proposed mechanism to identify changes in consciousness may be through recognition of normal sleep–wake cycles. Studies have demonstrated the presence of sleep–wake cycles similar to a healthy population in MCS patients.[14] This contrasted with patients in UWS that had observable behavioral periods of eye-opening and eye-closing, but their EEGs failed to show any resemblance to normal sleep patterns. Further studies elucidating EEG's ability to record response to stimuli are warranted.

TREATMENT INTERVENTIONS

The primary goal of DOC rehabilitation programs is to promote arousal while preventing secondary medical complications. Although there are no consensus treatment guidelines for DOC patients, there are several pharmacologic and nonpharmacologic treatments available.

Pharmacologic Treatment

Amantadine

Dopamine agonists and N-methyl-D-aspartate antagonists have been used in DOC for hypoarousal. In a large, multicenter, double-blind, placebo-controlled trial, the ability of Amantadine versus placebo to accelerate functional recovery among patients with nonpenetrating TBI in UWS or MCS was studied. A total of 184 patients were treated for 1 month, in the period between 4 and 16 weeks after severe TBI while also receiving inpatient rehabilitation (IPR). The rate of functional recovery was measured by the Disability Rating Score (DRS), and there was a statistically significant rate of weekly improvement of 0.24 (P5 .007) compared with the placebo group. Regardless of the interval since injury, the benefit of Amantadine appeared consistent.[39] Furthermore, although the rate of recovery diminished after a washout period, gains were sustained after cessation of the drug. Amantadine is recommended for patients with UWS or MCS 4 to 16 weeks after injury.

Modafinil

Modafinil's exact mechanism of action is unknown, but it is thought to stimulate adrenergic, histaminergic, glutaminergic activity and cause decreased gamma aminobutyric acid (GABA) activity in the brain. In a single-center, double-blind, placebo-controlled trial to evaluate modafinil in the treatment of excessive daytime sleepiness in patients with chronic TBI, there was no clear evidence between treatment with modafinil versus placebo.[40] Little evidence for its use in DOC post-TBI currently exists, and more research is warranted.

Bromocriptine

A direct agonist at the D2 receptor has limited information regarding its use in patients with DOC. A 5 patient case review series involving patients in UWS who were administered bromocriptine 1 month after TBI exhibited encouraging results. When compared with a literature-based control group at 3, 6, and 12 months, there was an improvement in the DRS and CRS scores.[41] This study, however, had a low sample size and a lack of experimental control, but additional studies with more robust patient populations have not been conducted.

Apomorphine

Apomorphine is a potent dopaminergic agonist acting directly at both the D_1 and D_2 classes of dopamine receptors, with higher affinity for D2 receptors.[42,43] The bioavailability, fast action, and subcutaneous administration of apomorphine allow for accurate, steady drug blood level. In a prospective double-blind randomized controlled trial being carried out by Sanz and colleagues,[43] patients diagnosed as in UWS or MCS will be administered apomorphine or placebo to assess changes in responsiveness and behavioral changes detected by CRS-R, NCS-R, MRI, PET, and high-density EEG.

Methylphenidate

Methylphenidate is a neurostimulant that acts synaptically by blocking the reuptake of dopamine and norepinephrine. A study conducted by Kim and colleagues,[44] suggested that methylphenidate may help to normalize cerebral glucose metabolism and neural circuits after brain injury on PET. If a patient does not respond to amantadine, a neurostimulant, like methylphenidate, is reasonable.[4] There are currently no data on adverse outcomes reported.

Zolpidem

Zolpidem is a sedative-hypnotic and GABA agonist. There have been several case studies in the literature describing a transient, paradoxic, awakening effect after administration of zolpidem.[45] A large, prospective, placebo-controlled, double-blind, single-dose, crossover study was designed to study the effects of zolpidem on recovery of consciousness in UWS and MCS patients. Of the 84 total participants, only 4 definite "responders" (5% of total) were identified, which had no demographic or clinic predictors of response. Further studies are warranted to identify why and how Zolpidem is active in such a selective manner.[46] Like methylphenidate, zolpidem is recommended on a trial basis for amantadine resistant patients.[4]

Levodopa

Levodopa is a precursor of the neurotransmitters dopamine, norepinephrine, and adrenaline. An 8 patient, prospective study of patients in a UWS, who were administered levodopa approximately 104 days after their TBI, was performed. All the patients made improvement in their consciousness, and 7 of 8 patients had full recovery of consciousness. Interestingly, gradual increases of levodopa doses were associated with increasing complexity of motor responses.[47] Although promising, more significantly powered studies are needed.

Nonpharmacolic Treatment

Nonpharmacologic treatments for DOC include neurorehabilitation with specially trained therapists, as well as noninvasive and invasive brain stimulation. Specialized neurorehabilitation programs in an IPR facility setting have shown improved emergence to consciousness, and more data about the benefits of early rehabilitation have emerged. Noninvasive brain stimulation and neurorehabilitation when used in conjunction have shown to enhance neuroplasticity more than either alone.[48,49]

Neurorehabilitation

Specialized rehabilitation protocols for DOC are essential for improving recovery and long-term care. In 2019, the National Institute on Disability and Rehabilitation Research and Traumatic Brain Injury Model Systems evaluated functional outcomes 10 years from patients admitted to IPR and unable to follow commands. Their study showed substantial proportions of the patients not following commands on admission to IPR recovered independent functioning over 10 years (88%–100% of patients in the early recovery group and 50%–75% of patients in the late recovery group), particularly if they followed commands before discharge (early recovery group).[50] Functional gains across year 1 to 2, 2 to 5, and 5 to 10 have been observed. Specialized, multidisciplinary rehabilitation with acute medical management and 90 minutes or more of therapy are likely to show improved consciousness and body function. Medical management can focus on prevention and/or treatment of medical complications of TBI, while neurorehabilitation should use standardized assessments for measurement of DOC level performed by trained interdisciplinary clinical teams to focus on recovery of consciousness, functional communication, and positioning/mobility.[51] The team consists of physicians, rehabilitation nursing, physical therapy, occupational therapy, speech language pathology, rehabilitation psychology, neuropsychology, case management, and social work. It has been seen that with specialized early treatment, including acute medical care and rehabilitation, patients may be able to transition to mainstream rehabilitation and emerge to consciousness.[51] Families who receive comprehensive education and hands on training with ongoing follow-up may be able to take care of patients with DOC at home versus facility placement.[51]

Music therapy

A study in 2020 by Carrière and colleagues[52] revealed that resting state fMRI functional connectivity increased among patients with DOC when listening to their favorite music compared to rest conditions. Beyond evidence about music therapy's utility as a treatment tool, there have been several studies validating the MATADOC's diagnostic and prognostic capabilities as a behavioral assessment.[31] Given its nonverbal and self-referential properties and emotional valence, further exploration of what music therapy offers as a unique diagnostic, prognostic, and interventional tool is needed.[53]

Transcranial direct current stimulation

Transcranial direct current stimulation (TDCS) is a form of neurostimulation that delivers a low constant current to an area of the brain using scalp electrodes. Anodal TDCS elicits prolonged increases in cortical excitability and facilitates underlying regional activity, while cathodal TDCS has the opposite effect.[54] Emerging data exist on the use of TDCS for transient improvement in consciousness in patients in MCS but not UWS.[55,56] Ease of use, minimal risk of harm, and portability make TDCS an encouraging intervention; however, more data are needed to create standardized protocols.[54]

Transcranial magnetic stimulation

Transcranial magnetic stimulation (TMS) provides neuromodulation with the application of rapidly changing magnetic fields to the scalp via a copper wire coil connected to a magnetic stimulator. Repetitive trains of TMS can suppress or facilitate cortical processes depending on stimulation parameters. The effect of TMS has been seen to have modulatory effects longer than the duration of the stimulation, thereby modulating neural plasticity. Case reports have been published that improved neural conduction mediates neurobehavioral gains in coma recovery.[57,58]

Deep brain stimulation
Deep brain stimulation is an invasive brain stimulation that requires surgical implantation of a deep brain stimulator. A multitude of targets have been tested, including the reticular formation, central nucleus of the thalamus, anterior intralaminar nuclei, and paralaminar areas, but neither the target of therapy nor frequency of stimulation have a clear impact on clinical response.[59]

Vagus nerve stimulation
Vagus nerve stimulation is a less invasive surgical alternative to DBS. While both the positive effect on reticular formation, thalamus, and forebrain metabolism and enhanced neuronal firing of the locus coeruleus have been documented, there is a need for more DOC-specific research to understand the potential therapeutic applications.[59]

CONSIDERATIONS

The care of each DOC patient is individual, there are patient populations that require special considerations. One such population is those who present with spasticity. Spasticity is a motor disorder arising from anarchic reorganization of the central nervous system, leading to hypertonia and hyperreflexia of affected muscle group.[60] Pediatric DOC patients are classified on the continuum of varying degrees of impaired arousal and awareness, like that of adults.[61] However, given the scarcity of neural correlates of consciousness, there is a lack of validated behavioral assessments and treatment options.

Spasticity
- Treatments are aimed at symptom management due to the lack of understanding regarding the pathophysiology
- Objective measures are needed; the Modified Ashworth Scale (MAS) is the most widely used clinical assessment tool for spasticity evaluation[62]
- Improvement in consciousness and functional behavior has been documented when treating spasticity early, rather than treating it as a secondary complication[60]
- Intrathecal baclofen (ITB) has been associated with improvements in MAS scores and cognitive recovery in several low powered studies[60]
- Pharmacologic therapies, including baclofen, dantrolene, phenol, and botulinum toxin, are considerations, but sedating effects should be considered for oral medications[60]
- Physiotherapy, soft-splinting, dynamic splinting, serial casting, and acupuncture have shown promise in reducing spasticity complications (loss of ROM, contractures, pain)[60]
- NCS-R could be used to detect presence of pain and assess efficacy of pain management regimen[62]

Pediatric DOC
- The sequential and ordered development of the brain should be accounted for when assessing developmentally appropriate behaviors[61]
- CRS-P use appears to be appropriate in patients as young as 12 months, and broader studies are currently being conducted[21]
- Music therapy, auditory stimulation, may be most appropriate assessment and intervention to meet a child's developmental needs[63]

- Both static and functional imaging techniques have shown promise as prognostic tools, but ongoing myelination in children and exposure to radiation must be considered when selecting an imaging modality[61]

SUMMARY

DOCs present scientific and clinical challenges for clinicians. Behavioral assessment remains the gold standard for diagnosis of these patients, but advanced neuroimaging and electrophysiological techniques present possibilities for improvement of the current diagnostic classification systems. Future studies need to focus on diagnostic, prognostic, and therapeutic interventions to aid in the management of DOC.

CLINICS CARE POINTS

Pearls
- CRS-R is gold standard of behavioral assessment
- Multimodal approach: appropriate behavioral assessments and imaging techniques, for diagnosis and prognosis is the preferred
- In prolonged DOC, amantadine improved functional recovery
- Early treatment of spasticity and consideration of ITB may prevent medical complications and improve recovery of consciousness

Pitfalls
- Reliance on imaging alone for diagnosis/prognosis due to limitations of access of current modalities
- Extensive training required to perform behavioral assessments
- Current lack of sensitivity and specificity data for behavioral assessments
- Scarcity of data related to pediatric DOC

DISCLOSURE

None.

REFERENCES

1. Maas A, Menon D, Adelson D, et al. The Lancet Neurology Commission Traumatic brain injury: integrated approaches to improve prevention, clinical care, and research The Lancet Neurology Commission. Lancet Neurol 2017;16:987–1048.
2. Faul M, Wald MM, Rutland-Brown W, et al. Using a cost-benefit analysis to estimate outcomes of a clinical treatment guideline: testing the Brain Trauma Foundation guidelines for the treatment of severe traumatic brain injury. J Trauma 2007;63:1271–8.
3. Gray M, Lai S, Wells R, et al. A systematic review of an emerging consciousness population: focus on program evolution. J Trauma 2011;71(5):1465–74.
4. Edlow BL, Claassen J, Schiff ND, et al. Recovery from disorders of consciousness: mechanisms, prognosis and emerging therapies. Nat Rev Neurol 2020; 17:135–56.
5. Giacino JT, Katz DI, Schiff ND, et al. Practice Guideline Update Recommendations Summary: Disorders of Consciousness. Arch Phys Med Rehabil 2018; 99(9):1699–709.
6. Elliott K, McVicar A. The impact of prolonged disorders of consciousness on the occupational life of family members. Neuropsychol Rehabil 2018;28(8):1375–91.

7. Plum F, Posner JB. The diagnosis of stupor and coma. Philadelphia: FA Davis; 1966. p. 5–6.
8. Koch C, Massimini M, Boly M, et al. Neural correlates of consciousness: progress and problems. Nat Rev Neurosci 2016;17(5):307–21.
9. Cavanna AE, Shah S, Eddy CM, et al. Consciousness: a neurological perspective. Behav Neurol 2011;24(1):107–16.
10. Snider SB, Edlow BL. MRI in disorders of consciousness. Curr Opin Neurol 2020; 33(6):676–83.
11. Cavanna AE, Ali F. Epilepsy: the quintessential pathology of consciousness. Behav Neurol 2011;24(1):3–10.
12. Giacino JT, Fins JJ, Laureys S, et al. Disorders of consciousness after acquired brain injury: the state of the science. Nat Rev Neurol 2014;10(2):99–114.
13. Laureys S, Owen AM, Schiff ND. Brain function in coma, vegetative state, and related disorders. Lancet Neurol 2004;3(9):537–46.
14. Landsness E, Bruno M-A, Noirhomme Q, et al. Electrophysiological correlates of behavioural changes in vigilance in vegetative state and minimally conscious state. Brain 2011;134(Pt 8):222232.
15. Schnakers C, Majerus S. Behavioral Assessment and Diagnosis of Disorders of Consciousness. In: Schnakers C, Laureys, editors. Coma and disorders of consciousness. 2nd edition. Springer; 2018. p. 1–13.
16. Sherer M, Katz DI, Bodien YG, et al. Post-traumatic Confusional State: A Case Definition and Diagnostic Criteria. Arch Phys Med Rehabil 2020;101(11):2041–50.
17. Giacino JT, Ashwal S, Childs N, et al. The minimally conscious state: definition and diagnostic criteria. Neurology 2002;58(3):349–53.
18. Giacino JT, Kalmar K, Whyte J. The JFK coma recovery scale-revised: measurement characteristics and diagnostic utility. Arch Phys Med Rehabil 2004;85(12): 2020–9.
19. Boltzmann M, Schmidt SB, Gutenbrunner C, et al. The influence of the CRS-R score on functional outcome in patients with severe brain injury receiving early rehabilitation. BMC Neurol 2021;21(1).
20. Løvstad M, Frøslie KF, Giacino JT, et al. Reliability and diagnostic characteristics of the JFK coma recovery scale-revised: exploring the influence of rater's level of experience. J Head Trauma Rehabil 2010;25(5):349–56.
21. Slomine BS, Suskauer SJ, Nicholson R, et al. Preliminary validation of the coma recovery scale for pediatrics in typically developing young children. Brain Inj 2019;33(13–14):1640–5.
22. Gill-Thwaites H, Munday R. The Sensory Modality Assessment and Rehabilitation Technique (SMART): a valid and reliable assessment for vegetative state and minimally conscious state patients. Brain Inj 2004;18(12):1255–69.
23. Gill-Thwaites H, Elliott KE, Munday R. SMART – Recognising the value of existing practice and introducing recent developments: leaving no stone unturned in the assessment and treatment of the PDOC patient. Neuropsychol Rehabil 2017; 28(8):1242–53.
24. Teasdale G, Jennett B. ASSESSMENT OF COMA AND IMPAIRED CONSCIOUSNESS. Lancet 1974;304(7872):81–4.
25. Rappaport M, Dougherty AM, Kelting DL. Evaluation of coma and vegetative states. Arch Phys Med Rehabil 1992;73(7):628–34.
26. McAleese A, Wilson CF, McEvoy M, et al. Comparison of SMART and WHIM as measurement tools in routine assessment of PDOC patients. Neuropsychol Rehabil 2016;28(8):1266–74.

27. Shiel A, Horn SA, Wilson BA, et al. The Wessex Head Injury Matrix (WHIM) main scale: a preliminary report on a scale to assess and monitor patient recovery after severe head injury. Clin Rehabil 2000;14(4):408–16.

28. Ansell BJ, Keenan JE. The Western Neuro Sensory Stimulation Profile: a tool for assessing slow-to-recover head-injured patients. Arch Phys Med Rehabil 1989; 70(2):104–8.

29. Giacino J, Whyte J. The Vegetative and Minimally Conscious States. J Head Trauma Rehabil 2005;20(1):30–50.

30. Pape TLB, Heinemann AW, Kelly JP, et al. A measure of neurobehavioral functioning after coma. Part I: Theory, reliability, and validity of the Disorders of Consciousness Scale. The Journal of Rehabilitation Research and Development 2005;42(1):1.

31. Magee WL, Siegert RJ, Taylor SM, et al. Music Therapy Assessment Tool for Awareness in Disorders of Consciousness (MATADOC): Reliability and Validity of a Measure to Assess Awareness in Patients with Disorders of Consciousness. J Music Ther 2015;53(1):1–26.

32. Day KV, DiNapoli MV, Whyte J. Detecting early recovery of consciousness: a comparison of methods. Neuropsychol Rehabil 2017;28(8):1233–41.

33. Schnakers C, Chatelle C, Vanhaudenhuyse A, et al. The Nociception Coma Scale: A new tool to assess nociception in disorders of consciousness. Pain 2010;148(2):215–9.

34. Sanz LRD, Thibaut A, Edlow BL, et al. Update on neuroimaging in disorders of consciousness. Curr Opin Neurol 2021;34(4):488–96.

35. Boly M, Faymonville M-E, Schnakers C, et al. Perception of pain in the minimally conscious state with PET activation: an observational study. Lancet Neurol 2008; 7(11):1013–20.

36. McLellan DL. Current priorities in the understanding and management of disorders of consciousness. Neuropsychol Rehabil 2018;28(8):1229–32.

37. Monti MM, Vanhaudenhuyse A, Coleman MR, et al. Willful modulation of brain activity in disorders of consciousness. N Engl J Med 2010;362(7):579–89.

38. Snider SB, Bodien YG, Frau-Pascual A, et al. Ascending arousal network connectivity during recovery from traumatic coma. Neuroimage Clinical 2020;28:102503.

39. Giacino JT, Whyte J, Bagiella E, et al. Placebo-controlled trial of amantadine for severe traumatic brain injury. N Engl J Med 2012;366(9):819–26.

40. Jha A, Weintraub A, Allshouse A, et al. A randomized trial of modafinil for the treatment of fatigue and excessive daytime sleepiness in individuals with chronic traumatic brain injury. J Head Trauma Rehabil 2008;23(1):52–63.

41. Passler MA, Riggs RV. Positive outcomes in traumatic brain injury-vegetative state: patients treated with bromocriptine. Arch Phys Med Rehabil 2001;82(3): 311–5.

42. Fridman EA, Krimchansky BZ, Bonetto M, et al. Continuous subcutaneous apomorphine for severe disorders of consciousness after traumatic brain injury. Brain Inj 2010;24(4):636–41.

43. Sanz LRD, Lejeune N, Blandiaux S, et al. Treating Disorders of Consciousness With Apomorphine: Protocol for a Double-Blind Randomized Controlled Trial Using Multimodal Assessments. Front Neurol 2019;10.

44. Kim YW, Shin J-C, An Y. Effects of methylphenidate on cerebral glucose metabolism in patients with impaired consciousness after acquired brain injury. Clin Neuropharmacol 2009;32(6):335–9.

45. Tucker C, Sandhu K. The effectiveness of zolpidem for the treatment of disorders of consciousness. Neurocrit Care 2016;24(3):488–93.

46. Whyte J, Rajan R, Rosenbaum A, et al. Zolpidem and restoration of consciousness. Am J Phys Med Rehabil 2014;93(2):101–13.
47. Krimchansky B-Z, Keren O, Sazbon L, et al. Differential time and related appearance of signs, indicating improvement in the state of consciousness in vegetative state traumatic brain injury (VS-TBI) patients after initiation of dopamine treatment. Brain Inj 2004;18(11):1099–105.
48. Page SJ, Cunningham DA, Plow E, et al. It takes two: noninvasive brain stimulation combined with neurorehabilitation. Arch Phys Med Rehabil 2015;96(4 Suppl): S89–93.
49. Estraneo A, Trojano L. Prognosis in Disorders of Consciousness. In: Schnakers C, Laureys, editors. Coma and disorders of consciousness. 2nd edition. Springer; 2018. p. 24–31.
50. Hammond FM, Giacino JT, Nakase Richardson R, et al. Disorders of Consciousness due to Traumatic Brain Injury: Functional Status Ten Years Post-Injury. J Neurotrauma 2019;36(7):1136–46.
51. Seel RT, Douglas J, Dennison AC, et al. Specialized early treatment for persons with disorders of consciousness: program components and outcomes. Arch Phys Med Rehabil 2013;94(10):1908–23.
52. Carrière M, Larroque SK, Martial C, et al. An Echo of Consciousness: Brain Function During Preferred Music. Brain Connect 2020;(10):385–95.
53. Magee WL. Music in the diagnosis, treatment and prognosis of people with prolonged disorders of consciousness. Neuropsychol Rehabil 2018;28(8):1331–9.
54. Demirtas-Tatlidede A, Vahabzadeh-Hagh AM, Bernabeu M, et al. Noninvasive brain stimulation in traumatic brain injury. J Head Trauma Rehabil 2012;27(4): 274–92.
55. Thibaut A, Bruno M-A, Ledoux D, et al. tDCS in patients with disorders of consciousness: sham-controlled randomized double-blind study. Neurology 2014; 82(13):1112–8.
56. Angelakis E, Liouta E, Andreadis N, et al. Transcranial direct current stimulation effects in disorders of consciousness. Arch Phys Med Rehabil 2014;95(2):283–9.
57. Louise-Bender Pape T, Rosenow J, Lewis G, et al. Repetitive transcranial magnetic stimulation-associated neurobehavioral gains during coma recovery. Brain Stimul 2009;2(1):22–35.
58. Bai Y, Xia X, Kang J, et al. Evaluating the effect of repetitive transcranial magnetic stimulation on disorders of consciousness by using TMS-EEG. Front Neurosci 2016;10:473.
59. Bourdillon P, Hermann B, Sitt JD, et al. Electromagnetic Brain Stimulation in Patients With Disorders of Consciousness. Front Neurosci 2019;13.
60. Martens G, Laureys S, Thibaut A. Spasticity Management in Disorders of Consciousness. Brain Sci 2017;7(12):162.
61. Ismail FY, Saleem GT, Ljubisavljevic MR. Brain Data in Pediatric Disorders of Consciousness: Special Considerations. J Clin Neurophysiol 2021;39(1):49–58.
62. Martens G, Foidart-Dessalle M, Laureys S, et al. How does spasticity affect patients with disorders of consciousness?. In: Schnakers C, Laureys, editors. Coma and disorders of consciousness. 2nd edition. Springer; 2018. p. 120–31.
63. Pool J, Magee WL. Music in the Treatment of Children and Youth with Prolonged Disorders of Consciousness. Front Psychol 2016;7:202.

Management of Medical Complications during the Rehabilitation of Moderate–Severe Traumatic Brain Injury

Derrick Allred, MD

KEYWORDS

- Traumatic brain injury • Complications • Paroxysmal sympathetic hyperactivity
- Hydrocephalus • Seizures • Agitation • Sleep • Spasticity

KEY POINTS

- Medical complications occur frequently in the acute rehabilitation period for patients who have sustained a moderate–severe traumatic brain injury (TBI). Medical providers caring for these patients must be able to readily recognize and treat them.
- Some of the more frequently encountered medical complications after a moderate–severe TBI include autonomic dysfunction, neurogenic bladder, agitation, sleep disturbances, seizures, hydrocephalus heterotopic ossification (HO), dizziness, neuroendocrine disorders, and venous thromboembolism.
- Prompt management of the medical complications encountered in a patient with moderate-to-severe TBI typically aids in improved overall functional outcomes.

INTRODUCTION

According to the Centers for Disease Control, in 2019, there were approximately 223,135 hospitalizations in the United States related to traumatic brain injury (TBI).[1] Improvement in overall outcomes has been in part due to improvement in the medical management of the diverse set of complications exhibited in this patient population. If not managed properly, these patients can suffer complications with significant negative implications with respect to morbidity, mortality, and long-term functional prognosis. It is imperative that medical providers who care for patients with TBI across the entire spectrum of care readily diagnose and treat the sequela associated with moderate–severe brain trauma. This article will focus on some of the key medical issues that providers may encounter during acute inpatient rehabilitation.

Department of Physical Medicine & Rehabilitation, University of Utah Health, 85 N Medical Drive, Salt Lake City, UT 84132, USA
E-mail address: derrick.allred@hsc.utah.edu

Phys Med Rehabil Clin N Am 35 (2024) 507–521
https://doi.org/10.1016/j.pmr.2024.02.004
1047-9651/24/© 2024 Elsevier Inc. All rights reserved.

AUTONOMIC DYSREGULATION

The body's mechanism for regulating subconscious neurologic and metabolic function is performed by the autonomic nervous system (ANS) which consists of the sympathetic and parasympathetic divisions. The ANS is essential in regulating multiple physiologic processes that include cardiopulmonary function, thermoregulation, gastrointestinal motility, and micturition. All of these functions are regulated without conscious thought.

During the early stages after sustaining a severe TBI, it is common in the acute and subacute phases to exhibit varying degrees ANS dysfunction, particularly uninhibited sympathetic outflow.[2] The paroxysmal nature of ANS dysfunction after brain injury is characterized by sympathetic hyperactivity resulting from dysregulation of cortical inhibitory pathways.[3] However, standardized diagnostic criteria and therapeutic interventions have historically been difficult to establish. In recent years, the term paroxysmal sympathetic hyperactivity (PSH) has been adopted, which is a more accurate and comprehensive name that has assisted to standardize efforts in its diagnosis and treatment. Presentation of PSH manifests in a transient manner with a combination of any of the following features of sympathetic and motor overactivity:

- Hypertension
- Tachycardia
- Tachypnea
- Elevated body temperature
- Diaphoresis
- Hypertonicity/posturing

Paroxysms of sympathetic hyperactivity can occur several times daily lasting from a few moments to an average of up to 30 minutes.[3] Diagnosis for PSH first begins with a process of exclusion of potential mimics that can include infections, drug withdrawal, serotonin syndrome, or neuroleptic malignant syndrome. If the diagnosis of PSH is considered, then identifying either external or internal factors that could be provoking the hypersympathetic response must be investigated prior to the use of medications. These can include (but are not limited to)

- Overstimulating environment
- Uncontrolled pain
- Intracranial changes such as a worsening hemorrhage, edema, or hydrocephalus
- Constipation
- Urinary retention
- Body malpositioning or occult injury
- Catheters or lines

A recent diagnostic tool that merits further research known as the Paroxysmal Sympathetic Hyperactivity Assessment Measure has been developed and shows potential as a means to standardize the diagnosis of PSH.[4]

Depending on the presenting signs or symptoms of PSH, medications including beta-blockers (propranolol and pindolol), alpha-agonists (clonidine), opioids, benzodiazepines, and other γ-aminobutyric acid type A (GABA-A) agonists (propofol), baclofen (oral and intrathecal), dopamine agonists (bromocriptine), neuropathic pain agents (gabapentin), or dantrolene have been used with varying degrees of evidence.[3] The choice of medication should be targeted at the specific clinical parameter the provider is attempting to treat. Patients with prolonged PSH generally have a more complicated medical course to include a higher infection rate, longer duration for ventilation, higher tracheostomy placement, and longer intensive care unit stays.[5] However, the sympathetic overactivity tends to diminish over time, but motor overactivity can continue to be a problem in the chronic phases of recovery. Severe PSH symptoms have also been shown to have worse functional outcomes.[6]

POSTTRAUMATIC SEIZURES

Seizures occurring after brain injury are one of the many complications that can be challenging to recognize but must be accurately diagnosed to ensure optimal neurorecovery during the rehabilitation period. The severity of the TBI has a correlation with the likelihood of developing a seizure disorder after injury, and posttraumatic seizures (PTS) can be associated with longer hospital admissions and ventilation as well as poorer outcomes and mortality.[7,8] PTS after a TBI are classified by the timing of onset from injury as follows:

- Immediate: within 24 hours
- Early: between 24 hours and 7 days
- Late: after 7 days

Posttraumatic epilepsy (PTE) is defined as more than one late seizure event after brain trauma separated by more than 24 hours. After a first late unprovoked posttraumatic seizure occurs, the prevalence of PTE can be as high as 86% within 2 years.[9] PTS frequently occurs in severe patients with TBI, especially those with risk factors such as premorbid alcohol abuse or epilepsy, loss of consciousness extending beyond 30 minutes, penetrating injuries, depressed skull fractures, intracranial hemorrhage, hydrocephalus, periods of posttraumatic amnesia (PTA) longer than 24 hours, and neurosurgical intervention.[10] During the acute phase of injury, other medical factors such as infection, hypoxic events, metabolic disturbances, and medications that lower the seizure threshold can further increase the likelihood of developing seizure activity. While PTS can include any type of seizure, including generalized tonic-clonic, the most common are partial seizures.[11] However, PTS can have diverse presentations depending on their foci of origin to include new neurologic changes on physical examination, altered mental status, behavior alterations and outbursts, auditory or visual disturbances, or motor overactivity. If any of these symptoms occur, the treatment team must retain PTS in the differential diagnosis and include this in the workup, which must involve electroencephalogram monitoring.[12]

There is no evidence that supports the use of antiepileptic medications (AEDs) in the prevention of late PTS. There is evidence to support medication usage in the prevention of early seizures, with phenytoin being the most studied AED.[13] However, given phenytoin's negative side effect profile, many providers opt to use different AEDs, such as levetiracetam or lacosamide, which in some studies have shown to be equally effective in the prevention of early PTS.[14] Despite this, there is significant variability across treating specialties regarding the use and duration of prophylaxis against PTS. This is likely due, in part, to the aforementioned negative side effects of AEDs, including cognitive blunting, mood disturbance, and somnolence. While patients who just demonstrate immediate PTS are not typically treated long term, those patients who do have early or late PTS are prescribed AEDs for active treatment typically in consultation with an epilepsy specialist. There is general consensus that patients who experience more than one early or late seizure event should be treated pharmacologically. However, AED initiation for treatment after just one early or late seizure is a topic of debate.

NEUROGENIC BLADDER

Urinary dysfunction after TBI is quite common and presents differently from patient-to-patient based on multiple factors to include the area of the brain injured, the patient's premorbid and comorbid medical conditions, and the patient's overall functional status. The central nervous system has a complex physiologic pathway to regulate urinary storage and micturition, with the brain containing 2 micturition centers within the frontal lobe and the pons. After a brief period of initial bladder areflexia postinjury, one of the most common presentations of neurogenic bladder in the TBI population is urinary incontinence which usually results from a combination of functional and physiologic factors.[15,16]

Suprapontine lesions will cause an uninhibited detrusor reflex pattern that results in a hypertonic bladder. This will present with an increase in urinary frequency and low-volume voids. Detrusor-sphincter dyssynergia may result from lesions at or inferior to the pontine micturition center as this region of the brain is thought to be a main contributor to coordination of bladder storage and voiding. If there is significant hypertonicity within the internal or external urinary sphincters, the patient may have difficulties with urinary retention. Apart from the neurophysiology of bladder control, in patients with TBI, there is functional component from the physical limitations sustained from the injury, as well as impaired awareness from the patient's cognitive dysfunction. Both can pose significant challenges in attaining urinary continence in patients with severe TBI.[15]

Usually during the acute phase post-TBI in an intensive care setting, neurogenic bladder is managed with an indwelling catheter to facilitate strict urine measurement and skin protection. However, once a patient has progressed to the rehabilitation phase, the assessment and management of neurogenic bladder progresses toward active management that will provide the patient with a successful bladder program as they eventually transition home. A comprehensive bladder program should be composed of the following when applicable.

- Strict fluid intake and output measurements where possible. This can be challenging in patients with incontinence, but the volume and frequency can lend insight into any degree of hypertonic bladder the patient may be exhibiting.
- For patients who are not able to void, an assessment for causes of urinary retention apart from the TBI must be considered to include urinary tract infection or benign prostatic hyperplasia. Clean intermittent catheterization in time intervals (every 4 to 6 hours) to maintain bladder volumes less than 500 cc is generally preferred to an indwelling catheter if it is not agitating to the patient. If the patient has the appropriate physical and cognitive capabilities, this is a skill that can be taught to them and replicated in a home environment.
- For patients who are urinating, it is important to ensure that they are not retaining too much urine by measuring postvoid residual volumes and performing intermittent catheterization when those volumes exceed 100 cc.
- For patients who are voiding and have the physical ability, a set voiding schedule every 4 hours can also be employed to decrease the frequency of incontinent episodes.
- The patient's medication list must be scrutinized for any agents that can potentially lead to urinary retention.
- Despite these aforementioned measures to enhance urinary continence, pharmacotherapy can be valuable to optimize the patient's physiology just so long as the side effects do not impede with functional progress. This can include the use of anticholinergics (oxybutynin) for hypertonic bladder, or alpha-1 blockers (tamsulosin) for urinary retention.

Urinary incontinence can be one of the most challenging issues to address in the rehabilitation of a patient with TBI, which, if not adequately managed, can lead to poor overall functional outcomes.[15]

SLEEP DISORDERS

Sleep disorders are prevalent among the patient population with severe TBI and can be among the most problematic during the acute and chronic phases postinjury causing negative effects on cognition and neurorecovery.[17–19] One cannot adequately address disorders of arousal, mood disturbances, or cognitive impairments until the patient is getting high-quality sleep. Sleep disorders are typically multifactorial involving environmental, behavioral, and physiologic variables that must be accounted for. Sleep patterns have shown to be altered post-TBI with less rapid eye movement (REM) sleep and poorer sleep efficiency. Patients with TBI also have low levels of melatonin which decreases REM sleep and affects daytime alertness.[20]

While patients with TBI are admitted in the hospital, attention must be given to external factors that could play a role in interfering with sleep. The simplest of these is to scrutinize the frequency and need of nighttime disturbances during typical sleep hours. These can include poorly scheduled medications, early laboratory draws, unnecessarily timed vitals, alarms, lights, and staff conversations. Medical complications including uncontrolled pain and infections can also interfere with sleep. While insomnia and excessive daytime sleepiness are the more commonly treated disturbance, post-traumatic sleep disorders may also include central or obstructive sleep apnea, circadian rhythm disorders, periodic limb movement in sleep, and narcolepsy. If any of these are suspected, these patients should undergo polysomnography if available.[20,21]

Despite the prevalence of sleep disorders in patients with severe TBI, significant research that assesses the utility of medication usage in this population is lacking. Much of the support for medication usage is from anecdotal experience or extrapolation of literature that supports medications is healthy in other populations with different diagnoses.[20] Care must be taken with all sleep aids to minimize the amount of drowsiness that may persist into the day after taking them the night prior. Some of these medications include

- Trazodone: Atypical antidepressant with anxiolytic and sedating properties
- Mirtazapine: Atypical antidepressant with sedating and appetite stimulating properties
- GABA-A agonists: Hypnotics like zolpidem and eszopiclone thought to be less addicting than benzodiazepines that may improve sleep onset
- Melatonin and ramelteon: Aids in re-establishing adequate circadian rhythms
- Atypical antipsychotics: Quetiapine or olanzapine which provide both sedating and neurobehavioral effects
- Tricyclic antidepressants: Can be used to treat insomnia, neuropathic pain, and headaches but can cause undesired anticholinergic effects[20]

AGITATION

Dysfunction in all cognitive domains can pose significant challenges to the medical management of a patient with severe TBI. This is particularly true when these patients exhibit agitation, which is most often due in part to a patient's impaired ability to process their internal and external environment, typically when they are in PTA.[22] Whether it be akathisia, emotional lability, or severe and violent outbursts, neurobehavioral dysfunction like agitation impedes medical interventions and functional recovery.[23–25]

The use of objective measures, such as the Agitated Behavioral Scale, can be effective in the assessment of agitation and the patient's response to treatment.[26] The mainstay of many treating providers outside the specialty of rehabilitation will rely principally on pharmacotherapy to quell neurobehavioral dysfunction. However, instead of merely attributing such behavior to their TBI broadly, the first matter that must be considered is to evaluate potential provocation in an agitated and cognitively impaired patient who has difficulty being redirected. Although more studies are needed to discern which nonpharmacologic methods are most effective in reducing agitation,[27] common considerations are as follows:

- Confusing surroundings: This can be addressed with the use of familiar objects such as family photos and frequent reorienting by the treatment team.
- Metabolic disturbances or infections.
- Uncontrolled somatic pain from concurrent injuries or centrally mediated neuropathic pain.
- Excessive ambient stimulation: This can include disturbing lighting in the room, simple conversation nearby, or a television in the room.
- Sleep-related issues that can be related to postinjury sleep disorders or unnecessary disruptions.
- Catheters or lines.
- Bowel or bladder incontinence.
- Excessive use of restraints: Often permissive restlessness monitored by staff in a safe environment can be effective.

Every circumstance surrounding an agitated patient is different, but often medications are needed and can be effective.[28] Benzodiazepines and typical antipsychotics are almost always uniformly discouraged due to their effects on recovery. The choice of medication should work to minimize undesired side effects and treat comorbid conditions. The following medications are the most commonly utilized classes:

- Beta-blockers (propranolol)
- Antiepileptics (valproic acid)
- Atypical antipsychotics
- Antidepressants (selective serotonin reuptake inhibitors [SSRIs], serotonin and norepinephrine reuptake inhibitors [SNRIs])
- Neurostimulants (amantadine)

Each class of medication poses advantages and disadvantages and should be utilized with the goal of eventually tapering off. As a patient's cognitive function improves, agitation also improves as there tends to be a relationship between PTA and the agitation exhibited by a patient with severe TBI.[29]

NEUROENDOCRINE DISORDERS

Posttraumatic pituitary dysfunction must be assessed for in both the acute and chronic phases of recovery after a TBI. Posttraumatic endocrinopathies are broadly estimated to occur in roughly 10% to 58% of patients with TBI.[30] Approximately two-thirds of patients who die from a severe TBI who undergo autopsy have been found to have structural abnormalities in the hypothalamus, pituitary stalk, and/or pituitary gland.[31] Hypopituitarism not only has negative consequences for metabolic process in the body but also has been shown to have significant implications in functional recovery within neurobehavioral and cognitive domains.[31,32] Due to its positioning within the sella turcica, the pituitary gland is susceptible to shearing injury during head trauma. Connected to the hypothalamus through the infundibulum, the pituitary gland is divided into an anterior and posterior lobe where several hormones are secreted for the regulation of multiple metabolic processes. Some key hormones are outlined as follows:

- Antidiuretic hormone (ADH): ADH regulates fluid balance within the body. It does this by controlling water loss in the kidneys by causing them to release less water in response to changes in fluid balance and osmolality. Disorders of ADH typically result in electrolyte disturbances involving serum sodium. If too much ADH is secreted irrespective of serum osmolality, this leads to water retention and hyponatremia in a condition known as the syndrome of inappropriate antidiuretic hormone secretion (SIADH). If the posterior pituitary gland decreases its ADH production, this can lead to a significant increase in hypo-osmolar urine output and polydipsia resulting in hypernatremia in a condition known as diabetes insipidus (DI). Standard treatment of SIADH involves fluid restriction, although it is customary in some clinical settings to use salt tablets or hypertonic saline as an adjunct. Centrally mediated DI can be treated with desmopressin. The third ADH-related condition to be aware of is cerebral salt wasting (CSW), which can cause significant hyponatremia. CSW differs from SIADH in that even though both manifest in the setting of elevated levels of ADH, in CSW, the body still excretes both sodium and fluids resulting in a true hypovolemic hyponatremia. As opposed to SIADH, CSW is treated with isotonic saline fluid administration. In all cases mentioned earlier, care must be taken to not to correct sodium disturbances too quickly as to avoid the central pontine myelinolysis.[33–36]
- Growth hormone (GH): GH deficiency is cited as the most common endocrinopathy after brain injury. GH deficiency or insufficiency can result in a myriad of symptoms to include mood disturbance, higher level of body fat and decreased lean muscle mass, impaired cognition, fatigue, and reduction in bone mineral density. Serum levels of insulin-like growth factor 1 (IGF-1) has traditionally been used as a screening test for GH deficiency, but recent evidence demonstrates that patients with TBI can be GH deficient with normal IGF-1 levels, thereby necessitating more dynamic testing. There are no consensus guidelines on GH replacement in patients with severe TBI. However, there are some recent studies to suggest it may be beneficial in treating certain functional domains such as cognition. However, GH deficiency is typically screened for in the chronic stages of recovery.[37,38]
- Thyroid-stimulating hormone: Hypothyroidism can cause cold intolerance, weight gain, fatigue, cognitive dysfunction, irregular menses in women, and hair loss. It is even postulated to increase late seizure risk. Screening for hypothyroidism is typically deferred until after the acute illness has improved. However, thyroid dysfunction can result in worse functional outcomes.[39]
- Adrenocorticotropic hormone (ACTH): ACTH stimulates the release of cortisol, mineralocorticoids, and androgens from the adrenal cortex. Lack of ACTH production can result in cortisol and mineralocorticoid deficiency which can ultimately be life-threatening if the body is unable to respond in instances of physiologic stress. It is imperative that this diagnosis remain on the clinician's differential in the event of hemodynamic instability, hyponatremia, and hypoglycemia. Adrenal insufficiency can also manifest as fatigue, weakness, anorexia, altered mental status, labile blood pressure, nausea, vomiting or diarrhea, and electrolyte disturbances. If adrenal insufficiency is suspected, a morning cortisol level or ACTH

stimulation test may be undertaken, but these tests can be unreliable in the acute postinjury period. If there is suspicion for adrenal insufficiency, stress dose steroids should not be delayed.[40]

SPASTICITY

Spasticity is a form of motor overactivity seen in central nervous lesions such as TBI or spinal cord injury which manifests as increased muscle tone that is velocity dependent to passive stretching. Despite this specific definition, the term spasticity is often used synonymously with other forms of hypertonicity. Spasticity can occur during any time of the acute or rehabilitative phases after TBI and must be managed appropriately to avoid short-term and long-term functional impairments. In the paretic upper limb, spasticity commonly presents with varying degrees of a flexor pattern of the fingers, wrist, and elbow with forearm pronation and shoulder adduction/internal rotation. In the paretic lower limb, the ankles can exhibit a plantar-flexed and equinovarus pattern, with the knees and hips flexed and leg adducted. As spasticity develops, the treatment team must make ongoing assessments as to whether the increase in muscle tone is beneficial or harmful. Functionally, patients may require some degree of spasticity in certain muscle groups to assist with tasks such as transfers or ambulation. However, spasticity can also pose significant challenges in patients with TBI by hindering activities of daily living, causing significant pain and affecting sleep.

A small degree of spasticity is often acceptable and can initially be managed through nonpharmacologic means such as routine stretching and range of motion exercises used in combination with bracing throughout the day. Other modalities such as ultrasound, transcutaneous electrical nerve stimulation, and extracorporeal shock wave therapy have been used with promising but mixed results.[41,42] If spasticity worsens, the medical provider must first assess for potential causes of acute provocation to include metabolic disturbances or infection, bowel or bladder distention, deep venous thrombosis (DVT), or other nociceptive input.[43]

Once potential provoking factors have been accounted for, and therapies and physical modalities have been optimized, such as casting, physiotherapy, splinting, tilt table, and electrical stimulation,[44] pharmacologic interventions are commonly employed. The most routinely prescribed oral medications with their mechanisms of action outlined as follows:

- Baclofen: GABA-B receptor agonist
- Diazepam: GABA-A receptor agonist
- Tizanidine: Alpha-2 receptor agonist
- Clonidine: Alpha-2 receptor agonist
- Dantrolene: Inhibits calcium release from the sarcoplasmic reticulum

Each of these medications has potential undesired side effects. All of the above medications can be sedating, even though dantrolene is thought to do so to a lesser degree due to its peripheral mechanism of action. Baclofen can have severe withdrawal symptoms if discontinued abruptly. Tizanidine and dantrolene (and baclofen to a lesser degree) can be hepatotoxic. Tizanidine and clonidine can cause significant hypotension. These are just a few of the more common side effects of these medications.[45]

Botulinum toxin is an effective injectable treatment of spasticity that works by blocking acetylcholine release at the neuromuscular junction in targeted muscles. It is a preferred treatment in patients with focal spasticity that can last anywhere between 2 and 4 months.[45] However, botulinum toxin is not typically used until the outpatient setting. This is due to the need for maximization of other treatment options and the delayed onset of the toxin's effect. In addition, there financial constraints imposed by insurance companies of using botulinum toxin it in the inpatient setting. The use of phenol for motor point or nerve blocks is a cheaper alternative with an immediate and longer lasting effect.

HETEROTOPIC OSSIFICATION

HO is the formation of mature lamellar bone in structures where bone does not exist. HO can form in practically any location throughout the body becoming problematic from a functional and pain standpoint.[46,47] HO typically develops during the first several months following a severe TBI and usually presents with pain, swelling, warmth, and decreased mobility in the affected body part. Diagnosing HO can be difficult because it mimics other common medical complications, such as a deep venous thrombosis or hypertonicity. Risk factors for the development of HO in patients with brain injury are typically associated with the severity of the TBI, such as prolonged coma, surgical procedures, spasticity in the affected limb, ongoing immobility and other injuries such as long-bone fractures. HO can affect any limb but is most commonly seen in the hip region in patients with TBI. If not accurately diagnosed and managed, HO can lead to worsening mobility as well as pain syndromes, osteoporosis, neurovascular entrapment, skin breakdown, or increased spasticity.[48–50]

The rehabilitation provider must maintain high clinical suspicion for HO in any patient who is complaining of ongoing joint or limb pain with restricted range of motion. An elevated alkaline phosphatase has traditionally been thought of as early laboratory finding in patients with HO, but it is extremely nonspecific, especially in patients with liver injury or polytrauma. Plain radiographs are often the first diagnostic measure undertaken, but they cannot typically detect the formation of HO for several weeks after its initial formation and deposition. Triple phase bone scan has been shown to be the most sensitive evaluation for early HO but may not be able to delineate between other potential causes of regional inflammation. Other imaging modalities such as MRI have shown potential in the diagnosis of early HO within days after symptom onset.[50]

Treatment of HO largely depends on the medical and functional implications for each individual patient. If found incidentally, and there is no associated medical complication, functional restriction or the potential for such, watchful waiting is sometimes undertaken. However, in cases where there is joint involvement, it is vitally important to maintain functional range of motion. Dedicated studies investigating the use of medications in the treatment of HO in the population with severe TBI are lacking. However, nonsteroid anti-inflammatory drugs (such as indomethacin) and bisphosphonates are the mainstay of pharmacotherapies to halt HO formation, but these are most effective if initiated in the early stages after visualization on bone scan, but before findings on plain films.[50] Often these drugs are avoided in patients with comorbid fractures for fear of preventing those injuries from healing. Surgical excision has traditionally been reserved for those patients who have matured HO and are 1.5 years postdiagnosis. However, there are studies suggesting the resection of immature HO may not increase recurrence rates.[50]

VENOUS THROMBOSIS

One of the most common and feared medical complications seen on a rehabilitation floor, especially in patients with TBI, is venous thromboembolism (VTE). Severe brain injury along with many of the accompanying medical complexities seen in these patients result in immobility and hypercoagulability that leaves patients susceptible to

VTE. If not recognized, pulmonary embolism can be life-threatening. There has been considerable debate regarding the safety of initiating pharmacologic prophylaxis in patients with brain injury. Historically, what has been practiced has varied across different providers due the array of presentations of intracranial hemorrhage and fear of causing worse bleeding.

One of the first considerations for initiating chemical prophylaxis is obtaining a medical history specific to coagulopathy and any blood thinning medications the patient may be prescribed. Obtaining baseline coagulation studies to include platelet count, international normalised ratio (INR), and prothrombin time (PT) and partial thromboplastin time (PTT) is also vital.

After this, the 2 biggest questions that arise in considering the safety of pharmacologic prophylaxis is how soon can it be initiated and what is the most appropriate medication to use? There are published estimates of upward of 54% of patients with TBI develop VTE without chemoprophylaxis and in 20% to 30% of patients even with the use of mechanical prophylaxis.[51]

Recent studies are beginning to indicate that in patients with head bleeds deemed stable on computed tomography (CT) initiating chemical prophylaxis may be safe after 24 to 72 hours after injury. However, some contend that earlier chemical prophylaxis can come with a risk of increased likelihood of repeat neurosurgical intervention.[52] The Berne–Norwood criteria, which are cited by the American College of Surgeons, suggest tiers for low, moderate, and high-risk categories for worsening bleeding and the initiation of chemoprophylaxis after 24 hours, 72 hours, or the need to place an inferior vena cava filter.[53] However, although there are some promising data within this topic, there is still a lack of consensus as to the timing and more research is needed. In addition, deciding which medication to use is also lacking consensus. It appears that low-molecular weight heparin may not pose a higher risk for worsening intracranial hemorrhage, but due to its shorter half-life, many providers still opt to use unfractionated heparin. The Brain Trauma Foundation does not currently endorse one over the other.[51]

POSTTRAUMATIC HYDROCEPHALUS

A posttraumatic complication that can easily go unrecognized is hydrocephalus. It is a condition characterized by dilation of the brain's ventricular system from excessive accumulation of cerebrospinal fluid (CSF) due to excessive production or outflow obstruction into the subarachnoid space. Hydrocephalus can be divided into communicating or noncommunicating depending on the CSF flow within the ventricular system. Most forms of posttraumatic hydrocephalus (PTH) are communicating due to blood product interference with CSF reabsorption through the arachnoid granulations. The most significant risk factors for the development of PTH are higher severity TBI, intraventricular hemorrhage, subarachnoid hemorrhage, intracranial infections such as meningitis, and having underwent a craniectomy.[54] Historically, hydrocephalus had been associated with the classic presenting triad of urinary incontinence, altered mental status, and motor disturbances such as ataxia. However, PTH should be part of the differential anytime a patient begins to show either slower-than-expected progression or functional regression. It can present with a myriad of signs and symptoms such as neurobehavioral or cognitive changes, decreased postural stability, worsening motor abnormalities to include gait disturbances or new spasticity, nausea and vomiting, or change or worsening in headache patterns. Some studies have suggested that a large proportion of patients who develop PTH occur during acute rehabilitation.[55] Therefore, it is imperative that treating providers are cognizant of risk factors and include this PTH as part of the differential when unexpected cognitive decline or plateau occurs during acute rehabilitation.[56] Untreated PTH is known to be associated with prolonged PTA and worse functional outcomes during inpatient rehabilitation.[57]

When hydrocephalus is suspected, brain imaging with either CT or MRI should be performed. However, the mere visualization of ventriculomegaly is often insufficient to determine whether a patient will respond to surgical intervention with shunting.[54] Specialized imaging modalities such as single-photon emission computed tomography have been investigated in assessing hydrocephalus.[58] However, regardless of imaging findings, invasive drainage of CSF is often employed to determine potential shunt responsiveness. This is accomplished either by a single lumbar puncture with removal of CSF or through a prolonged drainage trial with a lumbar catheter over the course of a few days. Neurologic response to these procedures should be closely monitored shortly thereafter and should involve cognitive and functional testing to include gait analysis if possible. If deemed to be appropriate, CSF diversion with shunting can improve outcomes.[57,59]

DIZZINESS

Dizziness can be one of the most debilitating and frustrating sequalae of TBI during a patient's rehabilitation and is a term used by patients to describe many issues such as imbalance, lightheadedness, or vertigo. While disruption of the vestibular system can be the etiology for such symptoms, it is essential to make a full assessment for post-TBI dizziness.[60] It is also important to keep dizziness as part of a differential for agitation as some patients, due to their cognitive disruption or aphasia, may not be able to articulate to their treatment team what they are experiencing.

Due to volume depletion, autonomic dysfunction, and antihypertensive medications, orthostasis is often a cause of dizziness. This can often be managed by fluid resuscitation and careful titration of cardioprudent medications. The donning of compression stockings or an abdominal binder before the start of a therapy can be effective as well. Pharmacologic agents such as midodrine or fludrocortisone can be used and titrated to maintain normotension and ameliorate orthostasis caused by autonomic dysfunction.

Dizziness may also be a result of visual impairment. Although it can be challenging if the patient is not able to fully cooperate, a vision screen should be undertaken to assess for issues such as visual field deficits, diplopia, or oculomotor convergence abnormalities—all of which can contribute to a feeling of dizziness. If available, vision specialists such as neuro-ophthalmologists or neuro-optometrists can provide early assessments and treatment plans such as the use of patches, prisms, or other forms of vision rehab.

Vestibular dysfunction can be either central or peripheral in etiology with the more common etiologies being vertebrobasilar insufficiency and benign paroxysmal positional vertigo (BPPV). Vestibular therapists can employ a comprehensive treatment plan which may include repositioning maneuvers in the setting of BPPV.[61] Pharmacotherapy often involves the use of anticholinergics such as scopolamine or meclizine, but medications such as these must be used with caution due to their side effect profiles.

SUMMARY

There are a number of brain-injury-specific medical complications that occur during inpatient rehabilitation including autonomic dysregulation, neurogenic bladder, sleep and behavioral disturbances, endocrinopathies, spasticity, HO, VTE, PTH, and dizziness. This is not a comprehensive list as every brain-injured patient presents with his or her own unique set of medical and behavioral challenges. However, the rehabilitation specialist must be able to identify these issues, and all others, to ensure optimal functional recovery.

CLINICS CARE POINTS

- The prompt identifcation of intrinsic and extrinic provoking factors in patients with severe traumatic brain sequelae, such as autonomic dysregulation, sleep disruption, agitation, and spasticity must be used in conjunction with medication management.

DISCLOSURE

None.

REFERENCES

1. TBI data. Centers for Disease control and prevention. Available at: https://www. cdc.gov/traumaticbraininjury/data/index.html. [Accessed 25 July 2023].
2. Zheng R-Z, Lei Z-Q, Yang R-Z, et al. Identification and management of paroxysmal sympathetic hyperactivity after Traumatic Brain Injury. Front Neurol 2020; 11. https://doi.org/10.3389/fneur.2020.00081.
3. Jafari AA, Shah M, Mirmoeeni S, et al. Paroxysmal sympathetic hyperactivity during Traumatic Brain Injury. Clin Neurol Neurosurg 2022;212:107081.
4. Samuel S, Lee M, Brown RJ, et al. Incidence of paroxysmal sympathetic hyperactivity following Traumatic Brain Injury Using Assessment Tools. Brain Inj 2018;32(9):1115–21.
5. Fernandez-Ortega JF, Prieto-Palomino MA, Garcia-Caballero M, et al. Paroxysmal sympathetic hyperactivity after traumatic brain injury: Clinical and prognostic implications. J Neurotrauma 2012;29(7):1364–70.
6. Totikov A, Boltzmann M, Schmidt SB, et al. Influence of paroxysmal sympathetic hyperactivity (PSH) on the functional outcome of neurological early rehabilitation patients: A case control study. BMC Neurol 2019;19(1). https://doi.org/10.1186/s12883-0191399-y.
7. Laing J, Gabbe B, Chen Z, et al. Risk factors and prognosis of early posttraumatic seizures in moderate to severe traumatic brain injury. JAMA Neurol 2022; 79(4):334.
8. Majidi S, Makke Y, Ewida A, et al. Prevalence and risk factors for early seizure in patients with traumatic brain injury: Analysis from National Trauma Data Bank. Neurocritical Care 2016;27(1):90–5.
9. Haltiner AM, Temkin NR, Dikmen SS. Risk of seizure recurrence after the first late posttraumatic seizure. Arch Phys Med Rehabil 1997;78(8):835–40.
10. Temkin NR. Risk factors for posttraumatic seizures in adults. Epilepsia 2003;44: 1820.
11. Agrawal A, Timothy J, Pandit L, et al. Post-traumatic epilepsy: An overview. Clin Neurol Neurosurg 2006;108(5):433–9.
12. Verellen RM, Cavazos JE. Post-traumatic epilepsy: An overview. Therapy 2010; 7(5):527–31.
13. Thompson K, Pohlmann-Eden B, Campbell LA, et al. Pharmacological treatments for preventing epilepsy following traumatic head injury. Cochrane Database Syst Rev 2015;2015(8). https://doi.org/10.1002/14651858.cd009900.pub2.

14. Kwon SJ, Barletta JF, Hall ST, et al. Lacosamide versus phenytoin for the prevention of early post traumatic seizures. J Crit Care 2019;50:50–3.

15. Chua K, Chuo A, Kong KH. Urinary incontinence after traumatic brain injury: Incidence, outcomes and correlates. Brain Inj 2003;17(6):469–78.

16. Lucke-Wold B, Vaziri S, Scott K, et al. Urinary dysfunction in acute brain injury: A narrative review. Clin Neurol Neurosurg 2020;189:105614.

17. Castriotta RJ, Wilde MC, Lai JM, et al. Prevalence and consequences of sleep disorders in traumatic brain injury. J Clin Sleep Med 2007;03(04):349–56.

18. Pattinson CL, Brickell TA, Bailie J, et al. Sleep disturbances following traumatic brain injury are associated with poor neurobehavioral outcomes in US military service members and Veterans. J Clin Sleep Med 2021;17(12):2425–38.

19. Zuzuárregui JR, Bickart K, Kutscher SJ. A review of sleep disturbances following traumatic brain injury. Sleep Science and Practice 2018;2(1). https://doi.org/10.1186/s41606-0180020-4.

20. Driver S, Stork R. Pharmacological management of sleep after traumatic brain injury. NeuroRehabilitation 2018;43(3):347–53.

21. Viola-Saltzman M, Watson NF. Traumatic brain injury and sleep disorders. Neurol Clin 2012;30(4):1299–312.

22. Lombard LA, Zafonte RD. Agitation after traumatic brain injury. Am J Phys Med Rehabil 2005;84(10):797–812.

23. Wang Z, Winans NJ, Zhao Z, et al. Agitation following severe traumatic brain injury is a clinical sign of recovery of Consciousness. Frontiers in Surgery 2021;8. https://doi.org/10.3389/fsurg.2021.627008.

24. Bogner JA, Corrigan JD, Fugate L, et al. Role of agitation in prediction of outcomes after Traumatic Brain Injury. Am J Phys Med Rehab 2001;80(9):636–44.

25. Phyland RK, Ponsford JL, Carrier SL, et al. Agitated behaviors following traumatic brain injury: A systematic review and meta-analysis of prevalence by post-traumatic amnesia status, hospital setting, and agitated behavior type. J Neurotrauma 2021;38(22):3047–67.

26. Amato S, Resan M, Mion L. The feasibility, reliability, and clinical utility of the agitated behavior scale in brain-injured rehabilitation patients. Rehabil Nurs 2012;37(1):19–24.

27. Carrier SL, Hicks AJ, Ponsford JL, et al. Effectiveness of non-pharmacological interventions for managing agitation during post-traumatic amnesia following traumatic brain injury: A systematic review protocol. JBI Evidence Synthesis 2020;19(2):499–512.

28. Rahmani E, Lemelle TM, Samarbafzadeh E, et al. Pharmacological treatment of agitation and/or aggression in patients with traumatic brain injury: A systematic review of reviews. J Head Trauma Rehabil 2021;36(4). https://doi.org/10.1097/htr.0000000000000656.

29. McKay A, Love J, Trevena-Peters J, et al. The relationship between agitation and impairments of orientation and memory during the PTA period after Traumatic Brain Injury. Neuropsychol Rehabil 2018;30(4):579–90.

30. Molaie AM, Maguire J. Neuroendocrine abnormalities following traumatic brain injury: An important contributor to neuropsychiatric sequelae. Front Endocrinol 2018;9. https://doi.org/10.3389/fendo.2018.00176.

31. Masel BE, Urban R. Chronic endocrinopathies in traumatic brain injury disease. J Neurotrauma 2015;32(23):1902–10.

32. Gray S, Bilski T, Dieudonne B, et al. Hypopituitarism after traumatic brain injury. Cureus 2019. https://doi.org/10.7759/cureus.4163.

33. T; SBL. Concurrence of inappropriate antidiuretic hormone secretion and cerebral salt wasting syndromes after traumatic brain injury. Front Neurosci 2017; 11:499. Available at: https://pubmed.ncbi.nlm.nih.gov/28932182/.

34. Dick M, Catford SR, Kumareswaran K, et al. Persistent syndrome of inappropriate antidiuretic hormone secretion following traumatic brain injury. Endocrinology, diabetes & metabolism case reports 2015;2015:150070. https://pubmed.ncbi.nlm.nih.gov/26527077/.

35. Capatina C, Paluzzi A, Mitchell R, et al. Diabetes Insipidus after traumatic brain injury. J Clin Med 2015;4(7):1448–62.

36. Cindi JC, Day MW. Central neurogenic diabetes insipidus, syndrome of inappropriate secretion of antidiuretic hormone, and cerebral salt-wasting syndrome in traumatic brain injury. Crit Care Nurse 2012;32(2). https://doi.org/10.4037/ccn2012904.

37. Kgosidialwa O, Hakami O, Zia-Ul-Hussnain HM, et al. Growth hormone deficiency following traumatic brain injury. Int J Mol Sci 2019;20(13):3323.

38. Gasco V, Cambria V, Bioletto F, et al. Traumatic brain injury as frequent cause of hypopituitarism and growth hormone deficiency: Epidemiology, diagnosis, and treatment. Front Endocrinol 2021;12. https://doi.org/10.3389/fendo.2021.634415.

39. Mele C, Pagano L, Franciotta D, et al. Thyroid function in the subacute phase of traumatic brain injury: A potential predictor of post-traumatic neurological and functional outcomes. J Endocrinol Invest 2021;45(2):379–89.

40. Mahajan C, Prabhakar H, Bilotta F. Endocrine dysfunction after traumatic brain injury: An ignored clinical syndrome? Neurocritical Care 2023. https://doi.org/10.1007/s12028-022-01672-3.

41. Mahmood A, Veluswamy SK, Hombali A, et al. Effect of transcutaneous electrical nerve stimulation on spasticity in adults with stroke: A systematic review and meta-analysis. Arch Phys Med Rehabil 2019;100(4):751–68.

42. Yang E, Lew HL, Özçakar L, et al. Recent advances in the treatment of spasticity: Extracorporeal shock wave therapy. J Clin Med 2021;10(20):4723.

43. Thomas AM, Joseph AP. Management of spasticity in adults. InnovAIT: Education and inspiration for general practice 2020;13(10):574–81.

44. Vasudevan V, Amatya B, Khan F. Overview of systematic reviews: Management of common traumatic brain injury-related complications. PLoS One 2022;17(9). https://doi.org/10.1371/journal.pone.0273998.

45. Chang E, Ghosh N, Yanni D, et al. A review of spasticity treatments: Pharmacological and interventional approaches. Crit Rev Phys Rehabil Med 2013;25(1–2): 11–22.

46. Huang H, Cheng W-X, Hu Y-P, et al. Relationship between heterotopic ossification and traumatic brain injury. Journal of Orthopaedic Translation 2018;12:16–25.

47. Simonsen LL, Sonne-Holm S, Krasheninnikoff M, et al. Symptomatic heterotopic ossification after very severe traumatic brain injury in 114 patients: Incidence and risk factors. Injury 2007;38(10):1146–50.

48. Wong KR, Mychasiuk R, O'Brien TJ, et al. Neurological heterotopic ossification: Novel mechanisms, prognostic biomarkers and prophylactic therapies. Bone Research 2020;8(1). https://doi.org/10.1038/s41413-020-00119-9.

49. Xu Y, Huang M, He W, et al. Heterotopic ossification: Clinical features, basic researches, and mechanical stimulations. Front Cell Dev Biol 2022;10. https://doi.org/10.3389/fcell.2022.770931.

50. Sullivan MP, Torres SJ, Mehta S, et al. Heterotopic ossification after central nervous system trauma. Bone Joint Res 2013;2(3):51–7.

51. Rappold JF, Sheppard FR, Carmichael SP II, et al. Venous thromboembolism prophylaxis in the Trauma Intensive Care Unit: An American Association for the surgery of trauma critical care committee clinical consensus document. Trauma Surgery & Acute Care Open 2021;6(1). https://doi.org/10.1136/tsaco-2020-000643.

52. Byrne JP, Witiw CD, Schuster JM, et al. Association of venous thromboembolism prophylaxis after neurosurgical intervention for traumatic brain injury with thromboembolic complications, repeated neurosurgery, and mortality. JAMA Surgery 2022;157(3). https://doi.org/10.1001/jamasurg.2021.5794.

53. ACS TQIP - The American College of Surgeons. Available at: https://www.facs.org/media/mkej5u3b/tbi_guidelines.pdf. [Accessed 29 July 2023].

54. Svedung Wettervik T, Lewén A, Enblad P. Post-traumatic hydrocephalus – incidence, risk factors, treatment, and clinical outcome. Br J Neurosurg 2021; 36(3):400–6.

55. Kammersgaard LP, Linnemann M, Tibæk M. Hydrocephalus following severe traumatic brain injury in adults. incidence, timing, and clinical predictors during rehabilitation. NeuroRehabilitation 2013;33(3):473–80.

56. Chen K-H, Lee C-P, Yang Y-H, et al. Incidence of hydrocephalus in traumatic brain injury. Medicine 2019;98(42). https://doi.org/10.1097/md.0000000000017568.

57. Kowalski RG, Weintraub AH, Rubin BA, et al. Impact of timing of ventriculoperitoneal shunt placement on outcome in posttraumatic hydrocephalus. J Neurosurg 2019;130(2):406–17.

58. Mazzini L, Campini R, Angelino E, et al. Posttraumatic hydrocephalus: A clinical, neuroradiologic, and neuropsychologic assessment of long-term outcome. Arch Phys Med Rehabil 2003;84(11):1637–41.

59. Weintraub AH, Gerber DJ, Kowalski RG. Posttraumatic hydrocephalus as a confounding influence on brain injury rehabilitation: Incidence, clinical characteristics, and outcomes. Arch Phys Med Rehabil 2017;98(2):312–9.

60. Chandrasekhar SS. The assessment of balance and dizziness in the TBI patient. NeuroRehabilitation 2013;32(3):445–54.

61. Harrell RG, Manetta CJ, Gorgacz MP. Dizziness and balance disorders in a traumatic brain injury population: Current clinical approaches. Current Physical Medicine and Rehabilitation Reports 2021;9(2):41–6.

Acute Concussion

Clausyl J. Plummer II, MD*, Nicholas Abramson, MD

KEYWORDS

- Concussion • Mild traumatic brain injury • Post-concussive syndrome
- Return to play • Return to work

KEY POINTS

- Concussions (or mild traumatic brain injury) are the most common head injuries.
- Concussions can cause multiple types of disturbances from a symptomatology standpoint.
- Concussions are a clinical diagnosis.
- Treatment plans should be personalized and should address category of symptoms.

INTRODUCTION/HISTORY/DEFINITIONS/BACKGROUND

A concussion or mild traumatic brain injury (mTBI) is defined as a "traumatically induced transient disturbance of brain function."[1] The WHO (World Health Organization) defines head trauma as an "acute brain injury to the head from external physical forces."[2] Traumatic brain injury remains a significant cause of death and debility worldwide and it is estimated that around 50 million individuals are affected annually by a new TBI.[2] Mild TBI remains the most common classification of TBI and accounts for around 90% of cases overall and are classified by initial GCS (Glascow Coma Scale) of 13 to 15, post-traumatic amnesia (PTA) duration between none and 24 hours, and duration of loss of consciousness (LOC) between none and 30 minutes.[2,3]

In addition to these classification systems, it is also recommended to consider the following when suspecting mild TBI: Any alteration in consciousness (confused state or disoriented state), transient focal deficits, headaches, new vestibular deficits, any change in behavioral status, or transient changes in visual function in the setting of head trauma.[3]

Pathophysiology

There are several steps to the neuro-metabolic cascade that are initiated after a mild TBI that are important to understand. It is thought that this complex cascade involves neuronal injury that results in neuronal membrane disruption, increased extracellular

---

Department of Physical Medicine and Rehabilitation, Vanderbilt University Medical Center, 2201 Children's Way, Nashville, TN 37212, USA
* Corresponding author. 2201 Children's Way Nahsville, TN 37212.
E-mail address: clausyl.j.plummer@vumc.org

Phys Med Rehabil Clin N Am 35 (2024) 523–533
https://doi.org/10.1016/j.pmr.2024.02.005
1047-9651/24/© 2024 Elsevier Inc. All rights reserved.

potassium release (indiscriminate ionic release), indiscriminate release of excitatory glutamate with eventual progression to mitochondrial dysfunction, and cell death (autophagy, apoptosis, and cell necrosis). Recent studies have also explored whether there is a component of triphasic hypoperfusion, hyperperfusion, and then hypoperfusion in the setting of mild TBI (has accepted with more severe head injuries).[4] This is not to be secondary to several mechanisms to include impaired autoregulation of cerebral blood-flow and vaso-reactive compromise.[4] As more is understood about the pathophysiology involved in concussion, more attempts are being made to correlate these molecular findings with clinical symptoms; particularly with advancements in functional MRI.

Persisting Symptoms After Concussion

The trajectory of recovery after concussion generally occurs over the course of 2 to 4 weeks post-injury and is observed in approximately 90% of individuals who have sustained a concussion. If recovery does not occur, 3 months post-injury, the patients are considered to develop persisting symptoms after a concussion (PSaC).[5] Of note, this was previously referred to post concussive syndrome but it is thought that the persisting symptoms after concussion more accurately illustrates that there can be symptoms that develop after a concussion that could be related to the concussion or not.[5] There are also recommendations to avoid using the term "persistent" and to replace it with "persisting" symptoms to avoid characterizing them as "unrelenting and unremitting."[5]

DISCUSSION
Diagnosis

Concussions/mild TBI remain a clinical diagnosis and can be very difficult to diagnose objectively.[3] There are several reasons for this, to include limitations in timing of the initial assessment, limitations in head imaging, biomarkers, and continued reliance on subjective reporting of symptoms.[6] Nonetheless, it is important to be aware of the more frequently used clinical modalities in the acute work-up of concussions.

It is important to note that a majority of individuals who have sustained a mild TBI do so in a non-sports setting.[7] Falls remain the most common cause of TBI in the United States (US) with motor vehicle accidents (MVA) being the second most common cause overall.[8] Many are initially evaluated by either primary care providers or in the emergency room setting.[8] It is in these settings that a thorough history should be gathered to determine mechanism of injury, duration of LOC, duration of alteration of consciousness (AOC), precipitating events leading up to head trauma, and degree of post traumatic symptoms. There should be screening for risk factors for prolonged recovery by way of a detailed review of systems. It has been identified that the most important risk factor for prolonged recovery is having multiple severe symptoms at the time of diagnosis.[6,9] Other risk factors for prolonged recovery include prior history of headaches, sleep disorders, mood disorders, and cognitive disorders.[6]

The common domains implicated after mTBI includes somatic/physical symptoms, cognitive symptoms, sleep issues, and mood related issues. At minimum, patients should be screened for issues in these domains during clinical evaluation.

While in-depth discussion on on-field assessments in sports concussions are beyond the scope of this article, it is worth noting that there are several assessments that can be used. It is recommended to consider on-field assessment such the SCAT-5(sports concussion assessment tool-5) if an on-field concussion is suspected.[8] Please see the dedicated article to sports-related concussions for more details.

Individuals who present develop symptoms after a concussion can develop the following types of symptoms (**Table 1**).

After gathering a detailed history, it is recommended that an extensive physical examination be completed. It is recommended that there be a thorough assessment of the patient's degree of alertness, orientation, GCS scoring, and current cognitive ability. There are several domains that are affected after concussion/mild TBI and these authors recommend utilizing the post concussive symptom checklist (or an equivalent assessment) to not only gather data on what symptoms are prevalent but also to track improvement during serial assessments.

The examination should also include a detailed assessment of the patient's cranial nerves to ensure there are no acute changes. This author recommends a thorough neurologic examination that includes sensory testing to the upper and lower extremities, reflexes for signs of upper/lower motor neuron derangements, and cerebellar sign testing. It is also important to conduct a full musculoskeletal examination to rule out issues with focal deficits in strength. Given the nature of this diagnosis, it is also important to perform cognitive screening in cases of suspected TBI. Cognitive screens such as the Montreal Cognitive Assessment, Trail making A and B, and the Mini Mental Status Examination can screen for common patterns of cognitive impairment after concussion such as inattention, short-term memory loss, and processing speed issues. It is also important to consider screening tools for mood disorders such as the patient health questionnaire (PHQ-9), generalized anxiety disorder (GAD-7) scale, or the post-traumatic stress disorder check list (PCL-5). These can help assess for degree of behavioral derangement and can be trended to assess interventions.

Imaging

Imaging considerations are important when conducting the medical work up after a concussion. It is important to understand that most head imaging will be negative for acute intracranial abnormalities after a concussion, especially when assessing with non-contrasted computated tomography (CT) scan of the head.[10,11] Of the

Table 1 Signs and symptoms	
Physical	Headache
	Cervical pain
	Nausea/vomiting
	Balance impairment
	Photosensitivity
	Phonosensitivity
	Diplopia
Cognitive	Inattention
	Short-term memory impairment
	Slowed processing speed
	Impaired ability to multi-task
Sleep	Insomnia
	Hypersomnia
	Circadian rhythm dysfunction
Mood	Depression
	Post-traumatic stress disorder (PTSD)
	Anxiety
	Irritability

various imaging modalities, the non-contrasted CT head is generally considered first line after head trauma to rule out acute intracranial pathology.[10] The CT head will assess for skull fractures and intracranial hemorrhaging (subdural, hematoma, epidural, hematoma, and subarachnoid hemorrhage).[10] An advantage of the CT head includes being able to rapidly assess for intracranial injury that could require surgical intervention. A limitation of the CT head is that it does not provide detailed assessment of brain parenchyma outside of bleeding.[10,11] This can present a challenge if there is concern for shearing injuries to the brain tissue.

Brain MRI is better able to assess brain parenchyma, contusions, and micro hemorrhaging after head trauma.[10,11] It is utilized in the acute setting after concussion and is generally considered after symptoms persist beyond 3 months.[12] There are several structural MRIs sequences that can be utilized after head trauma and include diffusion tensor imaging (DTI), gradient echo imaging (GRE), diffusion weighted imaging (DWI), and susceptibilities weighted imaging (SWI).[10–12] Limitations with brain MRI include longer time intervals to complete the study, cost, and availability of different sequences.[11] Studies have demonstrated that the susceptibility weighted image are thought to be the most sensitive to diffuse axonal injury (DAI).[10]

Functional brain MRIs are also being explored for clinical application after concussion.[10] The most common types of functional brain MRIs are task-based fMRI and resting state fMRI.[11] There have been several studies to suggest differences in BOLD signaling on both task-based and resting state fMRIs when comparing individuals with concussion versus healthy control groups.[11]

Its utilization remains mostly experimental in the concussion/mTBI population.

Skull X-rays are not considered routine after a concussion but can be used in the acute setting after head trauma to assess for skull fractures.[10]

Biomarkers

There have been several biomarkers currently being studied to both identify and stratify severity of brain injury.[13,14] Blood, cerebrospinal fluid, saliva, and urine have all been studied in the setting of head trauma to better understand the degree of injury.[13] The goal has been to better establish more objective ways to not only confirm brain injury (predictive biomarkers) but also to quantify degree of head trauma (prognostic biomarkers).[13,14] Another goal with biomarkers after brain injury would be to better predict/monitor response to therapies (predictive biomarkers).[13] One of the major challenges surrounding routine use of biomarkers after head trauma involves the fact that most of them are nonspecific.[13,14]

Blood

Blood biomarkers remain the most common biofluid biomarker and typically our focus within the first 24 hours after injury.[13] The 3 most common serum biomarkers used in TBI are glial fibrillary acidic protein (GFAP), S100 B, and Ubiquitin Carboxyl terminal hydrolase L1 (UCH-L1).[13–15] GFAP is a cytoskeleton proteins that is released after cell death and that typically peaks 20 hours after TBI.[13] S100 B is a protein that is implicated in cytotic calcium binding.[15] UCH-L1 has enzymatic properties and helps remove abnormal neuronal proteins.[16] Studies have examined these biomarkers and have noted association with concussion. For example, a prospective study conducted by McCrea and colleagues 2020 found that collegiate athletes with concussion also had elevated GFAP when compared to their pre-season baseline levels and when compared to contact sport controls acutely and at 24 hours.[17] This study also demonstrated an increase in serum GFAP level in the concussion group that had LOC and post traumatic amnesia (PTA) when check at the acute, 24 hour, and at the asymptomatic time point.[17] Another study showed that UCH-L1 was elevated in individuals with symptoms from a concussion when checked at the 4 hour mark. This was in comparison to patients who sustained a concussion at the same interval but did not have symptoms.[18] Finally, a review of literature on S100 B highlighted that it could be helpful in exclusion of an intracranial hemorrhage after mTBI.[15]

Cerebrospinal Fluid

Biomarkers found in the cerebral spinal fluid (CSF) have also been implicated in the setting of TBI given their proximity to the brain. There have been several studied exploring the association between TBI and changes in biomarkers in the CSF; include UCH-L1, Microtubule associated protein (MAP-2), and S100 B. A review completed by Santacruz and colleagues 2021 demonstrated that UCH-L1 and microtubule associated protein – 2 (MAP-2) elevation were associated with lower GCS scores on admission after TBI and with worse functional outcomes.[19] This study also illustrated association between S100 B elevation in individuals who have sustained subarachnoid hemorrhages and worsened functional outcomes at the 3 to 6 month mark.[19]

Further studies are needed to explore both sensitive and specific biomarkers unique to TBI.

Salivary Fluid

Salivary biomarkers are also being studied after post traumatic head injury. While both serum and CSF based biomarkers have been validated after TBI, they remain more invasive, in terms of collection.[20] Salivary testing is considered faster and significantly less invasive.[20]

Mavroudis and colleagues cited multiple studies that demonstrated association between elevated salivary S100 B levels and TBI when compared to control groups.[20]

Salivary S100 B and Neurofilament light chains (NfL) were also investigated in a study conducted by Monroe and colleagues and demonstrated that salivary NfL was elevated in water polo participants post tournament.[21] The same study also highlighted a link between NfL elevation and head impact frequency/magnitude.[21]

Initial management

Early evaluation and monitoring are critical following a suspected injury. Individuals should be assessed by a healthcare provider (HCP) as early as possible. Details of the event such as the time and mechanism of the injury, loss of consciousness, and reported symptoms should be recorded and provided to the HCP.

If there is concern that a concussion was sustained during sport, the player should be immediately removed from play and evaluated. Specific signs that raise concern for a possible concussion include loss of consciousness, confusion, memory changes, as well as deficits in coordination and balance. In the presence of any suspicion, it is essential that the individual refrains from returning to play and instead undergoes careful observation and evaluation over the subsequent hours to days.

There are a number of tools readily available to help HCPs detect signs and symptoms of a concussion. These include the CDC's HEADS UP Concussion Signs and Symptoms Checklist, as well as the Concussion in Sport Group's Sport Concussion Assessment Tool (SCAT5).

It is important to note that symptoms and signs of a concussion may not always manifest immediately. Therefore, vigilance and continued monitoring are necessary even if initial assessments do not reveal obvious indications. Further guidance regarding criteria for head imaging or additional laboratory testing can be found in the preceding section.

Education is a key at this stage. Healthcare providers should emphasize to patients the importance of striking a balance between avoiding intensive exercise and cognitive work while also avoiding complete cessation of all activity.

The belief that complete rest is beneficial following a concussion continues to be extremely common but is not supported by current evidence. Strict rest following a concussion is no longer considered beneficial, and may in fact lead to prolonged recovery. Instead, relative rest is recommended immediately and for the first 2 days post-concussion. This entails reducing exercise and screen time while continuing Activities of Daily Living (ADLs).[22] However, reducing screen time beyond the initial 24 to 48 hours does not demonstrate benefits in terms of shortening the duration of symptoms.[23,24]

Rest and graduated return to activity should be discussed with the patient. Moderate levels of both physical and cognitive rest may be associated with better outcomes than immediate return to higher levels of activity.[25]

In neurocognitive evaluation following concussion, athletes between the ages of 13 and 18 displayed more robust recovery percentiles in the visual memory and reaction time categories when engaged in school and light activities at home such as slow jogging and lawn mowing. This outcome was observed in comparison to both more intensive activity, such as school and sports practice, and less intensive activity, such as complete rest or no athletic activity.[26]

Exercise modalities such as moderate intensity stationary cycling and walking are ideal, however the risk of falling or subsequent head injury should be minimized.

Early activity following injury

Resumption of light activity in the days following an injury may be beneficial, and pace of return should ultimately be guided by overall symptom burden. The goal of management at this stage should be to detect symptoms early and work to reduce their severity and frequency. Each patient's activity tolerance and symptom distribution will be different, so education about concussion, symptoms, and symptom-guided return to activity is helpful.

Following concussion, early subthreshold aerobic activity has been associated with a reduction in time to symptom-free recovery compared to placebo. Subthreshold aerobic activity may be defined as exercise up to that, which worsens symptoms compared to a patient's pre-injury baseline.[27]

Patients can begin engaging in light exercise on their own within 1 to 2 days after the injury so long as it does not worsen their symptoms.

If exercise testing is available, subthreshold aerobic exercise therapy is safe to initiate as early as 2 to 10 days post-injury. Patients can begin light exercise 1 to 2 days post-injury so long as it does not worsen symptoms.[22] One of the most common tools to assess symptom return during exercise is the Buffalo Concussion Treadmill Test (BCTT), which employs a 1-to-10 point Visual Analog Scale to assess symptom severity and a 6 to 20 point Borg scale to rate perceived exertion. Resting heart rate is obtained prior to initiation. Treadmill incline and speed are slowly increased. Test is terminated if or when the patient notes a 3 point or more increase on their VAS, or when exhaustion or 90% rate of percieved exertion (RPE) is reached.

Athletes and individuals involved in aerobic activities post-injury should receive counseling regarding the risk of Second Impact Syndrome (SIS). While rare, SIS can occur when a person in concussion recovery sustains a second head injury. This syndrome involves the potential development of sudden, rapid, and potentially catastrophic brain edema, leading to significant morbidity and mortality.[28]

Return-to-play

The speed of symptom-free recovery following a concussion can vary significantly. Therefore, when beginning the return-to-play process, it is essential to adopt a graded and tiered approach. Providers should refrain from advocating strict rest and instead recommend a gradual increase in the level of activity.

The 2023 *Consensus Statement on Concussion in Sport* emphasizes a stepwise approach to recovery.[22] Athletes should start with gentle activity, such as Activities of Daily Living, within the first 24 hours post-injury. Advancement to the next stage of activity should be done no earlier than 24 hours so long as it does not provoke a return of symptoms.[22]

Levels of activity progress as follows: (i) symptom-limited activity (ii) light to moderate aerobic activity, (iii) individual sport-specific training that does not risk head impact, (iv) non-contact training drills, (v) full contact practice, and (vi) return to normal game play.[22]

For steps 1 to 3, if the patient experiences more than mild exacerbation of symptoms, exercise should be halted for the day. For steps 4 to 6, any return of symptoms necessitates a return to step 3. On average, it takes about 2 weeks for a patient (child or adult) to achieve symptom-free recovery. The average duration to return to sport is approximately 20 days.[29]

If symptoms do not improve or worsen within the expected time frame, further evaluation may be necessary.[22] It is common for neurosensory changes to develop in the acute to post-acute phase of concussion. Therefore, new and persistent symptoms should be closely monitored, and if necessary, re-evaluation and therapy referral should be considered.

Return to learn and work

Similar to the return-to-play approach, a gradual and tiered system should be implemented for students and individuals whose work involves substantial concentration and focus. This structured process allows for a step-by-step reintegration into school and employment activities, ensuring that cognitive demands are managed appropriately to support recovery and minimize symptom exacerbation. The overarching goal of this process should be to detect and reduce symptom burden while incrementally resuming tasks and responsibilities.

During the return-to-school process, students should follow a gradual increase in cognitive load, progressing through different stages: typical non-school activities, school-adjacent activities like homework, part-time school attendance, and finally full-time classwork. Close monitoring of symptoms is crucial, and if there is more than mild exacerbation of symptoms, the speed of return should be slowed down to ensure a safe and successful transition.[22]

School staff should actively participate in addressing barriers to the return-to-learn process. Students can benefit from academic supports such as additional time for tests and assignments, as well as potential accommodations like delaying testing and homework to allow time for proper recovery.

To this author's knowledge, there are no clinical practice guidelines regarding return to the workplace following mTBI. Returning to work can be challenging, especially given variations in what falls under work-related tasks. Patients may benefit from a gradual, symptom-guided return to workplace responsibilities. Accommodations such as decreased hours, reduced scope of responsibilities, and modified working conditions may be helpful.

Neurosensory deficits

Neurosensory deficits can manifest during the acute to post-acute phase following an injury and can pose significant challenges to recovery. They may include vestibular changes, visual dysfunction, auditory processing, tolerance difficulties, mood, and sleep changes. It is common for patients to develop these changes in the days to weeks following mTBI. The emergence of new symptoms should prompt evaluation by a healthcare provider and, if necessary, referral to therapy.

Vestibular dysfunction

Vestibular dysfunction can manifest as dizziness, loss of balance, discomfort with head motion, and postural instability. Examination may reveal the presence of nystagmus. Posture maintenance is a complex process involving various factors, including input from the semicircular canals and the cerebellum to the lateral vestibulospinal tract. Disruption or absence of sensory input can lead to postural instability as the brain fails to activate antigravity muscles effectively.

The differential diagnosis for vestibular dysfunction is wide-ranging, as the mechanism of injury may raise concern for a structural cause. In the context of mTBI, Benign Paroxysmal Positional Vertigo (BPPV) is frequently observed. Recent reviews have reported incidence rates of BPPV ranging from 8.5% to 39.7% across all severities of TBI.[30,31]

Treatment for BPPV involves otolith repositioning within the semicircular canals. The most common maneuver for this is known as the Epley maneuver.

Vestibular dysfunction can also originate centrally from injuries affecting the cerebellum and fusiform gyri.[32] Additionally, direct injury to the vestibular nerve can contribute to dysfunction. If there is suspicion of a structural cause, surgical referral may be necessary for further evaluation and management.

Vestibular rehabilitation can play a crucial role in improving patients' ability to compensate for sensory or central dysfunction. This form of therapy often includes exercises to train balance, stabilize gaze, and address fall risk. Although evidence for vestibular therapy regimens is varied, it appears to support faster return-to-play and return-to-learn outcomes, as well as improvements in balance and subjective dizziness.[33,34]

Light aerobic exercise may also be helpful in reducing the time it takes for individuals to become symptom-free.[35]

Visual dysfunction

Visual dysfunction is highly prevalent in individuals who have experienced mTBI. Accommodation dysfunction and convergence insufficiency may be present in up to greater than half of patients. However, visual field loss and visual acuity loss are relatively rare in this population.[36] As changes in visual field and acuity are less commonly reported they may require further workup including imaging or ophthalmologic evaluation.

Visual and oculomotor rehabilitation techniques are heterogenous, and there is currently inconclusive and mixed evidence for their effectiveness. Techniques include convergence and accommodation exercises, pursuit exercises, binasal occlusion, light filtering glasses, and prisms.[37]

Sleep dysfunction

After mTBI, alterations in sleep patterns may arise and pose a substantial obstacle to the recovery process. Sleep-wake disturbances may persist for months after injury and manifest in various ways. These changes may present as insomnia, hypersomnia, daytime fatigue, and may arise as a result of disturbance to sleep modulatory centers of the brain in the hypothalamus, forebrain, and brainstem.[38] A substantial percentage of patients report sleep changes following concussion, and in 1 study examining sport-related concussion in teens, up to 34% reported sleep disturbances.[39]

The focus of treatment should be identifying and addressing specific barriers to sleep. Patient education and cooperation are crucial in this process. Specific strategies may include: keeping a consistent sleep schedule, eliminating distractions such as TV and devices late at night, avoiding caffeine, and daytime naps (especially long ones). In the case of persistent sleep-wake disruptions even following lifestyle and schedule adjustments, use of medication to aid in sleep may be appropriate. However, use of benzodiazepines and antipsychotic agents should be avoided due to their potential negative effects on cognitive recovery.

SUMMARY

In summary, it is very important to understand the key components of identifying and treating individuals who have sustained a concussion acutely. It is important to know that concussions are the most common type of TBI and that they result from external force (direct and indirect) to the head that causes neuro-metabolic dysfunction. This can lead to a conglomeration of symptoms in various domains, to include physical, cognition, mood, and sleep. It is for this reason that concussions are considered clinical diagnoses. It is still important to rule out acute intracranial pathology and this can be done through detailed history-gathering and physical examination with special consideration toward head imaging. Treatment should be individualized and multifaceted.

CLINICS CARE POINTS

- Concussions (or mTBI) are the most common type of TBI.
- It is important to identify and track the various domains of symptoms after concussion.
- It is important to rule out acute intracranial pathology and imaging modalities should be considered, particularly if red flags are present.
- Concussions are still considered a clinical diagnosis.
- Treatment plans should be personalized and should address category of symptoms.

DISCLOSURE

No commercial or financial conflicts of interest and no external funding sources.

REFERENCES

1. Jackson WT, Starling AJ. Concussion Evaluation and Management. Med Clin 2019;103(2):251–61.
2. Lefevre-Dognin C, Cogné M, Perdrieau V, et al. Definition and epidemiology of mild traumatic brain injury. Neurochirurgie 2021;67(3):218–21.
3. Levin HS, Diaz-Arrastia RR. Diagnosis, prognosis, and clinical management of mild traumatic brain injury. Lancet Neurol 2015;14(5):506–17.
4. Romeu-Mejia R, Giza CC, Goldman JT. Concussion Pathophysiology and Injury Biomechanics. Curr Rev Musculoskelet Med 2019;12(2):105–16.

5. Broshek DK, Pardini JE, Herring SA. Persisting symptoms after concussion: Time for a paradigm shift. PM&R. 2022;14(12):1509–13.

6. Scorza KA, Cole W. Current concepts in concussion: Initial evaluation and management. Am Fam Physician 2019;99(7):426–34.

7. Concussion StatPearl, Available at: https://www.ncbi.nlm.nih.gov/books/NBK537017/. Accessed September 8, 2023.

8. *CDC report to congress*, 2015. Available at: https://www.cdc.gov/traumatic braininjury/pdf/TBI_Report_to_Congress_Epi_and_Rehab-a.pdf. Accessed September 2, 2023.

9. Scorza KA, Cole W. Current Concepts in Concussion: Initial Evaluation and Management. Am Fam Physician 2019;99(7):426–34. Available at: http://www.ncbi.nlm.nih.gov/pubmed/30932451.

10. Zetterberg H, Winblad B, Bernick C, et al. Head trauma in sports - clinical characteristics, epidemiology and biomarkers. J Intern Med 2019;285(6):624–34.

11. Lunkova E, Guberman GI, Ptito A, et al. Noninvasive magnetic resonance imaging techniques in mild traumatic brain injury research and diagnosis. Hum Brain Mapp 2021;42(16):5477–94.

12. Hageman G, Hof J, Nihom J. Susceptibility-Weighted MRI and Microbleeds in Mild Traumatic Brain Injury: Prediction of Posttraumatic Complaints? Eur Neurol 2022;85(3):177–85.

13. Wilde EA, Wanner IB, Kenney K, et al. A Framework to Advance Biomarker Development in the Diagnosis, Outcome Prediction, and Treatment of Traumatic Brain Injury. J Neurotrauma 2022;39(7–8):436–57.

14. Swaney EEK, Cai T, Seal ML, et al. Blood biomarkers of secondary outcomes following concussion: A systematic review. Front Neurol 2023;14. https://doi.org/10.3389/fneur.2023.989974.

15. Oris C, Kahouadji S, Durif J, et al. S100B, Actor and Biomarker of Mild Traumatic Brain Injury. Int J Mol Sci 2023;(7):24. https://doi.org/10.3390/ijms24076602.

16. Ghaith HS, Nawar AA, Gabra MD, et al. A Literature Review of Traumatic Brain Injury Biomarkers. Mol Neurobiol 2022;59(7):4141–58.

17. McCrea M, Broglio SP, McAllister TW, et al. Association of Blood Biomarkers With Acute Sport-Related Concussion in Collegiate Athletes: Findings From the NCAA and Department of Defense CARE Consortium. JAMA Netw Open 2020;3(1):e1919771.

18. Papa L, Zonfrillo MR, Welch RD, et al. Evaluating glial and neuronal blood biomarkers GFAP and UCH-L1 as gradients of brain injury in concussive, subconcussive and non-concussive trauma: a prospective cohort study. BMJ Paediatr Open 2019;3(1):e000473.

19. Santacruz CA, Vincent JL, Bader A, et al. Association of cerebrospinal fluid protein biomarkers with outcomes in patients with traumatic and non-traumatic acute brain injury: systematic review of the literature. Crit Care 2021;25(1):278.

20. Mavroudis I, Petridis F, Balmus IM, et al. Review on the Role of Salivary Biomarkers in the Diagnosis of Mild Traumatic Brain Injury and Post-Concussion Syndrome. Diagnostics 2023;13(8). https://doi.org/10.3390/diagnostics13081367.

21. Monroe DC, Thomas EA, Cecchi NJ, et al. Salivary S100 calcium-binding protein beta (S100B) and neurofilament light (NfL) after acute exposure to repeated head impacts in collegiate water polo players. Sci Rep 2022;12(1):3439.

22. Patricios JS, Schneider KJ, Dvorak J, et al. Consensus statement on concussion in sport: the 6th International Conference on Concussion in Sport-Amsterdam, October 2022. Br J Sports Med 2023;57(11):695–711.

23. Macnow T, Curran T, Tolliday C, et al. Effect of Screen Time on Recovery From Concussion: A Randomized Clinical Trial. JAMA Pediatr 2021;175(11):1124–31.
24. Cairncross M, Yeates KO, Tang K, et al. Early Postinjury Screen Time and Concussion Recovery. Pediatrics 2022;150(5). https://doi.org/10.1542/peds.2022-056835.
25. McLeod TCV, Lewis JH, Whelihan K, et al. Rest and Return to Activity After Sport-Related Concussion: A Systematic Review of the Literature. J Athl Train 2017; 52(3):262–87.
26. Majerske CW, Mihalik JP, Ren D, et al. Concussion in sports: postconcussive activity levels, symptoms, and neurocognitive performance. J Athl Train 2008;43(3): 265–74.
27. Leddy JJ, Haider MN, Ellis MJ, et al. Early Subthreshold Aerobic Exercise for Sport-Related Concussion: A Randomized Clinical Trial. JAMA Pediatr 2019; 173(4):319–25.
28. McLendon LA, Kralik SF, Grayson PA, et al. The Controversial Second Impact Syndrome: A Review of the Literature. Pediatr Neurol 2016;62:9–17.
29. Putukian M, Purcell L, Schneider KJ, et al. Clinical recovery from concussion-return to school and sport: a systematic review and meta-analysis. Br J Sports Med 2023;57(12):798–809.
30. Šarkić B, Douglas JM, Simpson A, et al. Frequency of peripheral vestibular pathology following traumatic brain injury: a systematic review of literature. Int J Audiol 2021;60(7):479–94.
31. Ahn SK, Jeon SY, Kim JP, et al. Clinical characteristics and treatment of benign paroxysmal positional vertigo after traumatic brain injury. J Trauma 2011;70(2): 442–6.
32. Alhilali LM, Yaeger K, Collins M, et al. Detection of central white matter injury underlying vestibulopathy after mild traumatic brain injury. Radiology 2014;272(1): 224–32.
33. Reneker JC, Hassen A, Phillips RS, et al. Feasibility of early physical therapy for dizziness after a sports-related concussion: A randomized clinical trial. Scand J Med Sci Sports 2017;27(12):2009–18.
34. Kleffelgaard I, Soberg HL, Tamber AL, et al. The effects of vestibular rehabilitation on dizziness and balance problems in patients after traumatic brain injury: a randomized controlled trial. Clin Rehabil 2019;33(1):74–84.
35. Chan C, Iverson GL, Purtzki J, et al. Safety of Active Rehabilitation for Persistent Symptoms After Pediatric Sport-Related Concussion: A Randomized Controlled Trial. Arch Phys Med Rehabil 2018;99(2):242–9.
36. Merezhinskaya N, Mallia RK, Park D, et al. Visual Deficits and Dysfunctions Associated with Traumatic Brain Injury: A Systematic Review and Meta-analysis. Optom Vis Sci 2019;96(8):542–55.
37. Subramanian PS, Barton JJS, Ranalli P, et al. Consensus Statement on Visual Rehabilitation in Mild Traumatic Brain Injury. Neurol Clin Pract 2022;12(6):422–8.
38. Baumann CR, Werth E, Stocker R, et al. Sleep-wake disturbances 6 months after traumatic brain injury: a prospective study. Brain 2007;130(Pt 7):1873–83.
39. Bramley H, Henson A, Lewis MM, et al. Sleep Disturbance Following Concussion Is a Risk Factor for a Prolonged Recovery. Clin Pediatr (Phila). 2017;56(14): 1280–5.

Rehabilitation of Persistent Symptoms After Concussion

Ashley Lujan, DO[a],*, Katherine Lin, MD[b]

KEYWORDS

- Postconcussive syndrome • Persistent symptoms • Headaches • Concussion
- Chronic

KEY POINTS

- Recognize that the multi-faceted nature of persistent symptoms after concussion is often influenced by the complex interplay of biological, psychological, and social factors.
- Early education that emphasizes clear recovery expectations and the high likelihood of full symptom resolution plays a crucial role in preventing persistent symptoms.
- Recommend an active approach for persistent symptoms by providing individualized guidance on gradual return to activity and early symptom-targeted interventions to improve outcomes.
- Headaches are the most common and frequently disabling persistent symptom after a mild traumatic brain injury.

INTRODUCTION

Persistent postconcussive syndrome (PPCS), also known as postconcussive syndrome (PCS), refers to a condition where symptoms associated with a concussion persist beyond the expected recovery period. These symptoms frequently encompass cognitive, physical, and somatic complaints, such as challenges with concentration, memory impairment, headaches, dizziness, and irritability.

The prevalence of PCS can vary depending on the population being studied (athletes, military personnel, general population) and the criteria used to define the condition. Estimates suggest that upwards of 15% of individuals who experience a concussion develop persistent symptoms that meet the criteria for PCS.[1] Determining the precise prevalence of PCS is challenging because of the variations in its definition and diagnosis (**Table 1**), as well as the influence of subjectivity and misattribution in self-reported symptoms.

[a] Department of Rehabilitation Medicine, South Texas VAHCS, 7400 Merton Minter, San Antonio, TX 78229, USA; [b] Department of Physical Medicine and Rehabilitation, Palo Alto VAMC, 3801 Miranda Avenue, Building 500, Palo Alto, CA 94304, USA
* Corresponding author.
E-mail address: Ashley.lujan@va.gov

Phys Med Rehabil Clin N Am 35 (2024) 535–546
https://doi.org/10.1016/j.pmr.2024.02.006
1047-9651/24/Published by Elsevier Inc.

Table 1
Highlights the differences between the DSM-IV, ICD-10, and DSM-V*

Criteria	ICD-10	DSM-IV	DSM-V
Terminology	Postconcussion syndrome	Postconcussion syndrome	[a]Mild neurocognitive disorder due to TBI
History of brain trauma required	Yes	Yes	Yes
Duration of symptoms	At least 4 wk	At least 3 mo	Not specified
Objective evidence of cognitive impairment required	Not specified	Yes	Yes

[a] Please note that the DSM-V no longer uses the term "post-concussion syndrome (PCS)" and instead introduces "Mild neurocognitive disorder due to TBI" based on performance-based quantifiable evidence of acquired cognitive deficit due to traumatic brain injury (TBI).

Abbreviations: *DSM-IV, diagnostic and statistical manual of mental disorders, fourth edition; DSM-V, diagnostic and statistical manual of mental disorders, fifth edition; ICD-10, 10th revision of the International Statistical Classification of Diseases.

The term "postconcussive syndrome" is a subject of controversy because these symptoms are not limited to patients with brain injuries; they are often found in healthy individuals without a history of mild traumatic brain injury (mTBI).[2,3] Furthermore, the severity of symptoms does not necessarily correlate with the severity of the injury, and the precise influence of brain structural damage on the persistence of symptoms remains uncertain.[4]

Persistent symptoms pose a significant threat to community reintegration, with studies showing reduced quality of life and decreased work re-entry.[5,6] Given the high prevalence of mTBI in the general population, PCS should be recognized as a major public health concern.

This chapter aims to improve understanding of the complex nature of persistent symptoms after mTBI, provide a general framework for approaching treatment, and provide targeted interventions for specific symptoms.

Key Takeaway

Controversy persists in postconcussion syndrome due to diagnostic challenges and symptom subjectivity. Nevertheless, persistent symptoms threaten community reintegration, underscoring the need for early recognition for positive long-term outcomes.

THEORY OF SYNDROME AND CO-CONTRIBUTING FACTORS

A latent model or common cause theory for PSC posits that there is a single underlying cause responsible for the development of persistent symptoms following a concussion. This perspective suggests that PCS is primarily driven by a biological factor, such as structural brain damage or a specific neurochemical imbalance. However, this viewpoint is inconsistent with the prevailing biopsychosocial model of PCS, which recognizes the multi-faceted nature of the condition.[7]

The biopsychosocial model emphasizes that PSC is influenced by the complex interplay of biological, psychological, and social factors.[4,7,8] It recognizes that while the initial injury may be a critical trigger, the persistence and severity of symptoms are also influenced by multiple factors. These can include pre-existing mental health conditions, coping strategies, emotional reactions, social support, access to healthcare, and environmental factors.[4] The model recognizes that the experience and impact of PCS are unique to each individual and cannot be solely explained by a single latent cause.

Several studies have aimed to establish prognostic multi-variable models for the development of PPCS.[9–12] No externally validated model exists at present. Robust predictors of prolonged recovery include preinjury mental health, postinjury symptoms of depression and anxiety, female gender, and early postconcussive symptoms.[8,13] Additional factors associated with the persistence of symptoms worth mentioning include the nocebo effect (adverse outcomes due to injury beliefs), good-old-days bias[14] (overestimating pre-post injury differences), and malingering.[15]

Key Takeaway

Adopting a broader biopsychosocial framework and recognizing prognostic factors for development of PCS can improve management and outcomes for individuals with persistent symptoms.

GENERAL TREATMENT APPROACH

The evidence in the form of randomized controlled trials (RCTs) guiding the treatment of postconcussion syndrome is limited. However, a review of the existing literature shows a relative expert consensus on appropriate treatment principles.[16–19] The approach to management has evolved from a more passive to an active stance.

In the past, management typically involved rest and symptom monitoring, with an expectation of spontaneous resolution over time.

Now, active management principles are emphasized, with a focus on *preventing* persistent symptoms through early intervention, education, and personalized treatment plans. The goal is to promote recovery and minimize harm to the patient's overall well-being.

Key Components of Early Intervention and Active Management

1. Early education: Mainstay of prevention of persistent symptoms
   - Provide information about expectations for recovery and symptom management.
   - Emphasize that most individuals will experience a full recovery of symptoms.[20]
2. Individualized treatment plan:
   - Create a personalized plan.
   - Provide guidance on a gradual return to activity. Historically rest was the cornerstone of treatment. The most recent Consensus Statement on Concussion in Sport (5th edition) states there is insufficient evidence to support the idea that complete rest promotes recovery. Instead, it is now recommended in the acute period to have 24 to 48 hours of relative rest followed by an individualized graded return to activity.[17]
   - Provide guidance on avoiding symptom exacerbation during the initial concussion management.
3. Identification and management of ongoing symptoms:
   - Schedule follow-up visits to reassess symptoms and track progress.
   - Utilize tracking tools (Neurobehavioral Symptom Inventory, Rivermead Post-Concussion Symptom Questionnaire, Concussion Symptom Checklist, Postconcussion Syndrome Checklist) to monitor symptom recovery process.

- Utilize a nonpharmacologic approach to address symptoms and tease out confounding factors.
  - i. Vestibular therapy, oculomotor vision therapy, and manual treatment of neck and back can help address any concomitant vestibular dysfunction or cervical soft-tissue strain resulting in "whiplash"-related symptoms.[8,18]
  - ii. A combination of psychoeducation, counseling, and cognitive behavioral therapy (CBT) can help address associated symptoms of depression, anxiety, and potential mal-adaptive behavioral patterns.[8,18]
- Implement Symptom Specific Treatments refer to "Symptom Specific" section below
4. Communication[21]:
- Use appropriate verbiage (ie, "concussion" instead of "brain injury") to avoid potential associations with ongoing disability.[22]
- Frame conversations in terms of multiple modifiable contributing factors.
- Validate symptoms without implying attribution or causation.

Caveats to Pharmacologic Intervention

Due to limited research on specific pharmacologic treatments for PCS, treatment decisions should be based on individual presentation and medical history. Careful assessment of benefits, side effects, drug interactions, risks of pain medication overuse, and duration of treatment is crucial.

Since postconcussive symptoms often cluster together (sleep, mood, concentration problems), caution is necessary to avoid polypharmacy.[22] It is recommended to prioritize the most bothersome symptom and consider medications that can address multiple symptoms simultaneously. For example, tricyclic anti-depressants may be used for mood symptoms, insomnia, and migraine prophylaxis. Close monitoring for potential side effects is important as many central nervous system (CNS)-acting medications can mimic other postconcussive symptoms. For example, topiramate, commonly used for headache prevention, can produce dizziness, "cognitive fog," and fatigue.

Shared decision-making and patient education on risks and benefits of pharmacologic management play a pivotal role in treatment. Clearly communicating measurable treatment goals and the intended duration of therapy to the patient is essential.

Key Takeaway

Early intervention plays a pivotal role in preventing the development of persistent postconcussion symptoms by providing education that emphasizes clear recovery expectations and the high likelihood of full symptom resolution.

We recommend early development of a personalized treatment plan, offering guidance on gradual return to activity and specific symptom-targeted treatments that may incorporate both pharmacologic and nonpharmacologic interventions.

SYMPTOM SPECIFIC
Headaches

Headaches are one of the most common complaints after a mTBI, occurring in approximately 25% to 78% of people following a mTBI, and posttraumatic headaches (PTHs) account for approximately 4% of all symptomatic headache disorders (**Table 2**).[23,24]

The International Classification of Headache Disorders defines PTHs as a secondary headache disorder attributed to head and/or neck trauma, with onset reported

Table 2 Classification of post-traumatic headache	
Acute posttraumatic headache:	Headache resolves within 3 mo or trauma exposure was <3 mo ago
Chronic posttraumatic headache:	Headache persists beyond 3 mo

within 7 days following trauma or injury, within 7 days after recovering consciousness, or within 7 days after recovering the ability to sense and report pain.[25]

PTH can be classified as acute or chronic. Acute PTH is defined as the headache resolving within 3 months or the trauma exposure was less than 3 months ago. Chronic PTH is defined by the headache disorder persisting beyond 3 months from the injury/trauma.

Migraine-like and Tension-type headaches are the most common headache phenotypes in PTH; however, there is significant variability in presentation. Other phenotypes may resemble cervicogenic headache, cluster headache, hemicrania among others. PTH does not have a uniform presentation and will generally present with overlapping features of other headache phenotypes.[26]

Risk factors for the development of PTH include female gender, prior headache history, adolescent age, and pertinent family headache history. In addition, studies have shown a higher rate of PTH following mild TBI events than following severe TBI (**Table 3**).[26]

Types of Post-traumatic Headaches

Tension type headaches, migraine headache, cluster headache, neuralgic headaches, cervicogenic headaches, and mixed headaches.

Management

Initial management of PTH should include education on brain injury and expectations based on the classification of the brain injury severity as well as a discussion on lifestyle modifications to include sleep, nutrition, hydration, stress management, identification and avoidance of triggers, and return to exercise and activity.

Nonpharmacologic management may utilize:[26]

- Lifestyle modifications: sleep hygiene/improve sleep, nutrition, improve hydration, identify and avoid triggers
- Physical therapy
- Return to physical activity with gradual and early exercise
- Neuromodulation: Repetitive transcranial magnetic stimulation, neurofeedback
- Cognitive and behavioral modification
- Acupuncture
- Hot/cold packs

Table 3 Abortive therapies	
Over the counter:	NSAIDS, acetaminophen, aspirin, aspirin plus caffeine plus acetaminophen
Prescription:	NSAIDS, ketorolac IM, triptans, antiemetics, butalbital plus caffeine plus acetaminophen or aspirin

Abbreviation: NSAID, nonsteroidal anti-inflammatory drugs.

- Cranial analgesic electrotherapeutic devices
- Massage therapy
- Stress management, relaxation training, mindfulness

Pharmacologic management

Pharmacologic management of PTH may include both medication-based therapies as well as interventional procedures to help alleviate headache symptoms. It is also important to be mindful that many traditional headache medications can contribute to unwanted side effects such as cognitive difficulties and fatigue. Clinicians should also be aware of medication overuse headaches which may result from the use of analgesics, opioids, ergot alkaloids, and triptans in the treatment of PTH.

Pharmacologic management of PTH can be divided into abortive and prophylactic therapies (**Box 1** and **2**).

Sleep

Sleep disturbances after a TBI are common, with estimates of post-TBI sleep disturbance occurring in over 50% of individuals.[30] Characteristics that may be seen include reduced total sleep time, poor sleep efficiency, and worse perceived sleep quality.[31] Sleep disturbances associated with TBI are broad and may include sleep disorders such as insomnia, hypersomnia, obstructive sleep apnea, narcolepsy, periodic limb movements, and complaints such as snoring, nightmares, and excessive daytime sleepiness. Sleep disturbances after TBI may also cause or worsen comorbidities, which may include depression, irritability, anxiety, pain, fatigue, cognitive deficits, and functional impairments.[32]

Poor-quality sleep during the acute phase after a concussion has been shown to predict persistent postconcussion symptoms, more mood disturbances, worse community reintegration, and more cognitive disability 1 year after injury in a study looking at sports-related concussions.[30]

Early education, recognition, and intervention of sleep disturbances can help improve a patient's clinical outcome. The treatment plan for sleep disturbances after TBI should be holistic and consider the possible comorbidities a patient may have such as posttraumatic stress disorder, pain, depression, obstructive sleep apnea, and apply targeted strategies.[16,33]

Management

Nonpharmacologic options to assist with improving sleep include.

- Sleep hygiene education
- Environmental modifications

Box 1
Prophylactic therapies:[27,28]

Antiepileptics (topiramate, Divalproex Sodium)

Beta blockers (propranolol, metoprolol)

Alpha blockers (prazosin)

Tricyclic antidepressants (TCAs) (amitriptyline, nortriptyline)

Supplements (magnesium oxide, vitamin B2)

Calcitonin gene-related peptide receptor antagonist (Anti-CGRP) monoclonal antibody (erenumab)

Box 2
Interventional procedures:[28,29]

Depending on the primary headache phenotype, injections may be an adjunct to consider. These may include.
   Greater and lesser occipital nerve blocks for occipital neuralgia
   Trigger point injections
   Facet medical branch blocks, pulsed or high-temperature radiofrequency ablation for cervicogenic headaches due to facet arthropathy
   Onabotulinumtoxin A for migraine headaches

- CBT
- Relaxation strategies
- Acupuncture
- Treatment of obstructive sleep apnea if present

Pharmacologic options include.

- Melatonin agonists (Melatonin, Ramelteon)
- Prazosin
- Antidepressants (Trazodone, TCAs, Doxepin, Mirtazapine)
- Hypnotics ("z" drugs Eszopiclone, Zaleplon, Zolpidem)
- Consideration of stimulant use in the daytime for Circadian Rhythm disorder

It is important to recognize that while sleep aids may be effective in some patients, others may find the side effects worsen other symptoms such as dizziness and cognitive complaints. In addition, the risk-benefit profiles of different pharmacologic options need to be evaluated along with the abuse potential and toxicity. It is recommended to utilize medications with the least side effects and pay close attention to dosing and response to therapy.

VISUAL DYSFUNCTION

Complaints of light sensitivity, blurry vision, eye fatigue, and eye strain may occur after mTBI, with most seeing recovery of those symptoms within minutes to hours.[16]

A vision-specific history and thorough eye examination are warranted for those with prolonged symptoms. Components of a thorough visual examination include assessment of visual acuity, smooth pursuit, ocular alignment, saccades, vestibulo-ocular reflex, and near point convergence.[34] Continued visual deficits can contribute to difficulty in return to school, work, and activity; thus, early identification and appropriate management are important to help in the recovery of symptoms after a mTBI.

Management

Initial symptom management for visual complaints after a concussion include reducing time spent on visual work and reading, limiting time on electronic screens, visual pacing, enlarged font or double spacing, and gradual return to full visual workload.[34]

Those with persistent visual symptoms should be evaluated by an optometrist, ophthalmologist, or vision rehabilitation specialist with a comprehensive visual examination. Therapies will vary depending on the findings of the eye examination but may include the use of prescription glasses with base-in prism to correct strabismus or refractive correction for visual accommodation.[34]

Audiological dysfunction

Hearing difficulties have been reported in over half of individuals who sustain blast-related mTBI, with hearing loss and tinnitus being the most common audiological complaints. Hearing loss, noise sensitivity, and tinnitus are typically self-limited after mTBI, and true pathology in central auditory acuity or processing is extremely rare after mTBI. Preinjury hearing deficits are common and should be considered.[16]

Management

Perform an otologic examination.

Review medications for agents that may cause ototoxicity.

Consider referral to an audiologist for objective evaluation, testing, and treatments.

Other options may include the use of white noise, tinnitus CBT, education, reassurance, and environmental modifications.

Vestibular Dysfunction

Dizziness and disequilibrium are symptoms that can present after a concussion and can be the result of inner-ear disorders, CNS disorders, psychological disorders, musculoskeletal disorders, and idiopathic disorders.[16]

Assessment

A comprehensive history and physical examination can help to guide the clinician in determining an etiology and developing a treatment plan. Physical examination components should include a neurologic examination, vision testing, orthostatic testing, a motor and musculoskeletal examination, vestibular examination, sensory testing, and auditory examination.

Careful review of a patient's medications is important as many medication classes can cause dizziness as a side effect. Common offending agents include TCAs, antiepileptic drugs, selective serotonin reuptake inhibitors (SSRIs), anticholinergics, benzodiazepines, beta blockers, and stimulants.

Management

Nonpharmacologic treatments include

- Vestibular and balance rehabilitation
- For those with symptoms of benign positional paroxysmal vertigo, recommend performing a Dix-Hallpike maneuver for assessment, and if positive, performing canalith repositioning maneuvers
- If someone is a fall risk due to their symptoms, recommend evaluation for adaptive equipment until their symptoms resolve to help prevent further injury

Pharmacologic treatments.

- Medications are generally not recommended after a concussion unless symptoms are causing a significant interference with functional activities. When indicated, a trial of meclizine or another vestibular suppressant may be considered. The use of benzodiazepines is not recommended due to their addictive and sedating effects.

MOOD

Preinjury depressed mood is a significant contributor to the severity of postinjury anxiety and postconcussion symptoms. In addition, depression has been tied to worse functional outcomes following mTBI.[35,36] Postinjury support and mental health interventions are necessary for optimizing outcomes in those with persistent postconcussion symptoms.[37] It is recommended to screen for mental health symptoms early and begin treatment when needed. It is also important to consider all the potential factors after a concussion that can contribute to mental health symptoms such as poor sleep, substance use, and pain and address them as part of a wholistic approach to care.

Management

CBT is recommended for the management of persistent mood symptoms after concussion. Complementary strategies such as biofeedback, acupuncture, breathing techniques, relaxation training, mindfulness, and cranioelectric stimulation may also be integrated into a patient's treatment plan to help with symptoms.

Pharmacologic options

When deciding which medication to add, it is important to review the side effect profile and avoid medications that are more sedating and have greater anticholinergic activity, as this can worsen fatigue and cognitive impairments. When beginning a medication, it is recommended to start at a low dose, and allow monitor efficacy and side effects. Common options include the use of SSRIs, serotonin and norepinephrine reuptake inhibitors and TCAs.

COGNITIVE SYMPTOMS

In those who report cognitive symptoms after mTBI, most improve within days to weeks; however, in a small subset, cognitive problems in attention, thinking speed, memory, and executive function may persist for months to years.[16]

Management

For those with persistence of cognitive complaints after concussion, a time-limited trial of cognitive rehabilitation, focusing on psychoeducation and strategies, may be helpful.[16] A referral for full neuropsychological evaluation can also assist in better characterizing current deficits and help guide treatment. Psychoeducation should focus on expected concussion trajectory, symptom validation, and the contribution of coexisting conditions like insomnia and depression and medication side effects.

SUMMARY

Persistent symptoms following mild TBI present treatment challenges and hinder community reintegration. Recognizing the multi-faceted nature of persistent symptoms, influenced by the complex interplay of biological, psychological, and social factors, can aid in developing an individualized treatment plan. The mainstay approach to prevention of persistent symptoms involves early education that manages expectations and emphasizes the high likelihood of full symptom resolution. Specific strategies can involve using terms like "concussion" instead of "brain injury" to avoid potential associations with ongoing disability and to validate symptoms without implying attribution or causation. Early active targeted symptom treatment, often necessitating a multi-disciplinary team, should be implemented. Prioritize nonpharmacological methods and try to avoid polypharmacy.

For further guidance, the following clinical practice guidelines are driven by evidence-based research and serve as a comprehensive resource for managing persistent symptoms after mTBI.

http://www.healthquality.va.gov/guidelines/Rehab/mtbi/

Management of Prolonged Symptoms | Living Concussion Guidelines (concussionsontario.org)

DISCLOSURE

The views, opinions, and/or findings expressed herein are those of the authors and do not necessarily reflect the views or the official policy of the Department of Veterans Affairs or US government.

REFERENCES

1. Rutherford WH, Merrett JD, McDonald JR. Symptoms at one year following concussion from minor head injuries. Injury 1979;10(3):225–30.
2. Meares S, Shores EA, Taylor AJ, et al. Mild traumatic brain injury does not predict acute postconcussion syndrome. J Neurol Neurosurg Psychiatr 2008;79:300–6.
3. Dean PJA, O'Neill D, Sterr A. Post-concussion syndrome: prevalence after mild traumatic brain injury in comparison with a sample without head injury. Brain Inj 2012;26(1):14–26.
4. Wäljas M, Iverson GL, Lange RT, et al. A prospective biopsychosocial study of the persistent post-concussion symptoms following mild traumatic brain injury. J Neurotrauma 2015;32(8):534–47.
5. Stalnacke BM. Community integration, social support and life satisfaction in relation to symptoms 3 years after mild traumatic brain injury. Brain Inj 2007;21: 933–42. https://doi.org/10.1080/02699050701553189.
6. Emanuelson I, Andersson Holmkvist E, Björklund R, et al. Quality of life and post-concussion symptoms in adults after mild traumatic brain injury: a population-based study in western Sweden. Acta Neurol Scand 2003;108:332–8.
7. Iverson GL. Network Analysis and Precision Rehabilitation for the Post-concussion Syndrome. Front Neurol 2019;10:489.
8. Polinder S, Cnossen MC, Real RGL, et al. A Multidimensional Approach to Post-concussion Symptoms in Mild Traumatic Brain Injury. Front Neurol 2018;9:1113.
9. Silverberg ND, Gardner AJ, Brubacher JR, et al. Systematic review of multivariable prognostic models for mild traumatic brain injury. J Neurotrauma 2015; 32(8):517–26.
10. Caplain S, Blancho S, Marque S, et al. Early Detection of Poor Outcome after Mild Traumatic Brain Injury: Predictive Factors Using a Multidimensional Approach a Pilot Study. Front Neurol 2017;8:666.
11. Falk H, Bechtold KT, Peters ME, et al. A Prognostic Model for Predicting One-Month Outcomes among Emergency Department Patients with Mild Traumatic Brain Injury and a Presenting Glasgow Coma Scale of Fifteen. J Neurotrauma 2021;38(19):2714–22.
12. Cnossen MC, van der Naalt J, Spikman JM, et al. Prediction of Persistent Post-Concussion Symptoms after Mild Traumatic Brain Injury. J Neurotrauma 2018; 35(22):2691–8.
13. Silverberg ND, Iaccarino MA, Panenka WJ, et al. American Congress of Rehabilitation Medicine Brain Injury Interdisciplinary Special Interest Group Mild TBI Task Force. Management of Concussion and Mild Traumatic Brain Injury: A Synthesis of Practice Guidelines. Arch Phys Med Rehabil 2020;101(2):382–93.
14. Lange RT, Iverson GL, Rose A. Post-concussion symptom reporting and the "good-old-days" bias following mild traumatic brain injury. Arch Clin Neuropsychol 2010;25:442–50. https://doi.org/10.1093/arclin/acq031.

15. Silver JM. Effort, exaggeration and malingering after concussion. J Neurol Neurosurg Psychiatry 2012;83:836–41. https://doi.org/10.1136/jnnp-2011-302078.
16. Management of concussion—mild traumatic brain injury (mTBI) (2021) - VA/DoD clinical practice guidelines. Available at: http://www.healthquality.va.gov/guidelines/Rehab/mtbi/. [Accessed 20 July 2023].
17. McCrory P, Meeuwisse W, Dvořák J, et al. Consensus statement on concussion in sport-the 5th international conference on concussion in sport held in Berlin, October 2016. Br J Sports Med 2017;51(11):838–47.
18. Rytter HM, Graff HJ, Henriksen HK, et al. Nonpharmacological Treatment of Persistent Postconcussion Symptoms in Adults: A Systematic Review and Meta-analysis and Guideline Recommendation. JAMA Netw Open 2021;4(11): e2132221.
19. Heslot C, Azouvi P, Perdrieau V, et al. A Systematic Review of Treatments of Post-Concussion Symptoms. J Clin Med 2022;11(20):6224.
20. Bell KR, Hoffman JM, Temkin NR, et al. The effect of telephone counselling on reducing post-traumatic symptoms after mild traumatic brain injury: a randomised trial. J Neurol Neurosurg Psychiatry 2008;79:1275–81. https://doi.org/10.1136/jnnp.2007.141762.
21. Tapia RN, Eapen BC. Rehabilitation of Persistent Symptoms After Concussion. Phys Med Rehabil Clin 2017;28(2):287–99. PMID: 28390514.
22. Wood RL. Understanding the 'miserable minority': a diathesis-stress paradigm for post-concussional syndrome. Brain Inj 2004;18(11):1135–53.
23. Seifert TD, Evans RW. Posttraumatic headache: a review. Curr Pain Headache Rep 2010;14(4):292–8.
24. Evans RW. The postconcussion syndrome and the sequelae of mild head injury. In: Evans RW, editor. Neurology and trauma. edition 2. New York: Oxford University Press; 2006. p. 95–128.
25. Ashina H, Eigenbrodt AK, Seifert T, et al. Post-traumatic headache attributed to traumatic brain injury: classification, clinical characteristics, and treatment. Lancet Neurol 2021;20(6):460–9.
26. Lee MJ, Zhou Y, Greenwald BD. Update on Non-Pharmacological Interventions for Treatment of Post-Traumatic Headache. Brain Sci 2022;12(10):1357.
27. Kamins J. Models for Treating Post-traumatic Headache. Curr Pain Headache Rep 2021;25(8):52.
28. Leung A. Addressing chronic persistent headaches after MTBI as a neuropathic pain state. J Headache Pain 2020;21:77.
29. Zirovich MD, Pangarkar SS, Manh C, et al. Botulinum Toxin Type A for the Treatment of Post-traumatic Headache: A Randomized, Placebo-Controlled, Crossover Study. Mil Med 2021;186(5–6):493–9. https://doi.org/10.1093/milmed/usaa391.
30. Mathias JL, Alvaro PK. Prevalence of sleep disturbances, disorders, and problems following traumatic brain injury: a meta-analysis. Sleep Med 2012;13(7): 898–905.
31. Grima N, Ponsford J, Rajaratnam SM, et al. Sleep disturbances in traumatic brain injury: a meta-analysis. J Clin Sleep Med 2016;12:419–28.
32. Singh K, Morse AM, Tkachenko N, et al. Sleep Disorders Associated With Traumatic Brain Injury-A Review. Pediatr Neurol 2016;60:30–6.
33. Kaleyias, Joseph, Kothare SV. Sleep Disorders in Traumatic Brain Injury. J Clin Neurophysiol 2022;39(5):356–62.
34. Master CL, Bacal D, Grady MF, et al. Vision and Concussion: Symptoms, Signs, Evaluation, and Treatment. Pediatrics 2022;150(2). e2021056047.

35. Scott KL, Strong CA, Gorter B, et al. Predictors of Post-concussion Rehabilitation Outcomes at Three-month Follow-up. Clin Neuropsychol 2016;30(1):66–81.
36. McCauley SR, Wilde EA, Miller ER, et al. Preinjury resilience and mood as predictors of early outcome following mild traumatic brain injury. J Neurotrauma 2013; 30(8):642–52.
37. Lambert M, Sheldrake E, Deneault AA, et al. Depressive Symptoms in Individuals With Persistent Postconcussion Symptoms: A Systematic Review and Meta-Analysis. JAMA Netw Open 2022;5(12). e2248453.

Sports Related Concussion

Scott R. Laker, MD*, Christian Nicolosi, MD

KEYWORDS

- Concussion • Sports concussion • Sports medicine • Traumatic brain injury

KEY POINTS

- Providers should know and follow state law and league policies and protocols when caring for athletes with sports-related concussions.
- Increasing evidence supports mouthguard use in ice hockey and policies disallowing bodychecking.
- Reduction of exposures, both overall (eg, reduction of contact practices) and in specific play circumstances (eg, kickoffs and home plate collisions) reduces concussion rates.

INTRODUCTION/HISTORY/EPIDEMIOLOGY

Sports-related concussions (SRC) have been a topic of interest for decades, though the roots can be traced back to ancient Greek medicine.[1,2] With the advent of American football in the early 19th century, severe traumatic brain injuries became more prominent, and athletes noticed the effects of head injury within the game. At that time, several felt fortunate having a "thicker head of hair" to soften the blow of head trauma in sport.[1,2] The understanding of concussions has evolved, as have our abilities to protect athletes from these injuries. Despite this, SRC continues to be a prevalent risk of sports participation. Recent studies estimate 1.0 to 1.8 million SRC for athletes between 0 and 18 years of age and roughly 400,000 per year in the high school athlete population.[3] The incidences of concussion has been steadily increasing over the last several decades, with some studies demonstrating a 4-fold increase.[4,5] This is in part due to the increasing awareness and identification of concussion symptoms amongst coaches, parents, and providers[6] and the mandated, medical return to play codified by concussion laws. Despite the increase in awareness, many athletes do not report their injury to their health care providers. In 2020, Gordon and colleagues found that 21.9% of the 2014 Canadian Community Health Survey respondents did not seek medical care within 48 hours after sustaining a concussion or other brain injury.[7] Other articles have identified underreporting as high as 50% even in situations where concussion education was provided.[8] It is well recognized that

Department of Physical Medicine and Rehabilitation, University of Colorado School of Medicine, 12631 East 17th Avenue, Mail Stop F493, Aurora, CO 80045, USA
* Corresponding author.
E-mail address: Scott.laker@cuanschutz.edu

Phys Med Rehabil Clin N Am 35 (2024) 547–558
https://doi.org/10.1016/j.pmr.2024.02.007
1047-9651/24/© 2024 Elsevier Inc. All rights reserved.

sports participation provides not only physical health benefits, but also social and psychological benefits.[9] While the risk of injury exists, participation in sports generally outweighs the risk of injury. The purpose of this article is to report the most up-to-date information on sports-related concussions and to discuss the most recent consensus statements for clinical care of athletes suffering from SRC. Given the complexity of management, the variability of symptoms, and the ever-evolving data regarding best practice guidelines, frequent updates to clinical care are necessary to provide high quality care for these athletes.

EPIDEMIOLOGY

Concussion epidemiology is a topic unto itself, but certain concepts are worth additional discussion. Collision sports (eg, American football, ice hockey, and wrestling) have higher rates than contact sports (eg, basketball, lacrosse, and soccer), which have higher rates than non-contact sports (eg, tennis, golf, track and field). Pierpont's 2021 article delineates current rates for high school and collegiate sports based on the High School Reporting Information Online (RIO) and the National Federation of State High School Associations databases.[6] It is important to clarify that no sport has a homogenous rate across all aspects of play. For example, it is consistently reported that competitions have higher rates of concussion than practice.[10,11] It is also well-understood that certain play scenarios have higher rates of concussions than others. For example, kickoffs in American football, plays at home plate in baseball, flyers, and stunting in cheerleading have higher rates within the individual sport. At this point, the epidemiology data can help determine the effectiveness of prevention efforts across sport and to identify trends within and across sports.

Certain ice hockey leagues and age groups have banned body-checking, and some soccer leagues have limited heading below a certain age.

At the time of this writing, the Centers for Disease Control and Prevention (CDC) is piloting the National Concussion Surveillance System to track concussions across the country. This database would help clarify the total number of concussions and the etiology of the injury. It would also allow more accurate tracking of sports concussions that occur outside of formal league settings.[12]

DEFINITION

Diagnostic criteria of concussion continues to be a debated topic, as many medical practitioners argue it is synonymous with mild traumatic brain injury (mTBI)[13] while others feel that it is the at the lowest end of the mTBI spectrum.[14,15] In 2001, the first Concussion In Sport Group (CISG) meeting was held to formalize the definition.[16] Since that time, the definition has been edited frequently to encompass the complexity of the diagnosis with the most updated data. Since its conception in 2001, there have been several editions of the definition, and during the 2022 annual meeting, a majority statement update garnered 78% agreement, falling 2% below the threshold to be recognized as a formal consensus agreement. Nonetheless, it provides impactful clarity on SRC definitions. The 2022 majority statement defines SRC as "a traumatic brain injury caused by a direct blow to the head, neck, or body resulting in an impulsive force being transmitted to the brain that occurs in sports and exercise-related activities". This initiates a neurotransmitter and metabolic cascade, with possible axonal injury, blood flow change, and inflammation affecting the brain. Symptoms may be present immediately, or evolve over minutes or hours, and commonly resolve within days, though, they may also be prolonged. No abnormality is seen on standard structural neuroimaging studies (computed tomography (CT) or MRI), but in the research setting, abnormalities may be present on functional, blood flow or metabolic imaging studies. Sport-related concussion results in a range of clinical symptoms that may or may not involve loss of consciousness. Other causes for the symptoms such as drug, alcohol, or medication use must be ruled out prior consideration of the diagnosis. Similarly, other diagnoses such as cervical spine injury or vestibular dysfunction should also be considered.[17] The Amsterdam Consensus Statement has used 'concussion' interchangeably with mTBI when neuroimaging is normal or not clinically indicated[17]". Thus, they can establish the definition in accordance with recent diagnostic guidelines for mTBIs. Recently, the American Congress of Rehabilitation Medicine (ACRM) established a new set of diagnostic criteria for mTBI. The ACRM describes a traumatic brain injury as an event that results from a transfer of mechanical energy to the brain from external forces resulting from the head being struck with an object; a head striking a hard object, or surface; from the brain undergoing an acceleration/deceleration movement without direct contact between the head and an object or surface; and/or forces generated from a blast or explosion.[18] In addition to a plausible mechanism, at least 1 additional clinical sign must be observed. Clinical signs include loss of consciousness immediately following injury, alteration of mental status, reduced responsiveness, inappropriate responses to external stimuli, complete or partial amnesia for events, or other neurologic symptoms. The diagnosis can be made in the absence of these clinical signs when at least 2 acute symptoms are found and at least 1 clinical or laboratory finding is also found. Acute symptoms include acute alteration in mental status, headache, nausea, dizziness, balance disturbance, vision problems, sensitivity to light, and/or sensitivity to noise. They also include cognitive symptoms (feeling slowed down, being in a mental fog, difficulty concentrating, and memory problems) and emotional symptoms (uncharacteristic emotional lability and or irritability). The ACRM diagnostic criteria incorporate clinical examination and laboratory findings for the first time. These examination findings include objectively measured cognitive impairment, balance impairment, oculomotor impairment, or symptom provocation in response to vestibular-oculomotor challenge on acute clinical examination. Neuroimaging is not required for the diagnosis.[18]

RECOGNITION OF CONCUSSIONS

There is increasing emphasis on the recognition of concussion symptoms at sporting events, and particular importance has been placed on the early recognition and removal from play.[19] Despite this, there are still identified knowledge gaps amongst coaches and sideline personnel.[20] Signs that warrant immediate removal from the field include actual or suspected loss of consciousness, seizure, tonic posturing, ataxia, poor balance, confusion, behavioral changes, and amnesia.[21] In 2006, the first Standardized Concussion Assessment Tool (SCAT) was introduced by the CISG as a method of assisting clinicians in diagnoses of concussions.[21] These tools have continued to evolve, with the most recent iteration being the 6th edition. Its utilization is most powerful within 72 hours of injury and begins to have diminished effects after 7 days. The SCAT is used to test the domains of symptoms, cognition, postural control, neurologic testing, and oculomotor/cervical/vestibular screens. Compared to previous iterations, the SCAT 6 looked to improve testing with regards to noted ceiling effects on the 5-word list. The newest update recommends including more challenging tasks such as a 10-word list. There were also several limitations identified such as its use in adolescent females, para-athletes, and children. The Child SCAT6 should be used in patients aged 8 to 12 years.[21] The evaluation process takes roughly 10 to 15 min and timing for proper evaluation should be allowed prior to the athlete's return to sport.

Evaluation continues outside of the playing field when the athlete returns for evaluation in the clinical setting. Tools such as the Sport Concussion Office Assessment Tool (SCOAT) were developed for the continued evaluation of concussion in the subacute phase. This tool is meant for ongoing evaluation for return-to-play (RTP) with a range of 72 hours post injury to several weeks.[22] These methods are helpful for RTP recommendations which will be discussed in the subsequent sections.

RETURN-TO-LEARN AND RETURN-TO-SPORT

Given the impact of concussion and its increasing prevalence, a tremendous effort has been made to improve guidelines regarding an athlete's RTP. This decision should not be taken lightly, as there are significant impacts of premature return, including severe brain injuries and death. An increasing emphasis on safe return to sport has been placed due to concerns about second impact syndrome, a potentially catastrophic complication repeat injury after concussion.[23] A second brain injury prior to recovering from the initial injury is rare, but the dysfunction of cerebral blood flow can lead to increased cerebral pressure with catastrophic complications.[24] In 2009, the ""Zackery Lystedt Law" was passed in the state of Washington, after Zackery Lystedt, a youth football player, suffered a severe brain injury after returning to play soon after sustaining closed head trauma. While Zackery survived, he suffered permanent disability as a result of his injuries.[25] Return to Sport (RTS) protocols have been intensely developed over the years in effort to ensure that athletes are not returned to sport prior to cessation of symptoms, and more importantly, returned in a time frame that allows them to avoid secondary severe injury.[26] The 2023 consensus statement updated a 6-step protocol for RTP with the end goal of a safe RTS. Each step of the RTS strategy typically takes a minimum of 24 hours. In step 1, the athlete performs symptom-limited activity, with daily activities that do not exacerbate symptoms. These should begin within the first 24 hours of injury and can proceed through the subsequent steps. The goal of step 1 is to reintroduce the athlete into work/school. In step 2, the athlete may begin aerobic exercise by performing first light (55% of max heart rate) then moderate (70% of max heart rate) in a manner that limits risk for reinjury. Max heart rate can be predicted as 220-the athletes age, a commonly used estimation in health care. Common methods used are stationary cycling or walking at a slow to medium pace with the goal of increasing the athlete's heart rate. In step 3, the athlete begins to work on individual sport-specific exercises. Notably, the athlete should be medically cleared if this level of participation place them at risk of head impact. Examples of this training include running and changing direction. If after progressing through steps 1 to 3 the athlete has complete resolution of symptoms, (including those after physical exertion) the athlete is then to progress through steps 4 to 6 of the RTS protocol. In step 4, the athlete begins non-contact training drills, where return to high intensity and technical drills can be performed in a team environment. This allows the athlete to resume typical intensity of exercise while working on regaining sport-specific coordination and cognitive processing. Following asymptomatic non-contact training, the athlete moves to step 5 and performs full contact practice without restriction. This is aimed to restore athletes' and coaches' confidence in sport-specific task completion. If the athlete continues to be asymptomatic, they are then cleared for full sport. It is important to note that mild and brief symptom exacerbation during the RTS protocol is acceptable. This is with the understanding that these symptoms do not exceed more than 2 points on a 10-point symptom scale, and that they last for less than 1 hour. If during steps 1 to 3 the athlete experiences prolonged or significant worsening of symptoms, they should repeat that step 24 hours after symptom exacerbation.[27,28]One major update to the consensus statement is the emphasis of early introduction in sub-symptomatic aerobic exercise.[29] Other interventions in the early hours of recovery include reduced screen time, which some data show may be beneficial immediately and for up to the first 2 days after injury.[29]

The consensus statement also identified the importance of structured and evidence-based recommendation for students (especially children, adolescents, and young adult athletes) to Return-to-Learn (RTL). Most concussed athletes return to learning with few complications, however, in some settings this can be much more difficult. Issues such as severe symptoms in the days and weeks following the injury, and previous learning difficulties can make RTL more challenging after concussion.[30] As recommended for RTS, those treating patients with concussions should not recommend strict rest in the first 24 to 48 hours, and instead focus on strategies to help promote RTL.[30] This includes environmental adjustments, including frequency of rest breaks from demanding cognitive tasks, reduced screen time, and consideration of modified attendance policies. Physical adjustments, such as avoidance of high-risk activities (eg, physical education class and after school activities), while still participating in tasks such as walking and other low risk activities. Accommodations such as extra time to complete assignments, pre-made notes, or allowing longer time for testing have been helpful in supporting RTL.[30] Step 1 of the return-to-learn protocol includes gradual return to typical activities with short bursts of learning (5–15 min) with an increase in time as symptoms allow. Steps 2 to 4 entail a stepwise return to school activities and return to part-time and full-time participation. Like RTS, progression through the stages should be slowed if symptoms increase by 2 points on a 10-point scale for more than an hour from baseline levels (**Table 1**).

Prevention

Concussion prevention is largely an effort to decrease the rates of concussion and the subsequent morbidity following concussion through policy changes, education, style of play changes, rule changes, and equipment evolution. Individuals reduce concussion risk by choosing sports with lower overall concussion risks (ie, trading soccer for basketball). Primary concussion prevention is defined by the CDC as "Intervening before health effects occur, through measures such as vaccinations, altering risky behaviors (poor eating habits and tobacco use), and banning substances known to be associated with a disease or health condition." Secondary prevention is screening to

Table 1
Return-to-learn and return-to-sport strategies[17]

Return-to-Learn	Return-to-Sport
• 4 step return-to-learn strategy	• 6 step return-to-sport strategy
○ Steps include progressing from symptoms that do not result in more than mild exacerbation of symptoms (eg, reading).	○ Steps include progressing from aerobic exercise, to sport specific training, non-contact training, full contact practice, and finally return to sport.
○ This is started at 5–15 min intervals. This progresses to school activities, then to part time school work with more frequent rest breaks if needed, and finally returned to full participation.	○ There must be 24 hrs between steps.
	○ Step 1 may start within 24 hrs of injury.
○ Athletes typically undergo a 24–48 h period of relative rest and are allowed to increase through each step assuming symptoms are not more than mildly exacerbated.	○ Mild exacerbation of symptoms is permitted without halting progression.
	○ More than mild exacerbation results in repeating step again the next day.

identify diseases at the earliest stages, before the onset of signs and symptoms, through measures such as mammography and regular blood pressure testing." (**Table 2**) All sports have a finite risk of concussion that can never be fully eliminated. The available literature on concussion prevention is focused on high school athletes, and additional work is needed around athletes aged under 14 years .[31] The Lystedt Law and the subsequent adoption of similar legislation across the United States is the broadest-sweeping attempt at identifying concussions. Increased identification of concussions, over the last 10 years, following these policy changes "increased" the rate of concussion.[32] This likely reflects increased diagnosis and awareness of concussion rather than an actual increase in the rates of concussion. Yang and colleagues observed increased new and recurrent concussions in the years following the implementation of the concussion laws. They also reported a significant decline in the rate of recurrent concussion 2.6 years after the laws went into effect.[33] (See **Table 2**)

Considerable research and development of improved equipment has been performed in an effort to decrease concussions. These equipment changes have multiple aims, including decreasing impact forces during helmet to helmet collisions. These studies offer promise, but have not definitively identified a superior brand or type of helmet. Proper fit and maintenance of helmets are clearly recommended. Other aims have been to document and identify forces during specific collision types and play situations. Headgear in soccer has also been studied and has not yielded definitive superiority.

The data on prevention is constantly evolving and individual studies often report conflicting results. Given this observation, the authors recommend the utilization of systemic review and meta-analysis to guide prevention strategies. The most recent meta-analysis from Eliason and colleagues makes several high-quality observations based on their systematic review. Mouthguards in ice hockey are associated with a 28% decrease in rates of concussion. The disallowing of body-checking in adolescent ice hockey is associated with a 58% decrease in the rate of concussion without an associated increase in concussion when subsequently participating in leagues with bodychecking. The limitation of contact practices is associated with a 64% reduction in concussion rates.[19] The.

Individual leagues have instituted a variety of interventions to decrease concussion. Major league baseball changed its rules around home plate collisions after identifying that catchers have the highest rate of concussions during plays at home plate.[34] The Ivy League's experience with kickoff rule changes led the NCAA to follow suit. Body checking in hockey has been identified as a risk factor for concussion. Several leagues have implemented rule changes, education, and increasing penalties for risky play. These changes highlight the importance of identification of the riskiest scenarios and targeted intervention.

Table 2
Examples of primary and secondary prevention in sports related concussion

Primary Prevention	Secondary Prevention

• Changing participation
• Exposure limitation
• Technique training
• Policy or rule changes
• Equipment implementation and advancement
	• Lystedt Law implementation
	  ○ Early recognition and removal from play
	  ○ Medically-supervised return to play protocols
	  ○ Education
	• Return-to-learn/work programs
	• Equipment implementation and advancement

IMAGING

Imaging in head injury is time-specific with recommendations changing based on chronology, history, and date of injury. There are multiple published guidelines for the utilization of brain imaging in the emergency literature that relate to acute head injury (eg, PECARN, New Orleans Head CT, and Canadian Head CT rules).[35–37] As discussed elsewhere in this publication, concussion and mTBI are not generally visible on standard imaging. Computed tomography is rapidly available, relatively inexpensive, and accurate in diagnosis skull fracture and intracranial hemorrhage. CT scan has limited utility in the ambulatory clinic setting, where MRI is favored.

The imaging management of subacute and chronic mTBI is more variable. MRI is less readily available, more expensive, though more sensitive to diffuse axonal injury and shear injury, especially when using diffusion weighted imaging (DWI).[38] Functional MRI show some promise in the evaluation of post-concussion syndrome and prolonged recovery situations.[39] Additionally, MRI in the subacute and chronic setting evaluates for alternative etiologies for symptoms. Advanced MRI techniques show non-specific microstructural and microvascular injury that could have relevance on long-term prognosis or earlier identification of neurodegenerative disease. However, this remains largely in the research phases, showing promise for in-vivo evaluation in the future.[40] An ideal imaging test for chronic mTBI would be inexpensive, reliable, sensitive, and specific, independently determine recovery, and offer insight into long-term prognosis.

Retirement from Sport

There is no evidence-based consensus for retirement from sport in the setting of concussion. Common clinical questions arise when counseling athletes with multiple concussions, severe symptoms, or prolonged recovery following a single concussion, concussions suffered at a young age, but also athletes that have suffered multiple head contacts without concussion. Wilson and colleagues published a summary of available retirement along with the considerations for retirement that is worth reviewing. These concepts include persistent symptoms, diminished academic or athletic performance, decreased injury threshold, persistent focal neurologic deficits, persistent neuropsychological deficits, TBI findings on imaging, and structural abnormalities found on imaging.[41] Retirement is always an individualized discussion that takes into account personal medical and neuropsychologic history, family history, age, playing level, and individual goals. For example, a high school athlete with no designs to play in college has a different time horizon than a Division I collegiate athlete with the potential for a long professional career that involves additional risk exposure. This framework allows the athlete and provider a more comprehensive understanding of the factors that are part of this decision. Modification of sport can also be a consideration. A change of position, limited exposure to year-round participation, moving to a non-contact league, or a lower competition level are all reasonable ways to balance the importance of physical activity with the risks of concussion in sport.

Providers and athletes should feel comfortable seeking additional expert opinions in these circumstances. The authors recommend in-depth, personalized neuropsychologic testing to evaluate cognitive functioning compared to averages or baseline, when available, to identify subclinical changes in functioning. All parties should be aware on the future risks, both known and unknown, when making these types of decisions. In most cases, the authors advocate for the involvement of a sports psychologist to partner with the athlete during and following these decisions. Additional concussions should be evaluated individually, and retirement conversations should be held as often as needed (**Box 1**).

Box 1
Factors to be considered when considering retirement

Retirement considerations
  Age of athlete
  Level of play
  Time horizon
  Personal and family psychiatric history
  Personal and family history of neurologic and neurodegenerative disease
  Number of concussions (diagnosed and suspected)
  Injury threshold
  Estimated number of collisions
  Recovery duration
  Severity of symptoms
  Neuroimaging results
  Neuropsychological testing results
  Neurologic examination

CHRONIC TRAUMATIC ENCEPHALOPATHY

The impacts of concussions on athletes goes beyond sport, as recent data suggest that 80% to 90% of athletes that undergo a typical recovery will still demonstrate persistent cognitive symptoms 3 or more months out from the initial injury.[42] Even more, there is some evidence that professional athletes with concussion history may have more severe presentations of chronic degenerative neurologic diseases like amyotrophic lateral sclerosis.[5] With the recent increase in coverage on SRC and its ramifications, particular attention has been placed on the diagnosis of Chronic Traumatic Encephalopathy (CTE). Recently, there has been increased emphasis on clarifying that CTE is not a clinical diagnosis, but instead one resulting from neuropathologic diagnosis with a new nomenclature of chronic traumatic encephalopathy neuropathologic change (CTE-NC). Namely, CTE-NC is thought to be associated with repetitive head impacts leading to an abnormal deposition of hyperphosphorylated tau proteins.[43] In 2021, a new consensus statement was published regarding a clinical diagnosis associated with CTE-NS[44] known as, Traumatic encephalopathy syndrome (TES). It requires substantial exposure to repetitive head impacts (RHI) from contact sports, military service, core clinical features of cognitive impairment (in episodic memory and/or executive functioning), and/or neurobehavioral dysregulation. It also must include progressive course; and that the clinical features are not fully accounted for by any other neurologic, psychiatric, or medical conditions. For those meeting criteria for TES, functional dependence is graded on 5 levels, ranging from independent to severe dementia. A provisional level of certainty for CTE pathology is determined based on specific RHI exposure thresholds, core clinical features, functional status, and additional supportive features, including delayed onset, motor signs, and psychiatric features.[44]

There has been recent investigation into the utility of identifying imaging modalities that may demonstrate evidence of CTE in living athletes.

MRI has been shown to demonstrate structural abnormalities including ventricular enlargement, cortical atrophy, as well as several other abnormalities. These findings of course, are not specific to the diagnosis of CTE, thus, MRI is mainly used to rule out other causes of brain injury in symptomatic athletes.[45] Interestingly, diffusion tensor imaging (DTI) has been shown to demonstrate physiologic changes seen in repetitive brain trauma in rats.[46] Other studies have demonstrated that anatomic MRI and F-Fluorodeoxyglucose positron emission tomography (PET), an imaging study that demonstrates the metabolic rate of glucose, have shown medial temporal lobe and frontal cortex neurodegeneration in high risk living participants.[47] There is growing excitement surrounding PET radiotracers for tau proteins, a microscopic hallmark of CTE.[48] Unfortunately, an optimal tau PET radiotracer with affinity for neurofibrillary tangles specific to those seen in CTE has yet to be discovered.[49] There is hope that a radiotracer specific to damage seen in CTE may be discovered to best optimize prevention strategies in high-risk populations.

CLINICS CARE POINTS

- Rule changes in specific sport scenarios show promise inconcussion reduction.
- There is no single test or symptom that reliable diagnsosis a concussion.
- Return to Learn and Return to Sport strategies should be implemented for successful recovery.
- There is no evidence-based consensus for medical retirement from sport due to concussion. Each situation is managed on a case-by-case basis.

DISCLOSURE

S.R. Laker, C. Nicolosi: Nothing to disclose.

REFERENCES

1. McCrory PR, Berkovic SF. Concussion: the history of clinical and pathophysiological concepts and misconceptions. Neurology 2001;57(12):2283–9.
2. Williams VB, Danan IJ. A Historical Perspective on Sports Concussion: Where We Have Been and Where We Are Going. Curr Pain Headache Rep 2016;20(6):43.
3. Bryan MA, Rowhani-Rahbar A, Comstock RD, et al. Sports- and Recreation-Related Concussions in US Youth. Pediatrics 2016;138(1).
4. Hootman JM, Dick R, Agel J. Epidemiology of collegiate injuries for 15 sports: summary and recommendations for injury prevention initiatives. J Athl Train 2007;42(2):311–9.
5. Iverson GL, Castellani RJ, Cassidy JD, et al. Examining later-in-life health risks associated with sport-related concussion and repetitive head impacts: a systematic review of case-control and cohort studies. Br J Sports Med 2023;57(12):810–21.
6. Pierpoint LA, Collins C. Epidemiology of Sport-Related Concussion. Clin Sports Med 2021;40(1):1–18.
7. Gordon KE. The Silent Minority: Insights into Who Fails to Present for Medical Care Following a Brain Injury. Neuroepidemiology 2020;54(3):235–42.
8. Beran KM, Scafide KN. Factors Related to Concussion Knowledge, Attitudes, and Reporting Behaviors in US High School Athletes: A Systematic Review. J Sch Health 2022;92(4):406–17.
9. Eime RM, Young JA, Harvey JT, et al. A systematic review of the psychological and social benefits of participation in sport for children and adolescents: informing development of a conceptual model of health through sport. Int J Behav Nutr Phys Act 2013;10:98.

10. Wasserman EB, Coberley M, Anderson S, et al. Concussion Rates Differ by Practice Type and Equipment Worn in an Autonomy Five Collegiate Football Conference. Clin J Sport Med 2020;30(4):366–71.

11. Zuckerman SL, Kerr ZY, Yengo-Kahn A, et al. Epidemiology of Sports-Related Concussion in NCAA Athletes From 2009-2010 to 2013-2014: Incidence, Recurrence, and Mechanisms. Am J Sports Med 2015;43(11):2654–62.

12. National Concussion Surveillence System: Centers for Disease Control and Prevention; 2024. Available at: https://www.cdc.gov/traumaticbraininjury/research-programs/ncss/index.html. and https://www.cdc.gov/traumaticbraininjury/research-programs/ncss/index.html. Accessed March 19, 2024.

13. Dwyer B, Katz DI. Postconcussion syndrome. Handb Clin Neurol 2018;158: 163–78.

14. Mayer AR, Quinn DK, Master CL. The spectrum of mild traumatic brain injury: A review. Neurology 2017;89(6):623–32.

15. Harmon KG, Drezner JA, Gammons M, et al. American Medical Society for Sports Medicine position statement: concussion in sport. Br J Sports Med 2013;47(1): 15–26.

16. Aubry M, Cantu R, Dvorak J, et al. Summary and Agreement Statement of the First International Conference on Concussion in Sport, Vienna 2001. Physician Sportsmed 2002;30(2):57–63.

17. Patricios JS, Schneider KJ, Dvorak J, et al. Consensus statement on concussion in sport: the 6th International Conference on Concussion in Sport–Amsterdam, October 2022. Br J Sports Med 2023;57(11):695–711.

18. Silverberg ND, Iverson GL, Cogan A, et al. The American Congress of Rehabilitation Medicine Diagnostic Criteria for Mild Traumatic Brain Injury. Arch Phys Med Rehabil 2023;104(8):1343–55.

19. Eliason PH, Galarneau JM, Kolstad AT, et al. Prevention strategies and modifiable risk factors for sport-related concussions and head impacts: a systematic review and meta-analysis. Br J Sports Med 2023;57(12):749–61.

20. Yeo PC, Yeo EQY, Probert J, et al. A Systematic Review and Qualitative Analysis of Concussion Knowledge amongst Sports Coaches and Match Officials. J Sports Sci Med 2020;19(1):65–77.

21. Echemendia RJ, Burma JS, Bruce JM, et al. Acute evaluation of sport-related concussion and implications for the Sport Concussion Assessment Tool (SCAT6) for adults, adolescents and children: a systematic review. Br J Sports Med 2023;57(11):722–35.

22. Patricios JS, Schneider GM, van Ierssel J, et al. Beyond acute concussion assessment to office management: a systematic review informing the development of a Sport Concussion Office Assessment Tool (SCOAT6) for adults and children. Br J Sports Med 2023;57(11):737–48.

23. Saunders RL, Harbaugh RE. The second impact in catastrophic contact-sports head trauma. JAMA 1984;252(4):538–9.

24. May T, Foris LA, Donnally IC. Second impact syndrome. StatPearls. Treasure Island (FL): StatPearls Publishing Copyright © 2023, StatPearls Publishing LLC.; 2023.

25. Adler RH, Herring SA. Changing the culture of concussion: education meets legislation. Pm r 2011;3(10 Suppl 2):S468–70.

26. Laurer HL, Bareyre FM, Lee VM, et al. Mild head injury increasing the brain's vulnerability to a second concussive impact. J Neurosurg 2001;95(5):859–70.

27. Leddy JJ, Haider MN, Ellis MJ, et al. Early Subthreshold Aerobic Exercise for Sport-Related Concussion: A Randomized Clinical Trial. JAMA Pediatr 2019; 173(4):319–25.

28. Leddy JJ, Master CL, Mannix R, et al. Early targeted heart rate aerobic exercise versus placebo stretching for sport-related concussion in adolescents: a randomised controlled trial. Lancet Child Adolesc Health 2021;5(11):792–9.

29. Leddy JJ, Burma JS, Toomey CM, et al. Rest and exercise early after sport-related concussion: a systematic review and meta-analysis. Br J Sports Med 2023;57(12):762–70.

30. Putukian M, Purcell L, Schneider KJ, et al. Clinical recovery from concussion-return to school and sport: a systematic review and meta-analysis. Br J Sports Med 2023;57(12):798–809.

31. Waltzman D, Sarmiento K. What the research says about concussion risk factors and prevention strategies for youth sports: A scoping review of six commonly played sports. J Saf Res 2019;68:157–72.

32. Bompadre V, Jinguji TM, Yanez ND, et al. Washington State's Lystedt law in concussion documentation in Seattle public high schools. J Athl Train 2014; 49(4):486–92.

33. Yang J, Comstock RD, Yi H, et al. New and Recurrent Concussions in High-School Athletes Before and After Traumatic Brain Injury Laws, 2005-2016. Am J Public Health 2017;107(12):1916–22.

34. Kriz PK, Roberts WO. Prevention of Sport-Related Concussion. Clin Sports Med 2021;40(1):159–71.

35. Kuppermann N, Holmes JF, Dayan PS, et al. Identification of children at very low risk of clinically-important brain injuries after head trauma: a prospective cohort study. Lancet 2009;374(9696):1160–70.

36. Stiell IG, Lesiuk H, Wells GA, et al. Canadian CT head rule study for patients with minor head injury: methodology for phase II (validation and economic analysis). Ann Emerg Med 2001;38(3):317–22.

37. Stiell IG, Clement CM, Rowe BH, et al. Comparison of the Canadian CT Head Rule and the New Orleans Criteria in patients with minor head injury. JAMA 2005;294(12):1511–8.

38. Pulsipher DT, Campbell RA, Thoma R, et al. A Critical Review of Neuroimaging Applications in Sports Concussion. Curr Sports Med Rep 2011;10(1):14–20.

39. Chen J-K, Johnston KM, Collie A, et al. A validation of the post concussion symptom scale in the assessment of complex concussion using cognitive testing and functional MRI. J Neurol Neurosurg Psychiatr 2007;78(11):1231–8.

40. Ware JB, Sandsmark DK. Imaging Approach to Concussion. Neuroimaging Clin N Am 2023;33(2):261–9.

41. Wilson JC, Patsimas T, Cohen K, et al. Considerations for Athlete Retirement After Sport-Related Concussion. Clin Sports Med 2021;40(1):187–97.

42. McInnes K, Friesen CL, MacKenzie DE, et al. Mild Traumatic Brain Injury (mTBI) and chronic cognitive impairment: A scoping review. PLoS One 2017;12(4): e0174847.

43. McKee AC, Cairns NJ, Dickson DW, et al. The first NINDS/NIBIB consensus meeting to define neuropathological criteria for the diagnosis of chronic traumatic encephalopathy. Acta Neuropathol 2016;131(1):75–86.

44. Katz DI, Bernick C, Dodick DW, et al. National Institute of Neurological Disorders and Stroke Consensus Diagnostic Criteria for Traumatic Encephalopathy Syndrome. Neurology 2021;96(18):848–63.

45. Dallmeier JD, Meysami S, Merrill DA, et al. Emerging advances of in vivo detection of chronic traumatic encephalopathy and traumatic brain injury. Br J Radiol 2019;92(1101):20180925.
46. Wright DK, Brady RD, Kamnaksh A, et al. Repeated mild traumatic brain injuries induce persistent changes in plasma protein and magnetic resonance imaging biomarkers in the rat. Sci Rep 2019;9(1):14626.
47. Lesman-Segev OH, Edwards L, Rabinovici GD. Chronic Traumatic Encephalopathy: A Comparison with Alzheimer's Disease and Frontotemporal Dementia. Semin Neurol 2020;40(4):394–410.
48. Hof PR, Bouras C, Buée L, et al. Differential distribution of neurofibrillary tangles in the cerebral cortex of dementia pugilistica and Alzheimer's disease cases. Acta Neuropathol 1992;85(1):23–30.
49. Alosco ML, Culhane J, Mez J. Neuroimaging Biomarkers of Chronic Traumatic Encephalopathy: Targets for the Academic Memory Disorders Clinic. Neurotherapeutics 2021;18(2):772–91.

Military Traumatic Brain Injury

Diane Schretzman Mortimer, MD, MSN[a,b,*]

KEYWORDS

- Military • Traumatic brain injury • Polytrauma • Rehabilitation

KEY POINTS

- Military TBI can differ from civilian injuries when it comes to mechanism of injury, diagnosis, treatment, and course of recovery.
- Unique physical and physiologic stressors in the military can lead to complex injuries, with the overlap between TBI, pain, and mental health conditions potentially confounding diagnosis and treatment.
- Military and veteran healthcare settings and programs attempt to address these complex and multifaceted situations, with the goal of optimizing recovery and function.

INTRODUCTION

Traumatic brain injuries (TBIs) are all-too common in the military. Service members (SMs) sustain injuries while deployed, in combat and noncombat situations, and in nondeployed roles. Members of the military can experience different injury mechanisms, symptoms, course, and recovery compared with civilians. SMs and veterans who have been affected by TBI benefit from dedicated efforts to optimize diagnosis, treatment, and overall function.

BRIEF HISTORY OF TRAUMATIC BRAIN INJURY IN THE MILITARY

Brain injuries have been an ongoing reality in wars and conflicts. During the Civil War, gunshot wounds to the head were significant causes of morbidity and mortality.[1] In World War (WW) I, SMs had stronger helmets to protect against at least some penetrating wounds, but they were still vulnerable to effects of blasts. WWI troops who were exposed to blasts were noted to have symptoms even when they did not have

[a] Department of Physical Medicine, and Rehabilitation, Inpatient Brain Injury/ Polytrauma Rehabilitation Center, Minneapolis VA Health Care System, 1 Veterans Drive, Mail Code 117, Minneapolis, MN 55417, USA; [b] Brain Injury Medicine Fellowship, Department of Rehabilitation Medicine, University of Minnesota
* Corresponding author. Department of PM&R, Minneapolis VA, 1 veterans Drive, # 117, Minneapolis, MN 55417.
E-mail address: Diane.mortimer@va.gov

Phys Med Rehabil Clin N Am 35 (2024) 559–571
https://doi.org/10.1016/j.pmr.2024.02.008
1047-9651/24/Published by Elsevier Inc.
pmr.theclinics.com

outwardly visible injuries. "Shell shock," as the phenotype came to be known, included problems with sleep, fatigue, cognition, vision, hearing, sensation, and tremor.[2]

In WWII, SMs with brain injuries had access to neurosurgical care acutely and to some rehabilitation services later. The Korean War saw a further improvement in neurosurgical care for injured troops. In the Persian Gulf War, more than 15% of all SM casualties were due to TBIs.[1]

TBI has featured prominently in the Global War on Terrorism: Operation Enduring Freedom (OEF), occurred in Afghanistan from 2001 to 2021, Operation Iraqi Freedom (OIF) in Iraq from 2003 to 2010, and Operation New Dawn (OND) in Iraq from 2010 to 2011. TBI is often called a signature wound of these conflicts. The constellation of warfare that involved blasts, modernized body armor and other equipment, and well-honed expertise in battlefield care, including mass casualty events and care in austere environments, led to unprecedented numbers of TBI survivors. TBI and polytrauma rehabilitation services have experienced corresponding expansion in availability and scope.[1,3,4]

DEFINITION

The Veterans Affairs (VA) and Department of Defense (DoD) define TBI as "traumatically induced structural injury and/or physiologic disruption of brain function as a result of an external force that is indicated by new onset of worsening of at least one of the following clinical signs.

- Any period of loss of decrease in level of consciousness
- Any loss of memory for events immediately before or after the injury
- Any alteration in mental state at the time of the injury (eg, confusion, disorientation, slowed thinking, alteration of consciousness/mental state)
- Neurologic deficits (eg, weakness, loss of balance, change in vision, praxis, paresis/plegia, sensory loss, aphasia, and so on) that may or may not be transient
- An intracranial lesion"[5]

Severity of brain injury has important implications for recovery, rehabilitation, and outcome. Injuries are classified into mild, moderate, or severe based on the factors listed in **Table 1**. Of note, VA and DoD use the terms "mild TBI" and "concussion" interchangeably.[5]

SIGNIFICANCE

TBI is a leading cause of morbidity and mortality among SMs injured in combat.[6] More than 400,000 US SMs sustained TBIs while deployed in support OEF, OIF, and OND. TBI thus affected at least 5%[7] and possibly as many as 20%[4,8] of the 1.6 million troops

Table 1 TBI severity[5]			
	Mild	**Moderate**	**Severe**
Structural imaging	Normal	Normal or abnormal	Normal or abnormal
Loss of Consciousness (LOC)	0–30 min	30 min-24 h	Over 24 h
Alteration in Mental Status (AMS)	Up to 24 h	Over 24 h	Over 24 h
Post-Traumatic Amnesia (PTA)	Up to 24 h	1–7 d	Over 7 d
Best Glasgow Coma Scale Score in First 24 h after Injury	13–15	9–12	8 or less

deployed. Nearly 90% of these injuries were mild in severity. The remainder were classified as moderate or severe.[7]

There was a 2% mortality rate for these SMs with TBI, including an 18% mortality rate for SMs with severe TBI.[7] Overall, one-third of battlefield deaths are attributable to TBI.[6]

TBI can be accompanied by polytraumatic injuries. Of the 80% of TBIs sustained in OEF/OIF/OND deployments which were classified as mild, approximately 55% were isolated mild TBIs. More than 30% were associated with minor systemic injuries, 9% were associated with moderate systemic injuries, and 4% were associated with severe to critical systemic injuries. More than 15% of SMs with severe TBI also experienced severe injury to at least one other body system.[6]

Military TBI has far-reaching effects on the SM, family, and beyond. The SM may have difficulty returning to the community and to prior roles.[9] Family roles can change significantly when the SM needs care in the short and long term. This change can be especially profound for military families with young children.[2,10]

ETIOLOGY/MECHANISM OF INJURY

Most military TBI cases occur in noncombat environments. Like their civilian counterparts, SMs sustain injuries in transportation mishaps, including crashes involving motor vehicles, motorcycles, and bicycles. Other injuries occur in recreational activities and sports. Of note, many SMs are male and between the ages of 18 and 24 years, demographic groups who are most at risk for these kinds of injuries.[7,11]

SMs can also be injured in activities that are related to their military occupations, while engaging in operational or training exercises. They routinely work with specialized equipment and perform maneuvers which are inherently dangerous. Heavy artillery, explosives, parachuting, and diving are just a few examples.[1,11,12]

TBIs sustained in combat environments can have multiple overlapping mechanisms. SMs may be injured in vehicle crashes or by blunt trauma. Blast-related TBIs and penetrating injuries are also often multidimensional.[2]

BLAST-RELATED TRAUMATIC BRAIN INJURY

Blasts, from artillery, improvised explosive devices, mines, rocket-propelled grenades, mines, and other powerful detonators, have been the leading cause of TBI during OEF/OIF/OND.[1,4,7] In these conflicts, where multiple blast exposures were common, an estimated 20% of deployed SMs experienced blast-related TBI.[1,4,12] Eighty percent of the combat-related TBIs involved blast exposures.[3] Morbidity is compounded by the fact that blast-related TBIs are frequently associated with additional physical injuries.[7,12] When blasts lead to severe injuries to the brain or other body systems, mortality rates approach 50%.[13]

Blasts lead to injury in several ways. The chemical reaction resulting in extreme heat powers the expulsion of an atmospheric pressure wave. Primary blast injuries occur when exposed individuals are injured by effects of the pressure wave on the body. Pressure can be especially traumatic to hollow organs. Hemotympanum, pulmonary barotrauma, and injuries to the globes of the eyes are some of the more common sequelae.[11,13]

Blasts cause secondary injuries by fueling the forceful scattering of fragments, debris, and other material. These items, which may have been inside the explosive device or in the affected environment, can cause blunt trauma to individuals they strike.[11,13]

Tertiary blast injuries occur when a person is displaced by the force of the explosion. Trauma can occur through effects of the acceleration and deceleration forces on the body. Injuries also occur when the individual forcefully lands on the ground or is thrown against other objects. Quaternary injuries result when the explosion's heat or fire causes damage or when individuals experience toxic exposures.[11,13]

Blast-related TBIs vary in severity and degree of damage. The blast wave can cause pressure changes and jarring that strew damage as the wave propagates through the brain. Shrapnel and other material can cause injuries to the skull and focal brain areas. The act of being thrown or colliding can lead to blunt force trauma. Resultant injuries can be widespread or focal. Diffuse axonal injury, resulting from large-scale shaking of the brain, involves cerebral white matter dysfunction. The resulting dysfunction is often transient but can last for minutes to hours or longer. More localized injuries affect certain brain areas, and their function, more than others.[1,13]

Most blast-related TBIs are characterized as mild in severity. It is crucial to note that blast-related mild TBIs have been shown to result in significant morbidity. Associated symptoms include problems involving vestibular, auditory, visual, cognitive, and language issues.[1] Despite these many symptoms, injuries can go undetected and undiagnosed in SMs.[2]

PENETRATING INJURIES

Penetrating injuries account for approximately 10% of military TBIs. Gunshot wounds and blast-related injuries are responsible for most penetrating TBIs, both in and out of combat. Seventy percent of penetrating injuries result from blasts, 30% from gunshot wounds, and less than 1% from knives or related objects.[3]

Bullets, shrapnel, and other skull-piercing materials can have devastating effects on the brain. Penetrating injuries are fatal more than half the time. Survivors experience persistent or permanent sequelae. Complications include infection and posttraumatic epilepsy. The degree of damage is directly related to the penetrating object's size and traveling velocity. The extent of impairments corresponds with location and amount of damaged brain tissue. Penetrating injuries often occur in association with other traumatic injuries, complicating recovery. These injuries are heterogeneous, with sequelae and outcomes that vary significantly between individuals.[12,14,15]

POLYTRAUMA

Polytrauma is defined as a serious injury to two or more body systems, with one being a brain injury. Co-occurring injuries and their sequelae can take many forms. Burns, abrasions, or other skin injuries can be associated with infection. Ocular injuries, and trauma to the face and orbits, are strongly associated with TBI. SMs may sustain fractures and other orthopedic or musculoskeletal injuries, including traumatic amputations and spinal cord injuries. Injuries to the chest and abdomen can also lead to damage to internal organs and the genitals.[9,11,12]

These injuries, and the complex constellation of associated symptoms, can lead to significant impairments in physical, emotional, and overall function. Pain is a particularly pervasive and troublesome symptom. Comorbid mental health conditions are also common. Given their proclivity to co-occur, some authors refer to TBI, pain, and mental health conditions as the "polytrauma clinical triad."[1,11]

There is some evidence that combat trauma resulting in severe injuries of any type can be associated with the development of chronic diseases like hypertension, diabetes, and heart disease. The reason is not certain. Proposed etiologies include exposures, stress, and side effects of treatment for the combat trauma. These chronic diseases can cause other health problems over time, so long-term comprehensive follow-up is warranted.[16]

MENTAL HEALTH

The interplay between mental health and TBI seems more complex for SMs and veterans than for civilians. TBI sequelae can manifest the same as conditions like post-traumatic stress disorder (PTSD), depression and other affective disorders, and anxiety. Symptoms like cognitive dysfunction, sleep problems, and neurobehavioral issues can reflect either TBI or mental health conditions, or both. Plus, TBI can mask the presence of mental health conditions or vice versa. Alternatively, TBI can compound the effects of a comorbid mental health problem. There may be some cumulative effect of symptom burden on overall functioning. The onset of mental health conditions can predate, co-exist with, or follow the injury.[12,17,18]

It is notable that TBI and PTSD are both considered signature injuries of the recent conflicts. PTSD's incidence has been estimated at up to 20% of OEF/OIF/OND combat veterans, 10% of Gulf War veterans, and 30% of Vietnam veterans.[19] Multiple studies have demonstrated that the risk of PTSD, and related symptoms, increases after TBI. This risk is even higher when the TBI is due to a blast, when sleep and pain issues co-occur, and when the SM was injured in combat.[12,17,20]

Other comorbid psychiatric conditions have similar relationships to TBI. Combat-related TBI has been associated with depression, anxiety, and severe stress.[21] TBI can also be associated with substance issues like alcohol use disorder (AUD).[22] Nearly 90% of veterans with TBI have at least one mental health comorbidity.[11] It is not certain which direction these associations follow, or whether relationships are bidirectional.[21,22]

Substance use disorders (SUDs), involving alcohol or other substances, are a formidable issue following TBI. SMs with SUDs at baseline have a more difficult time recovering from TBI. It has been postulated that AUD is more common in the military than among civilians, with more than 10% of SMs screening positive at any point. The incidence of AUD and opioid use disorder increases after combat traumatic experiences.[23,24] SUDs, which affect up to 15% of OEF/OIF/OND veterans, can negatively affect both reintegration after deployment and difficulties with interpersonal relationships or vocational pursuits. It is also notable that TBI is also a risk factor for the development of SUDs.[24]

Suicide can be a devastating consequence. TBI is associated with at least some increase in risk for suicidal ideation. This risk seems higher in military and veteran populations than among civilians.[24] This increase in suicide risk is a multilayered problem, with potential contributions from PTSD, depression, SUD, and pain, but TBI itself does seem to be an independent risk factor.[22,25]

Treating mental health in SMs can be complicated. The interplay with TBI can be one confounder. Another issue is that some SMs report feeling a stigma surrounding talking about mental health issues. In this population, there may be some reluctance to attribute problems to mental health or to seek care and treatment.[11,13] Clinicians can provide welcoming environments as they openly and competently discuss these vital issues.[22,25]

PAIN

The intersection of pain and TBI also seems to complicate recovery and subsequent function. SMs are at risk of developing pain due to any injuries they might experience. In a recent study of SMs and veterans, TBI was an independent risk factor for the development of chronic pain and pain-related disability diagnoses. The risk of developing chronic pain after TBI was highest when individuals were also experiencing PTSD and depression.[17]

MILD TRAUMATIC BRAIN INJURY (CONCUSSION)

There are important differences between concussions in the military and injuries of similar severity affecting civilians. In combat, 80% of concussions are related to blasts. SMs are much more likely than civilians to sustain polytraumatic injuries at the time of concussion.[12,13]

Some symptoms are more prevalent in SMs than in civilians. Hearing abnormalities, including tinnitus, affect at least 75% of individuals exposed to loud blasts.[9] Compared with civilians, SMs report higher rates of hearing loss and tinnitus after concomitant TBI.[17]

Mild TBI (mTBI) diagnosis is complicated because symptoms can be nonspecific. Problems with sleeping, headache, dizziness and vestibular issues, visual changes, cognitive symptoms, and neuropsychiatric symptoms like anxiety and low frustration tolerance are generally more subjective than objective.[4,11,13]

The deployed environment can itself play a role in clouding diagnosis of mTBI. Deployments have been associated with stressors and health effects. Issues can include physical stress related to the demands of the mission, alteration in sleep patterns, musculoskeletal stress, exposure to toxins, hyperarousal, feelings of isolation from friends and family, and other psychological stressors. These can overlap with mTBI symptoms, further delaying or confounding diagnosis.[12,13]

For concussions sustained during a combat situation, diagnosis can be obfuscated by surrounding circumstances, including need to engage in combat, attend to wounded colleagues, and mobilize.[13] Even outside of combat, military culture may influence an SM to continue working or to downplay symptoms he or she might be experiencing, and that can delay identifying an injury.[18,19]

Recovery from mTBI in military can be more complicated than for civilians. SMs may be at risk of persisting symptoms, including pain and impaired cognition, following concussion. The overlap between mental health, pain, and other conditions can negatively affect recovery.[11,18]

DIAGNOSING TRAUMATIC BRAIN INJURY IN THE MILITARY

mTBIs, with their nonspecific symptoms and complex interaction with mental health and pain conditions, pose diagnostic challenges to clinicians. Like civilian counterparts, if SMs have concussions that are not diagnosed and symptoms that are not addressed and treated, persisting sequelae can result. Furthermore, individuals recovering from a concussion, even one that has not been formally diagnosed, are at risk of second-impact syndrome if they sustain another concussion before the first one has healed.[18]

For injuries that are not diagnosed acutely, but likely occurred based on history, diagnosis depends heavily on attempts to discern whether an injury occurred. In this retrospective process, where TBI is essentially a historical diagnosis, added complexity arises from situations that cloud history or affect recall, such as traumatic events and acute stress.[11]

Assessment Tools

Military acute concussion evaluation
The Military Acute Concussion Evaluation (MACE) was developed and first used at Landsduhl Regional Medical Center in Germany in 2006 to facilitate rapid screening and diagnosing concussions in the military. It has become a part of the standard and mandatory evaluation for any SM who is suspected of having a concussion. The MACE is administered by clinicians at all locations, from the field to hospitals.[18]

The current version, MACE 2, includes multiple modalities of assessment. It describes red flag symptoms, like deteriorating neurologic examination, which should trigger transfer to higher level of care. The concussion screen then asks about the injury event, any loss of consciousness, posttraumatic confusion or amnesia, and current symptoms. If that screening demonstrates a concussion did not likely occur, the SM is put on 24-hour rest and re-evaluated later. If the screening points to a concussion having occurred, additional testing is implemented. The MACE 2 includes a brief cognitive and neurologic evaluation and visual oculomotor testing. After a diagnosis of concussion is made, SMs are placed on a program that includes rest and re-evaluation.[26]

For SMs who are injured in austere environments and other places where computed tomography (CT) scans are not readily available, clinicians must prioritize potential evacuations based on often incomplete evidence. Noninvasive field-deployable equipment that could accurately predict which SM would benefit from higher level of care and imaging could be very helpful.

Eye-tracking devices
Eye tracking has been postulated as a method for diagnosing TBI. Visual and binocular visuo-motor dysfunction commonly accompanies TBI. When the eyes are not working together normally, abnormal eye movements can result. Abnormal convergence occurs when the eyes are not fixating on the same target at the same time. Resultant symptoms can include blurriness, diplopia, easy fatiguability of eyes, difficulty reading, and dizziness.[27,28]

Eye-tracking devices can detect and quantify these abnormalities. These devices can be small enough to be portable. They are not yet stand-alone diagnostic tools but may add some important information for clinicians in both acute and sub-acute situations.[28]

Infrared spectroscopy
Infrared spectroscopy technology has been proposed as a method to identify intracranial injuries and thus aid in decisions regarding evacuation and whether to obtain imaging. The "Infra scanner, Brain Scope One" uses near-infrared spectroscopy to identify superficial intracranial injuries. The device is more sensitive for bleeds that are within 2 cm of the brain surface and have volume of at least 3 mL. Information from a tool like this could help guide the decision on when to send SMs for CT.[29]

Serum biomarkers
When neuronal or glial cellular structures are injured, corresponding substances are released. When these substances can be measured in the blood, the substances can serve as biomarkers of injury. Ubiquitin C-terminal hydrolase-L1 (UCH-L1) is released when there is injury to the neuronal cell body. Glial fibrillary acidic protein (GFAP) is released when astroglial cells are injured. The presence of UCH-L1 and GFAP in blood is associated with positive findings on head CT and can be an important factor in care decisions. Laboratory tests for both substances are Food and Drug Administration-approved but not yet widely used. In the future, a panel of biomarkers may be used to detect damage to neurons and glial cells and may help clinicians measure and track changes in these cells over time.[30,31]

Later diagnosis. It is vital to diagnose concussions, even after they have occurred, to ensure that SMs and veterans receive appropriate follow-up care. The military and VA have developed tools and programs to diagnose concussions by history.

The DoD's Post-Deployment Health Assessment, which is completed within 1 month of return from deployment, includes a review of health, mental health, and psychosocial issues. Deployment-related occupational and environmental exposures are also reviewed. The Post-Deployment Health Assessment and Reassessment (PDHRA) is completed within 3 and 6 months of return from deployment. The PDHRA reviews any health issues, including those affecting mental health, that emerged during the interim time after deployment.[11,18]

Veterans Health Administration (VHA), the VA's health care arm, implemented a national clinical reminder for TBI screening in 2007. Any provider seeing a SM or veteran following deployment asks about potential TBIs. Questions focus on the injury event, whether there was any immediate loss or alteration of consciousness, whether there were any immediate or acute concussion symptoms, and whether there are any current symptoms. The screen is positive if all four questions are answered in the affirmative.[8,9,11,18]

If the TBI screen is positive, the SM or veteran is referred to a TBI specialist for a comprehensive TBI evaluation (CTBIE). This evaluation includes discussion about the injury event and any potential exposure to blasts, targeted review of systems, including the use of the Neurobehavioral Symptom Inventory, and a focused physical examination. Goals of the CTBIE are to confirm the diagnosis of TBI and institute an appropriate plan for treatment.[8,11]

TREATMENT CONSIDERATIONS
Return to Activity and Work

Decisions regarding return to duty and other activities can be significantly more complicated in the military than for civilians. SMs with mTBI go through a progressive return-to-duty protocol. They have a rest period of at least 24 hours, followed by gradually advancing into activities with more physical and cognitive exertion.[2,18]

For injuries that occur during deployment, or combat, recommendations may need to be adjusted to ensure the SMs have the ability to recover in as safe an environment as possible. For those who are deployed or nondeployed, SMs' daily activities, including occupation, can involve significant risk, which could put them at risk of additional injuries. Careful consideration is warranted.[18]

In TBI rehabilitation, an interdisciplinary approach can help address symptoms, even if these are persisting, and resultant functional impairments. Team members include physiatrist, neuropsychologist, social worker, occupational therapist, physical therapist, speech language pathologist, recreation therapist, and psychiatrist. A comprehensive, individualized approach to addressing symptoms can help optimize function going forward.[5,32]

CARE SETTINGS

Military and veteran healthcare settings play a crucial role in optimizing TBI diagnosis, treatment, and outcomes. For battlefield injuries that include severe TBI, timely access to neurosurgical procedures can be lifesaving.[6] SMs with less-severe brain injuries also benefit from effective diagnosis and treatment. Healthcare systems in the military and at the VA are working to provide the best possible care to SMs and veterans with TBI. The military's Joint Trauma System is summarized in **Table 2**.[7,29]

The Defense and Veterans Brain Injury Program was launched in 1992 as a collaboration between DoD, VA, and civilian partners. The program's goals included developing exceptional TBI care and facilitating research and education about TBI, with a particular focus on SMs and veterans. The program was subsequently named the Defense and Veterans Brain Injury Center and is now called the Traumatic Brain Injury

Table 2
Military health system for trauma care–joint trauma system[7,29]

Level of Care		Type of Setting	
Level I	Battlefield aid, immediate lifesaving measures, and evacuation	Role 1	First responder care. Can be aid station or in field
Level II	Forward surgical team and division-level medical facilities. Goal is to access and stabilize	Role 2a	Light and mobile medical facility. Can provide damage-control resuscitation and stabilization
		Role 2b	Can provide damage- control surgery
Level III	In-theater hospital. Goal is to control wounds	Role 3	Large hospital, in theater. Has capability to do surgery, some imaging, and some specialty care.
Level IV	Nontheater hospital. Goal is to optimize wounds.	Role 4	Tertiary care hospitals, either in or outside continental US
Level V	US military hospital. Goal is to provide definitive care.		

Center of Excellence.[1,18,29] Other organizations that track military TBIs include Armed Forces Health Surveillance Center, Joint Trauma System Analysis and Prevention of Injury in Combat,[18] and National Intrepid Center of Excellence.[12]

The VA's Polytrauma System of Care (PSC), depicted in **Fig. 1**, was established by Congress in 2005 with the goal of providing care to the unprecedented numbers of survivors of TBI and polytraumatic injuries. These injured SMs required care that

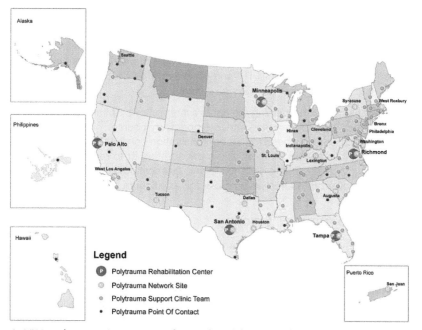

Legend

- Ⓟ Polytrauma Rehabilitation Center
- ◎ Polytrauma Network Site
- ◦ Polytrauma Support Clinic Team
- • Polytrauma Point Of Contact

Fig. 1. VHA polytrauma/TBI system of care. (Available at: Polytrauma/TBI System of Care Home (va.gov). Accessed July 30, 2023.)

included prolonged and protracted rehabilitation and recovery for complex, multifaceted courses. The PSC provides an organized and coordinated approach to providing acute medical and rehabilitation care. It also includes research and education efforts.[29] The VA and DoD have a memorandum of agreement which allows SMs with TBI and polytrauma to receive care at the VA.

The rehabilitation model, with a focus on function and an interdisciplinary approach, has been an apt care paradigm for this unique population. Services span from the time of injury through recovery. When necessary, services are also available on a chronic basis. The care is individualized, patient and family sensitive, and consistent with a biopsychosocial framework. A chronic care model is also appropriate, since veterans receive care at the VA indefinitely.[12]

The PSC comprised four levels of care.

1. Polytrauma Rehabilitation Centers (PRCs): regional referral centers that provide comprehensive acute medical and rehabilitation care for patients with severe TBI and polytrauma. They also provide education and engage in research. They offer specialized care in both disorders of consciousness rehabilitation and residential rehabilitation. PRCs also offer Intensive Evaluation and Treatment Programs for SMs who have persisting symptoms and suboptimal functioning after TBI. PRC services are certified by the Commission on Accreditation of Rehabilitation Facilities and meet criteria to be considered Centers of Excellence within the VA. PRCs are located in Palo Alto, CA; Richmond, VA; Minneapolis, MN; San Antonio, TX; and Tampa, FL.[1,11]
2. Polytrauma Network Sites (PNS): There are 23 PNS locations, one in each Veterans Integrated Service Network (VISN). PNS provide inpatient, outpatient, and postacute rehabilitation care. They also coordinate veterans' TBI and polytrauma care within their VISN.[1,11]
3. Polytrauma Support Clinic Team (PSCT): These are distributed across the national VHA system. PSCTs provide outpatient interdisciplinary rehabilitation care within their catchment areas. They coordinate and facilitate access to specialized rehabilitation services which are close to the veterans' home communities.[11]
4. Polytrauma Points of Contact (PPOC): PPOC team members manage consults for veterans with needs related to TBI and polytrauma. PPOCs can refer veterans for appropriate programs and services as indicated.[11]

Case management underpinning the entire system allows SM and veterans to move between different settings over the intricate postinjury course.[22] Tools like telehealth can be used to optimize access to these rehabilitation services. Telehealth can allow patients to continue seeing a provider in a prior setting or to receive care from providers who might be located a distance away. Telehealth also allows providers and care teams to collaborate effectively across this continuum.[8]

PREVENTION AND FUTURE DIRECTIONS

Recent, current, and future projects are working to develop new prevention, diagnosis, and treatment strategies for military TBI. Prevention programs have added coordinated campaigns. For example, the Department of Defense's TBI Center of Excellence (formerly called Defense and Veterans Brain Injury Center) has a program called "A Head for the Future," to increase awareness and provide education about TBI for SMs, veterans, and families.[18]

Research efforts are also underway. In 2011, DVBIC launched a longitudinal study, scheduled to last at least 15 years, to examine effects of TBI in OEF/OIF/OND SMs and veterans. Participants undergo imaging and neuropsychological testing at periodic intervals.[18] The Chronic Effects of Neurotrauma Consortium (CENC), coordinated through DoD, VA, and civilian sites, is working to identify and address potential long-term effects of concussion, including repeated injuries. CENC is also investigating treatment and rehabilitation strategies with the goal of optimizing function and quality of life.[17,18]

TBI diagnosis and treatment will continue to evolve. Future battlefields will likely be different from past ones. Military operations may occur on smaller scale and in more austere environments. More time may be spent at point of injury before evacuation to higher level of care. Care settings and systems will require adjustment so that SMs and veterans can continue achieving optimal recovery and functional status after TBI.[17]

CLINICS CARE POINTS

- Military TBI can differ from civilian injuries when it comes to mechanism of injury, diagnosis, treatment, and course of recovery.
- Unique physical and physiologic stressors in the military can lead to complex injuries, with the overlap between TBI, pain, and mental health conditions potentially confounding diagnosis and treatment.
- Military and veteran healthcare settings and programs attempt to address these complex and multifaceted situations, with the goal of optimizing recovery and function.

DISCLOSURE

The author has no financial relationships to disclose. She works at for the federal government as a VA employee.

REFERENCES

1. Cifu DX, Choen SI, Lew HL, et al. The history and evolution of traumatic brain injury rehabilitation in military service members and veterans. J Phys Med Rehabil 2010;89:688–94.
2. Robinson-Freeman KE, Collins KI, Garber B, et al. A decade of mTBI experience: What have we learned? A summary of proceedings from a NATO lecture series on military mTBI. Front Neurol 2020;11:1–12.
3. Lindberg MA, Martin EMM, Marion DM. Military traumatic brain injury: The history, impact, and future. J Neurotrauma 2022;39:1133–45.
4. Shively SB, Perl DP. Traumatic brain injury, shell shock, and posttraumatic stress disorder in the military: Past, present, and future. J Head Trauma Rehabil 2012; 27:234–9.
5. Veterans Health Administration Management and Rehabilitation of Post-Acute Mild Traumatic Brain Injury Work Group. VA/DoD Clinical Practice Guidelines: management and Rehabilitation of post-acute mild traumatic brain injury, version 3. Washington DC: VHA; 2021.
6. Shackleford SA, Del Junco DJ, Reade MC. Association of time to craniectomy with survival in patients with severe combat-related brain injury. Neurosurg Focus 2018;45:1–9.
7. Dengler BA, Agimi Y, Stout K, et al. Epidemiology, patterns of care and outcomes of traumatic brain injury in deployed settings: Implications for future military operations. J Trauma Acute Care Surg 2021;93:220–8.

8. Martinez RN, Hogan TP, Lones K, et al. Evaluation and treatment of mild traumatic brain injury through the implementation of clinical video telehealth: Provider perspectives from the Veterans Health Administration. PM&R 2017;9:231–40.

9. Hao AY, Eapen BC, Bowles AO. Treatment and rehabilitation services for mild to moderate traumatic brain injury in the military. In: Zollman FS, editor. Manual of traumatic brain injury: Assessment and management. 3rd edition. New York: Springer; 2022. p. 565–73.

10. Brickell TA, French LM, Gartner RL, et al. Factors related to perceived burden among caregivers of service members/veterans following TBI. Rehabil Psychol 2019;64:307–19.

11. Armistead-Jehle P, Soble JR, Cooper DB, et al. Unique aspects of traumatic brain injury in military and veteran populations. Phys Med Rehabil Clin 2017;28:323–37.

12. French LM, Lippa SM. Military traumatic brain injury: Special considerations. In: Zasler ND, Katz DI, Zafonte RD, editors. Brain injury medicine: principles and practice. 3rd edition. New York: Demos/Springer; 2022. p. 462–74.

13. Rigg JL, Mooney SR. Concussions and the military: Issues specific to service members. PM&R 2011;3:S380–6.

14. Lange RT, Lippa SA, French LM, et al. Long-term behavioral symptom reporting following mild, moderate, severe, and penetrating traumatic brain injury in U.S. military service members. Neuropsychol Rehabil 2019;30:1762–85.

15. Lippa SM, French LM, Brickell TA, et al. United States military service members demonstrate substantial and heterogeneous long-term neuropsychological dysfunction after moderate, severe, and penetrating traumatic brain injury. J Neurotrauma 2020;37:608–17.

16. Stewart IJ, Poltavskly E, Howard JT, et al. The enduring health consequences of combat trauma: A legacy of chronic disease. J Gen Intern Med 2020;36:713–21.

17. Cifu DX. Clinical research findings from the long-term impact of military-relevant brain injury consortium- Chronic Effects of Neurotrauma Consortium (LIMBIC-CENC) 2013-2021. Brain Inj 2022;36:587–97.

18. Helmick KM, Spells CA, Malik SZ, et al. Traumatic brain injury in the US military: Epidemiology and key clinical and research programs. Brain Imaging Behav 2015;9:358–66.

19. Ross PT, Ravindranath D, Clay M, et al. A greater mission: Understanding military culture as a tool for serving those who have served. J Grad Med Educ 2015;7:519–22.

20. Walker LE, Watrous J, Poltavskiy E, et al. Longitudinal mental health outcomes of combat-injured service members. Brain Behav 2021;11:e02088.

21. Vasterling JJ, Aslan M, Proctor SP, et al. Long-term negative emotional outcomes of warzone TBI. Clin Neuropsychol 2020;34:1088–104.

22. Pugh MJ, Swan AA, Amuan ME, et al. Deployment, suicide, and overdose among comorbidity phenotypes following mild traumatic brain injury: A retrospective cohort study from the Chronic Effects of Neurotrauma Consortium. PLoS One 2019;14:e0222674.

23. Alcover KC, Poltavskiy EA, Howard JT, et al. Post-combat opioid prescription and alcohol use disorder in the military. Am J Prev Med 2022;63:904–14.

24. Teeters JB, Lancaster CL, Brown DG, et al. Substance use disorders in military veterans: Prevalence and treatment challenges. Subst Abuse Rehabil 2017;8:69–77.

25. Howlett JR, Nelson LD, Stein MB. Mental health consequences of traumatic brain injury. Biol Psychiatry 2022;91:413–20.

26. Military Health System Traumatic Brain Injury Center of Excellence. Mace 2: military acute concussion evaluation. Washington DC: DoD; 2021.

27. Urosevich TG, Boscarino JJ, Hoffman SN, et al. Visual dysfunction and associated co-morbidities as predictors of mild traumatic brain injury seen among veterans in non-VA facilities: Implications for clinical practice. Mil Med 2018;183: e564–70.

28. Hussain SF, Raza R, Cash ATG, et al. Traumatic brain injury and sight loss in military and veteran populations: A review. Mil Med Res 2021;8:42–56.

29. Lazarus R, Helmick K, Malik S, et al. Continuum of the United States military's traumatic brain injury care: Adjusting to a changing battlefield. Neurosurg Focus 2018;45:E15–22.

30. Giza CC, McCrea M, Huber D, et al. Assessment of blood biomarker profile after acute concussion during combative training among US military cadets: A prospective study from the NCAA and US Department of Defense CARE Consortium. JAMA Netw Open 2021;4:0377311–5.

31. Helmrich IR, Czeiter E, Amrein K, et al. Incremental prognostic value of acute serum biomarkers for functional outcome after traumatic brain injury (CENTER-TBI): An observational cohort study. Lancet Neurol 2022;21:792–802.

32. Silverberg ND, Iccarino MA, Panenka WJ, et al. Management of concussion and mild traumatic brain injury: A synthesis of practice guidelines. Arch Phys Med Rehabil 2020;101:382–93.

Management of Pain and Headache After Traumatic Brain Injury

Udai Nanda, DO[a,b],*, Grace Zhang, MD[b], David Underhill, MD[b],
Sanjog Pangarkar, MD[b,c]

KEYWORDS

- Traumatic brain injury • Pain • Chronic pain • Headache • Post-traumatic headache
- Secondary headache • Rehabilitation

KEY POINTS

- External forces leading to traumatic brain injury can result in injuries to multiple body regions, with chronic pain being a common sequela.
- Posttraumatic headache has been described as the most prevalent type of pain attributed to mild traumatic brain injury, followed by pain in the neck, shoulders, back, and upper and lower limbs.
- The combination of chronic pain, headache, and other conditions related to traumatic brain injury, such as cognitive impairment and psychiatric disorders, creates obstacles to rehabilitation and recovery.
- Due to the complexity of pain and headache after traumatic brain injury, a multidisciplinary team-based approach is recommended.

INTRODUCTION

Individuals who have sustained a TBI often experience acute and chronic pain as a sequela of their injuries. As such, pain is a positive predictor of physical and functional impairment and occurs frequently in those with a history of TBI.[1] TBI is also a common cause of injury-induced disability in certain populations, including the military, and may influence other aspects of health, including trauma-related disorders such as post-traumatic stress disorder (PTSD). For example, soldiers that have suffered a

[a] Department of Physical Medicine and Rehabilitation, Pain Management, Headache Center of Excellence, VA Greater Los Angeles Healthcare System, Los Angeles, CA, USA; [b] Division of Physical Medicine and Rehabilitation, Department of Medicine, UCLA David Geffen School of Medicine, Los Angeles, CA, USA; [c] Department of Physical Medicine and Rehabilitation, Pain Management, VA Greater Los Angeles Healthcare System, Los Angeles, CA, USA
* Corresponding author. Department of Physical Medicine and Rehabilitation, Pain Management, Headache Center of Excellence, VA Greater Los Angeles Healthcare System, 11301 Wilshire Boulevard (W117), Los Angeles, CA 90073.
E-mail address: udai.nanda@va.gov

Phys Med Rehabil Clin N Am 35 (2024) 573–591
https://doi.org/10.1016/j.pmr.2024.02.009
1047-9651/24/Published by Elsevier Inc.

mild TBI (mTBI) with loss of consciousness (43.9%) also often meet the criteria for PTSD and are more likely to miss workdays, have a higher number of medical visits, and have physical symptoms.[2] TBIs are also more likely to be fatal in the male population and twice as likely to lead to hospitalization when compared with females.[3,4]

Prevalence of Traumatic Brain Injury and Pain

The Centers for Disease Control and Prevention (CDC) estimates approximately 220,000 TBI-related hospitalizations in 2019 and 69,000 TBI-related deaths in 2021. TBI most commonly affects patients older than 75 years of age and disproportionately affects racial and ethnic minorities, people who experience homelessness, and military members.[3,5] While some studies have shown rates of chronic pain to be as high as 80% in veterans with a history of polytrauma, the prevalence of TBI-related pain may be even higher due to frequent under-reporting of mTBI in the military.[6] In a VA pilot study, over half of veterans with a history of TBI reported pain at least 3 days a week. The most frequently endorsed types of pain included headache, back pain, and other musculoskeletal/joint pain.[7] TBI is often accompanied by other pain diagnoses, such as upper or lower limb fractures. In fact, in a retrospective assessment of patients with isolated limb fractures, the incidence of mTBI was 23.5%.[8] Mild TBI is more likely to present with concomitant pain syndromes, with chronic pain occurring 75% of the time, compared to moderate and severe TBI, where prevalence rates are closer to 32%.[9]

Evaluation of Pain in the Traumatic Brain Injury Patient

In the acute setting, pain assessment after TBI is often complicated by communication barriers. Self-reported pain scores may be difficult to obtain with varying levels of consciousness or sedation due to medications. In these scenarios, it is important to monitor for nonverbal signs of discomfort and other pain behaviors. These can include, but are not limited to, hypertension, tachycardia, agitation, increased muscle tone, and diaphoresis.[10] Additionally, patients might display changes in facial expressions, such as grimacing, or demonstrate verbal cues, such as increased sighing or moaning.[11] Scales, such as the Behavior Pain Scale or Critical-Care Pain Observation Tool, are useful for documenting pain-related behaviors. Monitoring for these clinical signs and symptoms is important when tapering medications, including opioids and sedative hypnotics.

Frequent and consistent pain assessments should be conducted in patients who are unable to communicate their pain. Serial physical exams should also be performed to check for pressure injuries or other external factors that may be contributing to pain in a critical setting. Patients' bowel and bladder function should be closely monitored for signs of urinary retention or constipation, which may also cause discomfort. Obtaining imaging may be beneficial if there is a suspicion of fractures or other traumatic injuries, as well as diffusion-weighted imaging (DWI) of the brain, which is a standard method for detecting diffuse axonal injury after TBI. DWI has shown a greater ability to detect DAI than T2-weighted images.[12,13]

Similarly, early mobilization may be beneficial for the functional recovery and reduction of contractures, but clinicians should be aware that routine therapy interventions, such as range of motion exercises, can be painful for individuals with a brain injury and subsequent disorder of consciousness (DoC). Difficulty in pain assessment may persist beyond the acute setting if those with moderate and severe TBI continue to have difficulty reporting or processing their symptoms.[9] Using a systematic multimodal approach to evaluate other factors that may influence pain perception, including biological, psychological, and social factors, is also important.

Headaches

The most commonly encountered the manifestation of pain after TBI is headache, with prevalence rates of 57.8%.[9] Risk factors include female gender, prior history of headache disorder, less severe injury, comorbid psychiatric disorders, sleep disturbance, and prior head trauma.[14] Headaches can be classified into primary and secondary headaches. Primary headaches have no attributive cause; in other words, they do not develop temporally in relation to the onset of another disorder. Examples include migraine, tension-type headache, and cluster headache. Secondary headaches are the result of a separate condition. Posttraumatic headaches (PTH) fall into the category of secondary headache disorders. It is important to note that while some PTH share a similar phenotype and symptom complex with primary headache disorders, they are categorized as secondary headaches due to the presence of (and temporal relation to) head trauma.

Secondary Headaches

Whiplash injury, striking the head with blunt trauma, blast injury, penetration by a foreign body, and headache attributed to craniotomy are all potential sources of PTH. Other sources include, but are not limited to, CSF leak, infection, and cerebral hemorrhage.[14]

PTH is the most common secondary headache disorder.[15] Exposure to head injury increases the risk of new onset headaches and can worsen underlying headache disorders.[16] Some studies suggest PTH is more common in mild TBI than severe TBI, which may arise from under-reporting in severe TBI due to communication deficits. In fact, longitudinal studies in the VA have shown no relation between acute PTH and increased severity of injury. It was noted, however, that 95% of those who reported headaches at 6 months continued to have headaches at 12 months.[17] Additional studies have shown that those with a history of headache tend to have worse pain outcomes compared with those without.[6]

Whiplash injuries can lead to cervicogenic headaches, another classification of secondary headaches. Cervicogenic headaches are headaches attributable to a disorder in the neck, such as the cervical spine or soft tissue. Patients may exhibit limited cervical range of motion and have referred pain to the head with the movement and manipulation of the neck. Targeted nerve blocks that alleviate the pain aid in diagnosis. Anesthetic blocks to the cervical zygapophyseal joints can localize the specific source of headache. Cervicogenic headaches attributable to zygapophyseal or facet joint disease typically originate from the C2-C3 level.[18] This joint is innervated by the deep and superficial medial branches of the C3 dorsal ramus. Damage of other structures, including the cervical intervertebral discs, greater occipital nerve, lesser occipital nerve, atlanto-occipital joint, and atlantoaxial joint are also sources of secondary headaches.

Pathophysiology of Posttraumatic Headaches

Injuries sustained at the time of trauma cause physical disruption to structures in the brain, including intracranial vasculature, brain parenchyma, and neurons, which can cause nociceptive pain. Proposed mechanisms for headache pain include cerebral metabolism alteration and axonal injury. Diffuse axonal injury induced after TBI has been shown to affect pain-relevant centers, which may subsequently lead to the development of chronic PTH.[6,19]

Like primary headaches, PTH is thought to occur in part due to an alteration in pain modulating systems, specifically descending the inhibition of the trigeminovascular pathway.[20] This pathway is also thought to play a role in chronic pain associated with stroke, postsurgical pain, and fibromyalgia.[6]

Under usual circumstances, alpha-2 adrenergic receptors inhibit pre- and post-synaptic neurons, which project into several areas of the central nervous system to inhibit pain. Additionally, norepinephrine release from neuron terminals in the locus coeruleus and the release of serotonin from neuron terminals in the rostroventral medulla can inhibit input from painful stimuli.[6] Alterations of these descending projections into the spinal cord after injury can lead to neuroinflammation and increased transmission of pain signals.[21]

Another suspected mechanism of PTH following blast-mediated TBI is dysregulated output of the periaqueductal gray (PAG), a major regulatory pathway affecting locus coeruleus activity.[6,22] Additional proposed pain mechanisms include damage to the spinothalamic tract and nuclei in the thalamus, as well as decreased dopamine signaling, which may enhance pain sensitivity.[6] Calcitonin gene-related peptide (CGRP) is suspected to mediate inflammatory pain in headaches due to its effect on neurotransmission in trigeminal nerve fibers[23,24] **(Fig. 1)**. Mouse studies have identified the role of CGRP in the development of centralized pain states after mTBI.[23] Some research suggests that damage to the glymphatic system after TBI, as well as posttraumatic sleep disruption, impairs the clearance of CGRP.[24]

Diagnostic Criteria of Posttraumatic Headache

While the International Classification of Headache Disorders, 3rd Edition (ICHD-3) criteria for PTH necessitates that headache develops within 7 days of the injury (or within 7 days of regaining consciousness), there has been some debate of this criterion. In a study conducted within the VA, up to one-third of veterans with clinically confirmed PTH reported the onset of headache after 7 days. These cases did not show any variability in phenotype compared with those who reported headache within 7 days of the injury.[25] Strict adherence to the ICHD-3 may cause some cases of PTH to be missed.

If patients have a pre-existing headache prior to trauma, the headache quality must significantly worsen (at least an increase of twice the usual frequency and/or severity) or become chronic to be classified as a PTH.[26] Acute headaches remit within 3 months of trauma, while persistent headaches continue beyond 3 months.

Clinical Presentation of Posttraumatic Headache

Symptoms of PTH present similarly to primary headaches, such as migraines, tension-type headaches, and trigeminal autonomic cephalalgias. However, the frequency, intensity, and duration of symptoms are poorly defined due to a lack of controlled trials.[26] Characteristics of migraine headaches include unilateral location, pulsating quality, nausea, vomiting, photophobia, and phonophobia, along with additional criteria related to intensity, duration, frequency, and aggravating factors. Tension-type headaches are bilateral and non-pulsating. They are often less intense than migraine headaches and are not accompanied by nausea or vomiting. Trigeminal autonomic cephalalgias, including cluster headaches and hemicrania continua, usually present with severe unilateral orbital, supra-orbital, or temporal pain and cranial autonomic features, such as conjunctival injection, nasal congestion, eyelid edema, miosis, and facial sweating, ipsilateral to the headache.[14]

PTH may present with associated symptoms such as autonomic dysfunction, particularly orthostatic intolerance, and urinary incontinence.[27] One prospective observational study of patients with PTH found nausea and photophobia/phonophobia in 42% and 55% of patients, respectively.[28] Physical activity was a common aggravating factor for PTH.

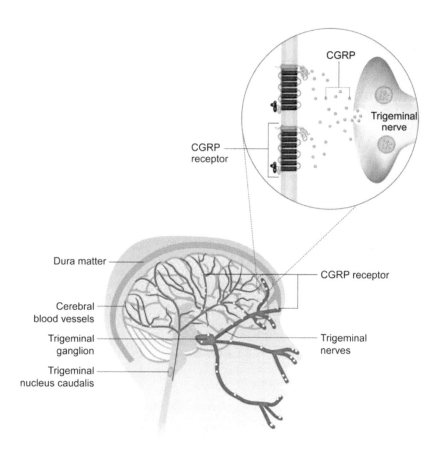

Fig. 1. The role of calcitonin gene-related peptide (CGRP) and the trigeminal system in headache pathophysiology. (Maureen Moriarty et al., Monoclonal Antibodies to CGRP or Its Receptor for Migraine Prevention, The Journal for Nurse Practitioners, 15 (10), 2019, 717-724.e1, https://doi.org/10.1016/j.nurpra.2019.07.009.)

Treatment Options for Posttraumatic Headache

Pharmacologic management

Current recommendations for the pharmacologic management of PTH are limited to expert opinion due to a lack of high-quality randomized controlled trials.[29] As such, treatment options for primary headaches are used for PTH. Identifying the PTH phenotype guides clinical decision-making (**Fig. 2**). Pharmacologic management is directed at the primary phenotype, the most common being PTH with a migraine phenotype followed by PTH with a tension-type headache phenotype.[27,30] Treatment can then be further divided into acute (abortive) or preventive (prophylactic) therapy.

Initial acute treatments, for both migraine and tension-type headache phenotypes, include simple analgesics such as nonsteroidal antiinflammatories (NSAIDs), aspirin, and acetaminophen.[30,31]

Second-line acute treatment incorporates combination analgesics, including acetaminophen, aspirin, and caffeine. For PTH with a migraine phenotype, triptans and gepants are also considered, with multiple triptan formulations available, including

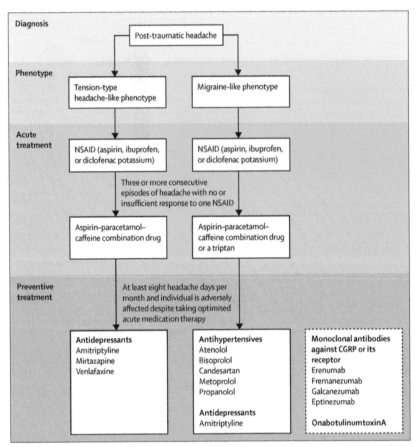

Fig. 2. Proposed pharmacologic treatment algorithm for posttraumatic headache attributed to traumatic brain injury. (Reprinted with permission from Elsevier. The Lancet Neurology, June 2021, 20 (6), 460-469.)

intranasal and subcutaneous options for headaches that peak rapidly [31]. Antiemetic medications also play a role, especially when nausea occurs with the headache. Intravenous ketorolac, metoclopramide, and ondansetron reduced pain scores in children presenting to the emergency department with PTH within 14 days of a mTBI.[32] A retrospective study of 21 patients with brain injury presenting to the ED showed IV metoclopramide 20 mg and diphenhydramine 25 mg to be effective treatments for PTH.[33]

It is important to note that regular, frequent use of acute medication treatment may cause medication overuse headaches, also referred to as rebound headaches. These can develop with greater than 3 months of regular, frequent use of certain acute medications. The definition of overuse varies based on medication class. For example, the use of opioids and triptans for more than 10 days per month constitutes medication overuse, while NSAID overuse is defined as use on more than 15 days per month.[34]

Specific criteria prompting preventive treatments vary slightly in the literature based on headache type and a variety of factors. Many of the principles of preventive therapy for primary headache disorders, such as migraine, can be applied to PTH. For example, preventive treatment is considered when acute medications provide inadequate relief, headaches occur with high frequency, headaches cause significant disability, and patients report frequent acute medication use, increasing their risk of developing medication overuse headaches.[31,35,36] In general, when selecting a preventive medication, the clinician should consider the side effect profile and a patient's comorbid conditions. When chosen appropriately, a preventive medication can provide dual benefits by treating the headache disorder and comorbid conditions.

Preventive medications used in the treatment of PTH with tension-type headache phenotype include amitriptyline, mirtazapine, and venlafaxine. For PTH with migraine phenotype, amitriptyline, candesartan, beta blockers (propranolol, metoprolol), and topiramate are considered.[31,37] PTH with migraine phenotype can also be treated with botulinum toxin injections or medications targeting CGRP signaling, such as CGRP monoclonal antibodies (mAbs) and CGRP receptor antagonists (gepants) (**Table 1**).[38]

As treatment recommendations are generally guided by headache phenotype, PTH-specific studies have yielded mixed results. A retrospective cohort study in 2019 showed that while gabapentin and tricyclic antidepressants decreased symptom burden in the short-term, long-term outcomes were similar between groups treated with either gabapentin, tricyclic antidepressants, or no medication.[39] In a retrospective study of soldiers with PTH, only topiramate demonstrated a significant decrease in headache frequency when compared to low-dose tricyclic antidepressants.[37] In the same study, 70% of subjects who used a triptan class medication experienced reliable headache relief within 2 hours compared to 42% of subjects using another abortive medication. Sumatriptan is widely regarded as the gold standard for oral migraine abortive therapy and acts through vasoconstriction as well as the prevention of neurotransmitter release at trigeminal nociceptive terminals.[40] Centrally acting drugs such as prazosin have also been identified as a potential preventive treatment for PTH by modulating posttraumatic glymphatic function.[25]

Intravenous infusion of CGRP may exacerbate migraine-like headaches in individuals with persistent PTH attributed to mild TBI and no pre-existing migraine.[29,30] Mouse studies have demonstrated the resolution of cephalic tactile pain hypersensitivity with sumatriptan or CGRP monoclonal antibodies following mTBI.[41] Further PTH-specific research is warranted to identify additional signaling molecules that contribute to the mechanism of PTH and help guide PTH-specific pharmacologic treatment.

Nonpharmacologic Management

Often, patients are dissatisfied with typical oral migraine therapeutics for PTH.[30] Utilizing an interdisciplinary approach with multimodal pain therapy has been shown to reduce the number of pain days for patients with TBI with chronic headache pain.[63] Nonpharmacologic approaches include psychotherapy, cognitive behavioral therapy, physical therapy, mindfulness and relaxation techniques, biofeedback, and cognitive restructuring.[24] Maintaining adequate sleep hygiene can also reduce headache frequency as up to 50% of individuals with TBI report sleep disturbances. Sleep disturbances are associated with PTH, likely due to elevation in proinflammatory cytokines during sleep deprivation[24,64]

For patients who are critically hospitalized, frequent repositioning, routine bowel and bladder programs, and close skin monitoring can help prevent, as well as modulate, pain.[10]

Interventional Options

Interventional procedures may have therapeutic effects for PTH that share phenotypes with occipital neuralgia or cervicogenic headaches. In a retrospective study of

Table 1
Medications commonly used in the treatment of posttraumatic headache

Medication	Mechanism of Action	Dose	Use	Side Effects
Common Non-Specific Acute Medications				
Acetaminophen	Central inhibition of COX1 & COX 2 - > Inhibits prostaglandin synthesis	PO: 500–1000 mg[42]	Abortive	• Liver Toxicity
Aspirin	Irreversibly binds COX1 & COX 2 - > Inhibits prostaglandin synthesis	PO: 500–1000 mg[43]	Abortive	• Renal Toxicity • GI Bleeding • Metabolic Imbalances
Ibuprofen	Central and peripheral Inhibition of COX1 & COX 2 - > Inhibits prostaglandin synthesis	PO: 200–800 mg[44]	Abortive	• Renal Toxicity • GI Bleeding
Diclofenac	Central and peripheral Inhibition of COX1 & COX 2 - > Inhibits prostaglandin synthesis	PO: 50–100 mg[45]	Abortive	• Renal Toxicity • GI Bleeding
Aspirin–paracetamol–caffeine combination drug	Central and peripheral Inhibition of COX1 & COX 2 - > Inhibits prostaglandin synthesis	Acetaminophen 250 mg/aspirin 250 mg/caffeine 65 mg: 2 tablets as a single dose	Abortive	• Liver toxicity • GI Bleeding • Renal Toxicity
Post-Traumatic Headache with Migraine Phenotype				
Metoprolol	Selective β1 blockade	PO: 100–200 mg/day in divided doses[46]	Preventive	• Bradycardia • Hypotension • Dyslipidemia
Propranolol	Non-selective β receptor blockade	PO: 40–160 mg/day in divided doses[47]	Preventive	• Bradycardia • Hypotension • Coronary Vasospasm
Amitriptyline	Inhibits 5HT & NE reuptake	PO: 10–50 mg QHS[48]	Preventive	• Arrhythmias • Postural hypotension • Anticholinergic effects

Drug	Mechanism	Dose	Type	Side effects
Topiramate	Blocks Na^+ channels, increases GABA transmission	PO: 50–200 mg/day in divided doses.[49]	Preventive	• Dose related dizziness, drowsiness • Increased risk of nephrolithiasis • Weight loss
Erenumab	Monoclonal Antibody to CGRP receptor	SubQ: 70–140 mg once monthly[50]	Preventive	• Hypertension (Obtain BP check 2–4 wk after initiation)
Fremanezumab	Monoclonal Antibody to CGRP	SubQ: 225 mg monthly or 675 mg every 3 mo[51]	Preventive	• Local Injection site irritation
Galcanezumab	Monoclonal Antibody to CGRP	SubQ: 240 mg as a loading dose, followed by 120 mg once monthly[52]	Preventive	• Local Injection site irritation
Sumatriptan	5-HT agonist - > prevents vasoactive peptide release - > cranial vasoconstriction	PO: 50–100 mg as a single dose.[53] May repeat after ≥2 h. Max dose: 100 mg/dose; 200 mg per 24 h (Also available in IV and Sub Q formulations)	Abortive	• Coronary vasospasm
Rizatriptan	5-HT agonist - > prevents vasoactive peptide release - > cranial vasoconstriction	PO: 5–10 mg as a single dose.[54] May repeat after ≥2 h. Max dose: 30 mg per 24 h	Abortive	• Coronary vasospasm • Dizziness
Zolmitriptan	5-HT agonist - > prevents vasoactive peptide release - > cranial vasoconstriction	PO: 2.5–5 mg as a single dose.[55] May repeat after ≥2 h. Max dose: 10 mg per 24 h (Also available in nasal formulation)	Abortive	• Coronary vasospasm • Dizziness
Metoclopramide	D2 Receptor Antagonist - > reduces nausea symptoms	IV, PO, SubQ: 10 mg as a single dose[56]	Abortive (Emergency setting) when headache associated with nausea	• Parkinsonian effects (high doses, contraindicated in Parkinson's) • Tardive dyskinesia • Restlessness • Fatigue • Diarrhea

(continued on next page)

Table 1
(continued)

Medication	Mechanism of Action	Dose	Use	Side Effects
Ubrogepant	CGRP receptor antagonist	PO: 50–100 mg as a single dose; if symptoms persist or return, may repeat dose after ≥2 h. Maximum: 200 mg per 24 h[57]	Abortive	• Nausea • Somnolence
Atogepant	CGRP receptor antagonist	PO: 10–60 mg/day[58]	Preventive	• Constipation • Weight loss
Rimegepant	CGRP receptor antagonist	Abortive: PO: 75 mg as a single dose. Maximum: 75 mg per 24 h[14] Preventive: PO 75 mg every other day[59]	Abortive & Preventive	• Abdominal pain
OnabotulinumtoxinA	Cleaves SNAP-25 - > blocks presynaptic acetylcholine release	Injectable: 5 units per site, 155 units every 12 wk[60]	Preventive	• Blepharoptosis • Distal spread to vascular resulting in systemic symptoms of dysphagia. & respiratory depression
Post-Traumatic Headache with Tension-Type Headache Phenotype				
Amitriptyline	Inhibits 5HT & NE reuptake	10–50 mg QHS[48]	Preventive	• Arrhythmias • Postural hypotension • Anticholinergic effects • Confusion in the elderly
Mirtazapine	α2 antagonist - > increases release of 5HT & NE; H1 antagonist	15-30 mg QHS[61]	Preventive	• Arrhythmias • Sedation • Increased appetite
Venlafaxine	Inhibits 5HT & NE reuptake	75-150 mg/day[62]	Preventive	• Hypertension • Bleeding risk • Serotonin syndrome

A phenotype-guided treatment approach is recommended for posttraumatic headache, whereby medications are selected based on the primary headache disorder that the patient's clinical features most closely resemble. The medication dosing recommendations in this table take into consideration the relevant evidence for the pharmacologic management of primary headache disorders and can be incorporated into the phenotype-guided pharmacologic treatment of posttraumatic headache.

children receiving greater occipital nerve block for acute PTH, 93% reported good therapeutic effect, and 71% reported complete headache resolution immediately following the intervention.[65] Cervical medial branch radiofrequency ablation for cervicogenic headaches may provide pain relief for several months to a year.[66]

Special Considerations for Traumatic Brain Injury Population

Drugs that impair neurocognitive recovery should be avoided or used with caution. These include drugs with sedative properties, anticholinergics, benzodiazepines, and dopamine agonists.[10] In addition, medications that lower seizure threshold, such as opiates, bronchodilators, tricyclics, tramadol, and bupropion should be avoided. Further, regularly monitoring for suicidality is recommended given the higher prevalence of suicidal ideation in the TBI population.[67] Pharmacologic prophylaxis of pain should also be considered in all persons with a disorder of consciousness (DoC), given the difficulty in assessing pain in this group.[10]

Musculoskeletal Pain

A common source of pain during early TBI recovery is from bone fractures (both axial and extremity) that may have occurred with the traumatic injury.[10] Following the acute period, chronic musculoskeletal pain can continue and has been reported in 79% of patients with TBI, some persisting more than 15 years after trauma.[68] Common sites include the neck, shoulders, back, and upper and lower limbs.[6] Approaches to musculoskeletal pain management should begin conservatively and focus on a multidisciplinary approach including physical therapy, stretching, heat therapy, cold therapy, bracing, and electrical stimulation.[69] Pharmacologic treatment should begin conservatively with non-opioid analgesics such as acetaminophen, low dose aspirin, or NSAIDs.[10]

In general, opioids should be avoided for chronic musculoskeletal pain, particularly in the TBI population which is disproportionately affected by substance use disorder.[70] It has been estimated that 10% to 20% of individuals with TBI develop substance use disorder following injury.[71] Multidisciplinary and multimodal therapies are strongly recommended in lieu of opioid therapy.[69] Providers may consider treating severe pain secondary to musculoskeletal injury with opioids after nonopioid pain medications have been adequately trialed, per CDC guidelines.[72]

In the United States, approximately half of the states have passed legislation recommending that opioid prescriptions for acute pain should be limited to 7 days.[73] Judicious utilization of opioids in the immediate postacute recovery phases should be practiced, as sedative side effects may impair executive functioning, which may already be compromised in patients with TBI.[55] If the sedative side effects of opioids impair a patient's cognitive functioning or ability to participate in rehab therapies, stimulants, such as methylphenidate, can be prescribed on an adjunctive basis to improve attention.[74]

Heterotopic Ossification

TBI is associated with the painful formation of extraskeletal bone in muscle and soft tissues. Affected sites include the hips, shoulders, elbows, and knees.[75] Symptoms include joint stiffness, pain, swelling, and warmth around the affected joint. This can result in decreased range of motion and painful resistance to the movement of the adjacent joint. Early mobilization and physical therapy can help minimize the risk of developing HO. Though prophylactic NSAIDs have shown benefit in preventing HO in patients with joint replacement and spinal cord injury, there has been no conclusive evidence to support this finding in patients with TBI.[76] Studies suggest surgical excision is the most effective treatment of HO after TBI.[77]

Neuromuscular Spasticity

Spasticity is defined as a velocity dependant increase in tone. It can occur both focally and diffusely and is more commonly seen in moderate to severe TBI. In general, spasticity is characterized by involuntary muscle contractions, stiffness, and tightness. In a sample of patients with DoC, spasticity was observed in 89% of subjects and was positively correlated with pain scores measured by means of the Nociception Coma Scale–Revised Scale (NCS–R).[78] Spasticity can be a primary generator of pain but also leads to painful conditions such as subluxation, tendonitis, and capsulitis.[79] More severe TBIs have an increased risk of developing spasticity and painful joint contractures. Spasticity can be managed through a variety of treatment approaches, including oral medications, chemodenervation, and physical therapy focused on stretching exercises. First line medications include oral baclofen and tizanidine. Botulinum toxin, phenol, and alcohol neurolysis are also used in targeted areas to improve focal spasticity. If conservative interventions fail, more invasive treatments are considered, including dorsal rhizotomy and intrathecal baclofen therapy.

Relationship Between Comorbid Psychiatric Disorders and Pain

Those with TBI, particularly veterans, are frequently diagnosed with PTSD and depression.[80] PTSD is particularly prevalent in patients who have experienced a mTBI.[6] The severity of PTSD and depression have been found to correlate with the intensity of pain experienced as well as the frequency of chronic pain. In a study comparing visual analog scale pain scores among veterans with PTSD, mTBI or both, pain intensity was highest in those with both PTSD and mTBI.[6] It must be noted, however, that intensity was found to be higher in PTSD alone compared with mTBI alone. This inability to cope with pain in PTSD may be due to the catastrophizing of such pain.[9] Likewise, there is a relationship between depression and pain intensity. Higher depressive symptoms during inpatient rehabilitation for TBI have been correlated with higher intensity of pain 1 year following discharge.[81]

Neuropathic Pain

The diagnosis of neuropathic pain requires a history of nervous system injury or disease and a neuroanatomically plausible distribution of the pain. Symptoms may vary but include positive symptoms such as a "burning" or "shocking" pain, tingling, or increased sensitivity to touch or temperature or negative symptoms such as decreased or lost sensation. Pain may be spontaneous or evoked, as an increased response to a painful stimulus (hyperalgesia) or a painful response to a normally nonpainful stimulus (allodynia). In 2015, the International Association for the Study of Pain (IASP) created a Task Force that worked in close cooperation with the World Health Organization (WHO) representatives to create an improved the classification of relevant pain syndromes in the preparation of the upcoming revision of the ICD-11.[82] This task force defined neuropathic pain as a lesion or disease of the somatosensory nervous system[83] and further subdivided conditions into the categories of central and peripheral neuropathic pain.

Central Neuropathic Pain and Development of Chronic Pain

Central neuropathic pain is chronic in nature and caused by a lesion or disease of the central somatosensory nervous system.[82] Patients with TBI are at risk for chronic pain that persists beyond the expected healing time of an injury. Per the IASP, chronic central neuropathic pain associated with brain injury is caused by a lesion or disease of the somatosensory cortex, connected brain regions, or associated pathways in the brain. Diagnosis requires a history of brain trauma, temporal onset of pain in relation to the trauma, and a pain distribution that is neuroanatomically plausible. Sensory signs or symptoms indicating brain involvement must be present in the body region corresponding to the brain injury.[84] The mechanisms underlying this disorder are complex but suggest that neuroinflammation, neurodegeneration, and synaptic dysfunction all play a role.[6]

Neuroinflammation

Mechanical injury to the brain results in a disruption of the blood brain barrier, allowing entry of neutrophils, lymphocytes, and macrophages to the site of injury. These cells release inflammatory mediators, which in turn activate microglia. This activation of microglia then leads to the production of multiple cytotoxic substances, including proinflammatory cytokines and oxidative metabolites. This cascade causes hyperexcitability of neurons and synaptic dysfunction, ultimately resulting in chronic changes that include reduced neurogenesis, neurodegeneration, and axonal degeneration[6,85] Cytokines of particular interest, TNFα and IL-1β, have been shown to be elevated following TBI in several pain centers including the thalamus, hippocampus, substantia nigra, and hypothalamus.[6,86] Paraspinal etanercept has been investigated, and one observational study involving 629 stroke and patients with TBI reported a statistically significant reduction in neuropathic pain, hyperesthesia, and allodynia measured by visual analog scale following 25 mg of paraspinal etanercept at 1 week and 3 week postinjection.[87]

Neurodegeneration

Neurodegeneration is a major consequence of TBI in which axonal dysfunction and neuronal death occur. Areas that are affected include but are not limited to the cortex, hippocampus, thalamus, amygdala, and brainstem. The changes to the pain pathways in analogous neurodegenerative diseases associated with chronic pain may inform our understanding of chronic pain in TBI. For example, in Parkinson's disease, alterations in the medial and lateral pain pathways and the basal ganglia lead to fundamental changes in the way pain-related and other sensory information is processed.[88]

Synaptic Dysfunction

Chemical and electrical impulses between synapses underlie the fundamental function of the brain. Following TBI, brain tissue from in vitro animal models has demonstrated synaptic dysfunction.[89] The development of chronic pain following TBI may be associated with synaptic dysfunction in pain-related centers, which has been demonstrated in studies of the hippocampus,[90] amygdala,[91] and cortex.[92]

Peripheral Neuropathic Pain

Peripheral neuropathic pain is due to a lesion or disease of the peripheral somatosensory nervous system.[84] Discreet occurrences of peripheral neuropathic pain may occur separately from TBI and include painful radiculopathy, polyneuropathy, traumatic neuropathy, trigeminal neuralgia, and postherpetic neuralgia. Specific peripheral neuropathic pain states can cooccur with TBI, including amputation related phantom limb pain, stump pain, or nerve damage, specifically in those in the military.[93] It is unclear whether peripheral neuropathic pain is worsened because of TBI, though mouse models suggest that neuropathic allodynia may be associated with synaptogenesis within the somatosensory cortex.[94]

CLINICS CARE POINTS

- Many individuals with TBI experience acute and chronic pain, which can lead to physical and functional impairment, as well as affect quality of life.
- The most common manifestation of pain after TBI is PTH. Treatment for PTH is guided by headache phenotype. Other sources of pain include musculoskeletal pain, heterotopic ossification, spasticity, and neuropathic pain.
- Patients with mTBI are more likely to develop chronic pain syndromes, which may occur from alterations in central pain modulating systems.
- First line pharmacologic agents that should be considered include nonopioid analgesics, for example, acetaminophen and NSAIDs. In general, opioids are not recommended for long-term use and should be closely monitored and prescribed at the lowest effective dose for the shortest period of time in the acute setting. Neuropathic medications, muscle relaxants, and interventional procedures can be considered depending on the etiology of pain. The effects of pharmacologic agents on neurocognitive recovery should be considered in the TBI population. Multimodal, interdisciplinary pain strategies should be used to address comorbid psychiatric and social contributors to pain.

DISCLOSURE

The authors have nothing to disclose.

REFERENCES

1. Kornblith ES, Langa KM, Yaffe K, et al. Physical and Functional Impairment Among Older Adults With a History of Traumatic Brain Injury. J Head Trauma Rehabil 2020;35(4):E320–9.
2. Hoge CW, McGurk D, Thomas JL, et al. Mild traumatic brain injury in U.S. Soldiers returning from Iraq. N Engl J Med 2008;358(5):453–63.
3. Centers for Disease Control and Prevention, Available at: https://www.cdc.gov/traumaticbraininjury/get_the_facts.html. Accessed June 16, 2023.
4. Peterson AB, Thomas KE and Zhou H. Traumatic Brain Injury-related Deaths by Age Group, Sex, and Mechanism of Injury, Centers for Disease Control and Prevention, National Center for Injury Prevention and Control, Available at: https://www.cdc.gov/traumaticbraininjury/data/index.html. Accessed June 16, 2023.
5. Stubbs JL, Thornton AE, Sevick JM, et al. Traumatic brain injury in homeless and marginally housed individuals: a systematic review and meta-analysis. Lancet Public Health 2020;5(1):e19–32.
6. Irvine KA, Clark JD. Chronic Pain After Traumatic Brain Injury: Pathophysiology and Pain Mechanisms. Pain Med 2018;19(7):1315–33.
7. King PR, Beehler GP, Wade MJ. Self-Reported Pain and Pain Management Strategies Among Veterans With Traumatic Brain Injury: A Pilot Study. Mil Med 2015; 180(8):863–8.
8. Jodoin M, Rouleau DM, Charlebois-Plante C, et al. Incidence rate of mild traumatic brain injury among patients who have suffered from an isolated limb fracture: Upper limb fracture patients are more at risk. Injury 2016;47(8):1835–40.
9. Nampiaparampil DE. Prevalence of chronic pain after traumatic brain injury: a systematic review. JAMA 2008;300(6):711–9.
10. Zasler ND, Formisano R, Aloisi M. Pain in Persons with Disorders of Consciousness. Brain Sci 2022;12(3):300.

11. Nazari R, Pahlevan Sharif S, Allen KA, et al. Behavioral Pain Indicators in Patients with Traumatic Brain Injury Admitted to an Intensive Care Unit. J Caring Sci 2018; 7(4):197–203.

12. Haacke EM, Duhaime AC, Gean AD, et al. Common data elements in radiologic imaging of traumatic brain injury. J Magn Reson Imaging 2010;32(3):516–43.

13. Le TH, Gean AD. Neuroimaging of traumatic brain injury. Mt Sinai J Med 2009; 76(2):145–62.

14. Headache Classification Committee of the International Headache Society (IHS). The international classification of headache disorders, (beta version). Cephalalgia 2013;33(9):629–808.

15. D'Onofrio F, Russo A, Conte F, et al. Post-traumatic headaches: an epidemiological overview. Neurol Sci 2014;35(Suppl 1):203–6.

16. Nordhaug LH, Hagen K, Vik A, et al. Headache following head injury: a population-based longitudinal cohort study (HUNT). J Headache Pain 2018;19(1):8.

17. Walker WC, Seel RT, Curtiss G, et al. Headache after moderate and severe traumatic brain injury: a longitudinal analysis. Arch Phys Med Rehabil 2005;86(9): 1793–800.

18. Pangarkar S, Pham QG, Eapen BC. Pain care essentials and innovations. 1st edition. Philadelphia, PA: Elsevier Health Sciences; 2020.

19. Defrin R, Riabinin M, Feingold Y, et al. Deficient pain modulatory systems in patients with mild traumatic brain and chronic post-traumatic headache: implications for its mechanism. J Neurotrauma 2015;32(1):28–37.

20. Ashina H, Porreca F, Anderson T, et al. Post-traumatic headache: epidemiology and pathophysiological insights. Nat Rev Neurol 2019;15(10):607–17.

21. Li J, Wei Y, Zhou J, et al. Activation of locus coeruleus-spinal cord noradrenergic neurons alleviates neuropathic pain in mice via reducing neuroinflammation from astrocytes and microglia in spinal dorsal horn. J Neuroinflammation 2022; 19(1):123.

22. Strigo IA, Spadoni AD, Lohr J, et al. Too hard to control: compromised pain anticipation and modulation in mild traumatic brain injury. Transl Psychiatry 2014;4(1): e340.

23. Navratilova E, Rau J, Oyarzo J, et al. CGRP-dependent and independent mechanisms of acute and persistent post-traumatic headache following mild traumatic brain injury in mice. Cephalalgia 2019;39(14):1762–75.

24. Piantino J, Lim MM, Newgard CD, et al. Linking Traumatic Brain Injury, Sleep Disruption and Post-Traumatic Headache: a Potential Role for Glymphatic Pathway Dysfunction. Curr Pain Headache Rep 2019;23(9):62.

25. McGeary DD, Resick PA, Penzien DB, et al. Reason to doubt the ICHD-3 7-day inclusion criterion for mild TBI-related posttraumatic headache: A nested cohort study. Cephalalgia 2020;40(11):1155–67.

26. Ashina H, Eigenbrodt AK, Seifert T, et al. Post-traumatic headache attributed to traumatic brain injury: classification, clinical characteristics, and treatment. Lancet Neurol 2021;20(6):460–9.

27. Howard L, Dumkrieger G, Chong CD, et al. Symptoms of Autonomic Dysfunction Among Those With Persistent Posttraumatic Headache Attributed to Mild Traumatic Brain Injury: A Comparison to Migraine and Healthy Controls. Headache 2018;58(9):1397–407.

28. Lieba-Samal D, Platzer P, Seidel S, et al. Characteristics of acute posttraumatic headache following mild head injury. Cephalalgia 2011;31(16):1618–26.

29. Larsen EL, Ashina H, Iljazi A, et al. Acute and preventive pharmacological treatment of post-traumatic headache: a systematic review. J Headache Pain 2019; 20(1):98.
30. Ashina H, Iljazi A, Al-Khazali HM, et al. Persistent post-traumatic headache attributed to mild traumatic brain injury: Deep phenotyping and treatment patterns. Cephalalgia 2020;40(6):554–64.
31. Ashina H, Dodick DW. Post-traumatic Headache: Pharmacologic Management and Targeting CGRP Signaling. Curr Neurol Neurosci Rep 2022;22(2):105–11.
32. Chan S, Kurowski B, Byczkowski T, et al. Intravenous migraine therapy in children with posttraumatic headache in the ED. Am J Emerg Med 2015;33(5):635–9.
33. Friedman BW, Babbush K, Irizarry E, et al. An exploratory study of IV metoclopramide+diphenhydramine for acute post-traumatic headache. Am J Emerg Med 2018;36(2):285–9.
34. Thorlund K, Sun-Edelstein C, Druyts E, et al. Risk of medication overuse headache across classes of treatments for acute migraine. J Headache Pain 2016; 17(1):1–9.
35. Estemalik E, Tepper S. Preventive treatment in migraine and the new US guidelines. Neuropsychiatr Dis Treat 2013;9:709–20.
36. Rapoport AM. Acute and prophylactic treatments for migraine: present and future. Neurol Sci 2008;29(Suppl 1):S110–22.
37. Erickson JC. Treatment outcomes of chronic post-traumatic headaches after mild head trauma in US soldiers: an observational study. Headache 2011;51(6):932–44.
38. Ailani J, Burch RC, Robbins MS, et al. The American Headache Society Consensus Statement: Update on integrating new migraine treatments into clinical practice. Headache 2021;61(7):1021–39.
39. Cushman DM, Borowski L, Hansen C, et al. Gabapentin and Tricyclics in the Treatment of Post-Concussive Headache, a Retrospective Cohort Study. Headache 2019;59(3):371–82.
40. Antonaci F, Ghiotto N, Wu S, et al. Recent advances in migraine therapy. SpringerPlus 2016;5:637.
41. Bree D, Levy D. Development of CGRP-dependent pain and headache related behaviours in a rat model of concussion: Implications for mechanisms of post-traumatic headache. Cephalalgia 2018;38(2):246–58.
42. Amar PJ, Schiff ER. Acetaminophen safety and hepatotoxicity–where do we go from here? Expert Opin Drug Saf 2007;6(4):341–55.
43. MacGregor EA, Dowson A, Davies PT. Mouth-dispersible aspirin in the treatment of migraine: a placebo-controlled study. Headache 2002;42(4):249–55.
44. Rabbie R, Derry S, Moore RA. Ibuprofen with or without an antiemetic for acute migraine headaches in adults. Cochrane Database Syst Rev 2013;2013(4): CD008039.
45. Acute treatment of migraine attacks: efficacy and safety of a nonsteroidal anti-inflammatory drug, diclofenac-potassium, in comparison to oral sumatriptan and placebo. The Diclofenac-K/Sumatriptan Migraine Study Group. Cephalalgia 1999;19(4):232–40.
46. Pringsheim T, Davenport W, Mackie G, et al. Canadian Headache Society guideline for migraine prophylaxis. Can J Neurol Sci 2012;39(2 Suppl 2):S1–59.
47. Linde K, Rossnagel K. Propranolol for migraine prophylaxis. Cochrane Database Syst Rev 2004;(2):CD003225.
48. Doyle Strauss L, Weizenbaum E, Loder EW, et al. Amitriptyline Dose and Treatment Outcomes in Specialty Headache Practice: A Retrospective Cohort Study. Headache 2016;56(10):1626–34.

49. Linde M, Mulleners WM, Chronicle EP, et al. Topiramate for the prophylaxis of episodic migraine in adults. Cochrane Database Syst Rev 2013;2013(6): CD010610.

50. Goadsby PJ, Reuter U, Lanteri-Minet M, et al. Long-Term Efficacy and Safety of Erenumab: Results From 64 Weeks of the LIBERTY Study [published online ahead of print, 2021 Apr 28]. Neurology 2021;96(22):e2724–35.

51. Dodick DW, Silberstein SD, Bigal ME, et al. Effect of Fremanezumab Compared With Placebo for Prevention of Episodic Migraine: A Randomized Clinical Trial. JAMA 2018;319(19):1999–2008.

52. Detke HC, Goadsby PJ, Wang S, et al. Galcanezumab in chronic migraine: The randomized, double-blind, placebo-controlled REGAIN study. Neurology 2018; 91(24):e2211–21.

53. Derry CJ, Derry S, Moore RA. Sumatriptan (oral route of administration) for acute migraine attacks in adults. Cochrane Database Syst Rev 2012;2012(2): CD008615.

54. Mannix LK, Loder E, Nett R, et al. Rizatriptan for the acute treatment of ICHD-II proposed menstrual migraine: two prospective, randomized, placebo-controlled, double-blind studies. Cephalalgia 2007;27(5):414–21.

55. Spierings EL, Rapoport AM, Dodick DW, et al. Acute treatment of migraine with zolmitriptan 5 mg orally disintegrating tablet. CNS Drugs 2004;18(15):1133–41.

56. Orr SL, Friedman BW, Christie S, et al. Management of Adults With Acute Migraine in the Emergency Department: The American Headache Society Evidence Assessment of Parenteral Pharmacotherapies. Headache 2016;56(6):911–40.

57. Dodick DW, Lipton RB, Ailani J, et al. Ubrogepant for the Treatment of Migraine. N Engl J Med 2019;381(23):2230–41.

58. Ailani J, Lipton RB, Goadsby PJ, et al. Atogepant for the Preventive Treatment of Migraine. N Engl J Med 2021;385(8):695–706.

59. Croop R, Lipton RB, Kudrow D, et al. Oral rimegepant for preventive treatment of migraine: a phase 2/3, randomised, double-blind, placebo-controlled trial. Lancet 2021;397(10268):51–60.

60. Blumenfeld A, Silberstein SD, Dodick DW, et al. Method of injection of onabotulinumtoxinA for chronic migraine: a safe, well-tolerated, and effective treatment paradigm based on the PREEMPT clinical program. Headache 2010;50(9): 1406–18.

61. Bendtsen L, Jensen R. Mirtazapine is effective in the prophylactic treatment of chronic tension-type headache. Neurology 2004;62(10):1706–11.

62. Adelman LC, Adelman JU, Von Seggern R, et al. Venlafaxine extended release (XR) for the prophylaxis of migraine and tension-type headache: A retrospective study in a clinical setting. Headache 2000;40(7):572–80.

63. Donath C, Luttenberger K, Geiß C, et al. Chronic headache patients' health behavior and health service use 12 months after interdisciplinary treatment - what do they keep in their daily routines? BMC Neurol 2022;22(1):149.

64. Herrero Babiloni A, Baril AA, Charlebois-Plante C, et al. The Putative Role of Neuroinflammation in the Interaction between Traumatic Brain Injuries, Sleep, Pain and Other Neuropsychiatric Outcomes: A State-of-the-Art Review. J Clin Med 2023;12(5):1793.

65. Dubrovsky AS, Friedman D, Kocilowicz H. Pediatric post-traumatic headaches and peripheral nerve blocks of the scalp: a case series and patient satisfaction survey. Headache 2014;54(5):878–87.

66. Silverman SB. Cervicogenic headache: interventional, anesthetic, and ablative treatment. Curr Pain Headache Rep 2002;6(4):308–14.

67. Cogan AM, Silva MA, Brostow DP. Low Back Pain and Traumatic Brain Injury. Arch Phys Med Rehabil 2021;102(7):1441–3.

68. Brown S, Hawker G, Beaton D, et al. Long-term musculoskeletal complaints after traumatic brain injury. Brain Inj 2011;25(5):453–61.

69. Trexler LE, Corrigan JD, Davé S, et al. Recommendations for Prescribing Opioids for People With Traumatic Brain Injury. Arch Phys Med Rehabil 2020;101(11): 2033–40.

70. Jacotte-Simancas A, Fucich EA, Stielper ZF, et al. Traumatic brain injury and the misuse of alcohol, opioids, and cannabis. Int Rev Neurobiol 2021;157:195–243.

71. Bjork JM, Grant SJ. Does traumatic brain injury increase risk for substance abuse? J Neurotrauma 2009;26(7):1077–82.

72. Dowell D, Haegerich TM, Chou R. CDC Guideline for Prescribing Opioids for Chronic Pain - United States, 2016 [published correction appears in MMWR Recomm Rep. 2016;65(11):295]. MMWR Recomm Rep (Morb Mortal Wkly Rep) 2016;65(1):1–49.

73. 59. National Conference of State Legislatures. Prescribing policies: states confront opioid overdose epidemic. Washington, DC: National Conference of State Legislatures; 2019. Available at: https://www.ncsl.org/research/health/prescribing-policies-states-confront-opioid-overdose-epidemic.aspx.

74. Huang CH, Huang CC, Sun CK, et al. Methylphenidate on Cognitive Improvement in Patients with Traumatic Brain Injury: A Meta-Analysis [published correction appears in Curr Neuropharmacol. 2016;14(6):662]. Curr Neuropharmacol 2016; 14(3):272–81.

75. Garland DE, Blum CE, Waters RL. Periarticular heterotopic ossification in head-injured adults. Incidence and location. J Bone Joint Surg Am 1980;62(7):1143–6.

76. Haran M, Bhuta T, Lee B. Pharmacological interventions for treating acute heterotopic ossification. Cochrane Database Syst Rev 2004;4:CD003321.

77. Aubut JA, Mehta S, Cullen N, et al, ERABI Group; Scire Research Team. A comparison of heterotopic ossification treatment within the traumatic brain and spinal cord injured population: An evidence based systematic review. Neuro-Rehabilitation 2011;28(2):151–60.

78. Thibaut FA, Chatelle C, Wannez S, et al. Spasticity in disorders of consciousness: a behavioral study. Eur J Phys Rehabil Med 2015;51(4):389–97.

79. Zafonte R, Elovic EP, Lombard L. Acute care management of post-TBI spasticity. J Head Trauma Rehabil 2004;19(2):89–100.

80. Taylor BC, Hagel EM, Carlson KF, et al. Prevalence and costs of co-occurring traumatic brain injury with and without psychiatric disturbance and pain among Afghanistan and Iraq War Veteran V.A. users. Med Care 2012;50(4):342–6.

81. Hoffman JM, Pagulayan KF, Zawaideh N, et al. Understanding pain after traumatic brain injury: impact on community participation. Am J Phys Med Rehabil 2007;86(12):962–9.

82. Treede RD, Rief W, Barke A, et al. A classification of chronic pain for ICD-11. Pain 2015;156(6):1003–7.

83. 64. International Association for the Study of Pain (IASP). Pain Terms. Available at: https//www.iasp-pain.org/terminology.

84. Schug SA, Lavand'homme P, Barke A, et al. The IASP classification of chronic pain for ICD-11: chronic postsurgical or posttraumatic pain. Pain 2019;160(1): 45–52.

85. Lyman M, Lloyd DG, Ji X, et al. Neuroinflammation: the role and consequences. Neurosci Res 2014;79:1–12.

86. Clausen F, Hånell A, Israelsson C, et al. Neutralization of interleukin-1β reduces cerebral edema and tissue loss and improves late cognitive outcome following traumatic brain injury in mice. Eur J Neurosci 2011;34(1):110–23.

87. Tobinick E, Kim NM, Reyzin G, et al. Selective TNF inhibition for chronic stroke and traumatic brain injury: an observational study involving 629 consecutive patients treated with perispinal etanercept. CNS Drugs 2012;26(12):1051–70.

88. Lawn T, Aman Y, Rukavina K, et al. Pain in the neurodegenerating brain: insights into pharmacotherapy for Alzheimer disease and Parkinson disease. Pain 2021; 162(4):999–1006.

89. Effgen GB, Vogel EW 3rd, Lynch KA, et al. Isolated primary blast alters neuronal function with minimal cell death in organotypic hippocampal slice cultures. J Neurotrauma 2014;31(13):1202–10.

90. Miyazaki S, Katayama Y, Lyeth BG, et al. Enduring suppression of hippocampal long-term potentiation following traumatic brain injury in rat. Brain Res 1992; 585(1–2):335–9.

91. Klein RC, Acheson SK, Qadri LH, et al. Opposing effects of traumatic brain injury on excitatory synaptic function in the lateral amygdala in the absence and presence of preinjury stress. J Neurosci Res 2016;94(6):579–89.

92. Cantu D, Walker K, Andresen L, et al. Traumatic Brain Injury Increases Cortical Glutamate Network Activity by Compromising GABAergic Control. Cereb Cortex 2015;25(8):2306–20.

93. Rauh MJ, Aralis HJ, Melcer T, et al. Effect of traumatic brain injury among U.S. servicemembers with amputation. J Rehabil Res Dev 2013;50(2):161–72.

94. Kim SK, Hayashi H, Ishikawa T, et al. Cortical astrocytes rewire somatosensory cortical circuits for peripheral neuropathic pain. J Clin Invest 2016;126(5):1983–97.

Neuropsychological Evaluation in Traumatic Brain Injury

Victoria O'Connor, PhD[a,b,c,]*, Robert Shura, PhD[a,b,c,d],
Patrick Armistead-Jehle, PhD[e], Douglas B. Cooper, PhD[f,g]

KEYWORDS

• Neuropsychology • Assessment • Traumatic brain injury • Concussion

KEY POINTS

• Neuropsychological evaluation involves the use of objective cognitive measures that have been validated; scores are converted to standardized scores based on the normal distribution and adjusted for various demographic features, most commonly age, gender, and education.
• Individuals with mild TBI typically make a fast and full recovery. In cases whereby there are chronic complaints, neuropsychological assessment can inform other factors that could be causal.
• Neuropsychological assessment in moderate and severe TBI injuries can be useful to track recovery in the subacute stage, inform rehab, and identify chronic deficits.

Traumatic brain injury (TBI) can lead to cognitive impairment, particularly moderate and severe injuries. Following TBI, a neuropsychological evaluation (NPE) can be helpful for quantifying the severity of cognitive impairment, tracking recovery, planning treatment, and identifying factors that might affect recovery. NPEs consist of a comprehensive clinical interview, a mental/neurobehavioral status examination,

---

[a] Department of Veterans Affairs, W. G. (Bill) Hefner VA Healthcare System, 1601 Brenner Avenue (11M), Salisbury, NC 28144, USA; [b] Veterans Integrated Service Networks (VISN)-6 Mid-Atlantic Mental Illness, Research Education and Clinical Center (MIRECC), Durham, NC, USA; [c] Wake Forest School of Medicine, Winston-Salem, NC, USA; [d] Via College of Osteopathic Medicine, Blacksburg, VA, USA; [e] Department of Veterans Affairs, Concussion Clinic, Munson Army Health Center, 550 Pope Avenue, Fort Leavenworth, KS 66027, USA; [f] Department of Psychiatry, University of Texas Health Science Center (UT-Health), South Texas VA Healthcare System, San Antonio Polytrauma Rehabilitation Center, 7400 Merton Minter Boulevard, San Antonio, TX 78229, USA; [g] Department of Rehabilitation Medicine, University of Texas Health Science Center (UT-Health), South Texas VA Healthcare System, San Antonio Polytrauma Rehabilitation Center, 7400 Merton Minter Boulevard, San Antonio, TX 78229, USA
* Corresponding author. Department of Veterans Affairs, W. G. (Bill) Hefner VA Healthcare System, 1601 Brenner Avenue (11M), Salisbury, NC 28144.
E-mail address: victoria.oconnor@va.gov

Phys Med Rehabil Clin N Am 35 (2024) 593–605
https://doi.org/10.1016/j.pmr.2024.02.010
1047-9651/24/Published by Elsevier Inc.

performance-based cognitive testing, a review of medical records, and when possible, a collateral interview. Interpretation of neuropsychological test scores are based upon an understanding of the psychometric properties and limitations of the tests, knowledge of brain-behavior relationships, and consideration of the impact of nonneurologic factors that may be associated with test performance. NPEs conducted in the acute recovery window are typically used to guide rehabilitation, whereas those conducted later are used to determine the level of chronic cognitive impairment and to distinguish from other potential sources of cognitive concern. NPEs can also inform psychiatric treatment and capacity decisions at any time along the recovery continuum.

In the acute recovery window, NPEs may be conducted in an inpatient setting and are typically briefer in duration. Beyond the acute recovery window, patients are referred for outpatient assessment, typically by a primary care provider, neurologist, or mental health provider. Referring providers submit a specific referral question, which neuropsychologists are tasked with answering. This referral question provides a target for neuropsychologists to structure their clinical interview and test selection. Thus, more specific referral questions generally result in improved assessments. Examples of referral questions include "does this patient have impaired cognitive functioning" or "does this person have dementia or depression," or "what are this person's cognitive strengths and weaknesses to aid in treatment planning?" In nonclinical settings, referral questions may focus on a person's ability to return to work, determine capacity to live independently or make medical decisions, or manage one's money. It is important to note that a neuropsychologist cannot conduct testing to determine if a person experienced a TBI, the existence of an injury can only be ascertained through gathering a detailed history. In other words, a TBI is a historic, injury event, and cognitive testing cannot confirm or rule out the occurrence of such an event.

The neuropsychological report is the product of an NPE. A report details the information gathered in the clinical interview (eg, details of the TBI, relevant medical and psychiatric conditions), explains the results of the cognitive testing, provides a diagnosis and summary, and provides recommendations for the patient and referring provider. Most importantly, the report should clearly answer the referral question. Report styles are variable; however, referring providers generally prefer reports that are brief (under 4 pages) and easily readable (bullet points and tables).

Objective testing includes measures of cognitive functioning that span numerous domains and include additional factors that influence performance on cognitive tests. The various cognitive domains and the tests typically used to assess them are presented in **Table 1**. The table is not all inclusive, but rather a sample of abilities tested and commonly available measures. There is no consensus regarding which tests to use for a given situation, what abilities belong under which domain, and which particular abilities each test actually samples. This lack of consensus is due, in part, the fact the no cognitive test is a pure measure of the targeted underlying construct. However, there is published guidance regarding common data elements for TBI specifically.[1,2] Although these elements were designed to inform research studies, the list is helpful in planning a battery clinically. In addition to objective tests, neuropsychologists may also include subjective, self-report measures assessing the patient's perception of their cognitive abilities, somatic and psychiatric symptoms, and personality traits.

Performance on cognitive tests is then compared with normative data matched by demographic factors known to affect performance, most commonly age, but also sex, education level, and race/ethnicity. Presented in **Fig. 1**, these comparisons are typically presented as standardized scores (StS; $M = 100$; $SD = 15$), T scores (T; $M = 50$, $SD = 10$), or age-corrected scaled scores (SS; $M = 10$, $SD = 3$) that explain

Table 1
Common cognitive domains of functioning with examples of common tests

Domain	Ability	Test Example
General	Mental Status	Montreal Cognitive Assessment
Motor	Fine Motor Speed	Finger Tapping Test
	Dexterity	Grooved Pegboard
	Strength	Hand Dynamometer
Processing Speed	Processing Speed	Symbol Digit Modalities Test
Complex Attention	Basic Attention	CPT-3, Omissions
	Sustained Attention	CPT-3, HRT Block Change
	Divided Attention	Trail Making Test
	Vigilance	CPT-3, HRT ISI Change
	Working Memory	WAIS-IV Digit Span
Language	Comprehension	Complex Ideational Material
	Repetition	Sentence Repetition
	Confrontation Naming	Boston Naming Test
Visual-Spatial	Visual Discrimination	Judgment of Line Orientation
	Construction	WAIS-IV Block Design
	Visual Problem Solving	WAIS-IV Visual Puzzles
Memory[a]	Learning	Rey Auditory Verbal Learning Test, 1–5 Total
	Delayed Recall	Rey Auditory Verbal Learning Test, Delayed Recall
	Recognition	Rey Auditory Verbal Learning Test, Recognition
Executive	Planning	D-KEFS Tower Test
	Set Shifting	Wisconsin Card Sorting Test
	Inhibition Control	CPT-3, Commissions
	Fluency	Controlled Oral Word Association Test
	Resistance to Interference	D-KEFS Color-Word Interference Test
	Abstraction	WAIS-IV Similarities
	Concept Formation	Category Test
Intelligence	Intellectual Ability	WAIS-IV
Emotional	Personality & Psychopathology	Minnesota Multiphasic Personality Inventory - 3

Note. CPT-3, conners continuous performance test-3; D-KEFS, Delis-Kaplan Executive Function System; HRT, hit reaction time; ISI, inter-stimulus interval; WAIS-IV, Wechsler Adult Intelligence Scale – Fourth Edition.
[a] Memory is typically evaluated for both auditory/verbal and visual tasks.

the individual's performance relative to that of their peers, with the assumption that cognitive abilities are normally distributed across the population. Typically, scores outside of two standard deviations are considered abnormal, and indicate impairment, though situations exist where a provider might lower this threshold.

MILD TRAUMATIC BRAIN INJURY

TBI severity is categorized as mild, moderate, and severe with the distinction based largely on the durations of unconsciousness and/or post traumatic amnesia. Subsequent to the injury, the patient can also be categorized as a function of time since the insult. While a universal timeline has never been adopted, the acute and postacute periods typically encompass the point of injury through 6 weeks and then 12 weeks,

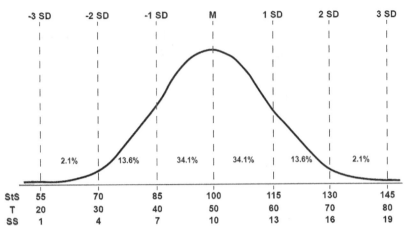

Fig. 1. Normal distribution with standard, T, and scaled scores. *Note.* SS, age corrected scaled scores; StS, standard scores; T, T scores.

respectively. Following 3 months, the concussive injury can be considered chronic in nature. NPE with the acute/postacute and chronic periods differs notably.

Within the acute and potentially the postacute phases, a range of symptoms that span somatic, cognitive, and affective domains are possible and expected. The vast majority of individuals who experience a mild TBI will recover to baseline functioning within a few days to a few months.[3] During this time (particularity within the first several days to weeks of injury) NPEs should be limited to focused and repeatable measures that can be used to track the anticipated course of recovery. Immediately following injury, NPE is appropriate, but typically takes place in the context of a larger concussion evaluation that is usually completed by a nonneuropsychologist. For instance, in the military setting the Military Acute Concussion Evaluation (MACE) is administered as soon after injury as possible, typically by medics or primary care providers. With sports related concussion, the Standardized Assessment of Concussion (SAC) is often administered on the field by training staff. These instruments include a cognitive component, but also assess vestibular, visual, and balance functioning and include a symptom report checklist. In the acute and postacute phases, computerized instruments of cognitive functioning are commonly used to track progress. In the military, the Automated Neuropsychological Assessment Metrics (ANAM) is used, while the ImPACT is popular within sports medicine. Within the acute and post-acute phases of concussion recovery, lengthy NPEs are not indicated and likely hold limited utility in most cases.

This however is not the case with chronic mild TBI. Within 3 months of injury, the majority of individuals will return to baseline functioning. For those that do not, NPE is indicated to verify objective cognitive deficits and psychological symptoms, and to assess for other factors that are contributing to the patient's presentation. NPE in the context of chronic mild TBI would include most cognitive domains, but a particular focus on those most susceptible to this injury would be appropriate. These include processing speed, memory, and attention. Owing to the role of psychological factors in protracted concussion recovery, a broad band measure of psychopathology (eg, PAI or MMPI-3) is also typically indicated. Finally, response validity must be established through the use of both performance and symptom validity measures. This is particularly true in cases where secondary gain is present, such as disability and legal evaluations.

MODERATE AND SEVERE TRAUMATIC BRAIN INJURY

Individuals who sustain moderate or severe TBI frequently have cognitive impairments that impact their ability to return to their preinjury level of functioning, and are more likely to require rehabilitation interventions, including inpatient brain injury rehabilitation, postacute residential treatment, and outpatient treatment and follow up. Neuropsychologists may encounter individuals with moderate or severe TBI in any of these settings. NPEs may be requested to assist with the determination of the course of recovery, the evaluation of cognitive strengths and weaknesses that might be the focus of rehabilitation interventions, and to assist with the determination of the need for ongoing restrictions/supervision, or the determination of an individual's ability to return to work, driving, or school.

Individuals who sustain moderate TBIs exhibit a slower rate of recovery of cognitive functioning and less uniform cognitive outcomes than individuals with mTBI. Following a moderate TBI, some individuals demonstrate complete cognitive recovery, and some individuals experience residual cognitive difficulties. The primary cognitive domains affected after a moderate TBI include speed and efficiency of cognitive processing, executive functions, and declarative memory.

Neuropsychological impairments are seen following severe TBI, and many individuals require serial NPEs across the course of their recovery. During the acute phase of recovery, individuals with severe TBI experience deficits in orientation, arousal, attention, behavior, mood, and perception often labeled posttraumatic amnesia (PTA). The assessment of the duration of PTA is often used along with other acute neurologic indicators, to predict long-term cognitive outcomes. The duration of PTA can be evaluated retrospectively by asking a patient about the first memory they can recall after their TBI. In inpatient or postacute residential settings, a more reliable assessment of PTA can be completed prospectively through the serial administration of standardized psychometric tests for evaluating PTA, such as the Orientation Log[4] or the Galveston Orientation and Amnesia Test.[5] A more extensive evaluation of cognitive functioning in an individual who is in PTA is unlikely to yield significant additional meaningful clinical information. Neuropsychologists working in inpatient/residential settings often provide consultation to the therapy team as well as education and support to family members during this stage of recovery.

Once an individual with a severe TBI clears from PTA, they may be appropriate for more comprehensive NPE. Neuropsychological test batteries in the subacute stage of recovery may be more protracted, focusing on cognitive domains that are most likely to be affected such as processing speed, attention, memory, and executive functioning. Determination about the scope of an initial NPE, depends largely on the setting, access to rehabilitation, and specific referral questions (eg, can this patient return to independent living?). Additionally, consideration should be given to including neuropsychological measures that can be repeated at a later time point, which may occur roughly 6 to 12 months later. Long-term neuropsychological impairments are common following severe TBI, with the widest range of deficits seen in individuals with the most severe injuries.

PREDICTORS OF NEUROPSYCHOLOGICAL OUTCOMES FOLLOWING TRAUMATIC BRAIN INJURY

There are a number of factors that are associated with neuropsychological outcomes following TBI (**Table 2**). Characteristics of the injury, age, and cognitive reserve predict the extent and timing of recovery. Psychiatric conditions are predictive of prolonged or incomplete recovery.[6,7] Symptom exaggeration is a factor, particularly in cases with

Table 2
Predictors of neuropsychological outcomes following TBI

Predictor	Details
Severity of injury	Greater injury severity is associated with worse outcomes.[45] There is a strong association between severe TBI and long-term cognitive deficits.[46]
Parenchymal volume	Greater atrophy is associated with poorer outcomes.[47]
Age	Age <40 y at the time of injury have better outcomes.[48,49]
Cognitive reserve	Cognitive reserve is a protective factor. Individuals with higher levels of cognitive functioning pre-injury have better outcomes, but this does not completely negate the effect of injury severity.[49,50]
Legal context	Individuals with an absence of litigation related to the injury (eg, disability claims) have better outcomes.[8,39,51]
Expectation of recovery	Expecting a fully recovery is associated with better outcomes, while expecting prolonged impairment is associated with worse outcomes.[52–54]
Psychiatric conditions	Psychiatric conditions that pre-date or develop after TBI are associated with poorer outcomes.[6,7,55–57]
Sleep disturbance	Sleep disturbance is associated with poorer outcomes.[58–60]
Pain	Greater pain intensity is associated with poorer outcomes.[55,56]

secondary gain.[8,9] The presence of a legal case relating to the TBI and the individual's expectation for their recovery also predict outcomes. An inaccurate perception of superior preinjury abilities has also been cited as a possible factor in subjective complaints in the context of chronic mild TBI (good old days bias).[10] Other factors to consider include dysregulated sleep (including insomnia and breathing related sleep disorders), chronic pain, medication side effects, and neuroendocrine and other metabolic dysfunction.

RISK OF DEMENTIA AND CHRONIC TRAUMATIC ENCEPHALOPATHY

At the more long-term, chronic stage, TBI may increase one's risk for developing neurodegenerative disorders. Brain reserve is the idea that those with greater brain functional capacity will have a higher threshold of neurologic injury needed prior to cognitive impairment emerging. Conceptually, any insult to brain tissue may lead to reduced brain reserve, and in turn an increased risk for later developing brain pathology, including proteinopathies present in neurodegenerative conditions. Numerous studies, reviews, and meta-analyses have found an association between having a history of TBI and an increased risk of developing neurodegenerative pathology and related neurocognitive disorders. For example, a recent meta-analysis of 32 studies found a 70% increased risk of developing dementia for those with a TBI history.[11] In contrast, although TBI has been associated with increased dementia risk, TBI did not affect the course of decline in one study.[12] In other words, although TBI is associated with an increased risk of developing dementia later in life, it does not affect the age of onset or speed of decline associated with dementia.

Traumatic Brain Injury Severity and Dementia

As described, mild TBI is functionally different than moderate/severe TBI, and the different severities carry different long-term prognoses. Conceptually, mild injuries do not increase the risk of dementia, given that there is no visible pathology on imaging and a fast recovery is expected. A systematic review did not find evidence to support an association between mild TBI and dementia or chronic cognitive impairment.[13] However, there were few studies that meet the inclusion criteria for the review. More recently, a study of postdeployment Veterans found a 3.77 greater chance of developing dementia for those with a history of moderate/severe TBI compared with those without; however, even for mild TBI, including those without LOC, there was a greater than 2 fold increase in dementia diagnoses compared with controls.[14] Other studies support later-life cognitive impairment in moderate/severe TBI, though results for mild TBI remain mixed, and some have highlighted the numerous methodological limitations in studies supporting the chronic effects of mild TBI.[15–17] Regardless, even for moderate/severe TBI, little is known about the neurobiological mechanism of how neurotrauma increases the risk of neurodegenerative pathology and neurocognitive disorders far later in life.[18]

Chronic Traumatic Encephalopathy

Related to dementia and TBI is the diagnosis of chronic traumatic encephalopathy (CTE), a degenerative disease initially called dementia pugilistica or "punch drunk" syndrome, and described by a forensic pathologist in a series of boxers.[19] The disease was found in a small percentage of boxers, involved primarily diffuse tauopathy and TDP-43, and clinically presented with both a dementia and a motor syndrome. Dementia pugilistica was later re-named CTE,[20] and in the past 20 years has received increasing attention due to professional sports, high profile litigation, and heavy media coverage. The diagnosis remains controversial, with some arguing against CTE as a disease distinct from other degenerative conditions,[21] and others pointing out numerous methodological flaws of available studies supporting CTE.[22,23] Nonetheless, at present CTE can only be diagnosed by a pathologist on autopsy,[24] and not by a neuropsychologist through clinical assessment, though various clinical criteria have been created.[25]

SPECIAL ISSUES RELATED TO NEUROPSYCHOLOGICAL ASSESSMENT
Repeat Assessment

A common occurrence, especially in rehab settings, is to complete repeated NPE in order to determine recovery following TBI. New results are compared with prior results to determine if cognitive abilities have improved, remained stable, or declined. If there is change, an examiner must somehow determine if the change is meaningful. A problem with making this determination is the occurrence of practice effects, which refer to the artificial improvement in scores on repeat testing due to familiarity with a test. One solution is using alternate forms of tests, where items are different but psychometrically equivalent. When alternate forms do not exist for a given test, various methods of statistical analysis are available, including deviation indices, reliable change indices, and regression formulae.[26] However, even when 2 scores are statistically different, they may not be clinically meaningful. Base rates can be useful when determining the clinical significance of change, if available. When not available, other information must be used, such as relying on a transition to a different score descriptor category (eg, improving from below average to average).

Symptom and Performance Validity

Performance validity tests are special measures that were designed to identify non-credible results on objective cognitive tests, whether due to uncooperativeness, malingering, or other factors. In contrast, symptom validity tests are measures that evaluate for response bias of self-report. Over the past 2 decades, much research has focused on validity measures, and a burgeoning selection of these measures are available. Several professional organizations within neuropsychology have highlighted the necessity of evaluating validity, regardless of the context of an evaluation.[27-29] Evaluation of validity is most important in cases involving litigation or disability, as nearly half of examinees will produce invalid data.[30] Mild TBI is one of the most common referrals for neuropsychologist in civil forensic settings,[31] highlighting the importance of validity assessment in TBI populations specifically.

Neurocognitive Assessment Tools

Computerized assessment of cognitive functioning has become increasingly popular. Preseason baseline testing is now common in a number of sports from high school to professional athletics. In the military setting, predeployment assessment is mandated and millions of administrations have been collected. Of the available NCAT instruments, the Immediate Post-Concussion Assessment and Cognitive Test (ImPACT) is most commonly used in sports settings, while the Automated Neuropsychological Assessment Metrics 4 (ANAM4) is the predominantly used measure in the military. Typically, such measures are used in the postacute phase of injury, and baseline testing is used for intra-individual comparison after an injury, with the intent of insuring a complete return to baseline functioning. When individual baseline testing is not available, demographically based normative data can be reliably used for comparison.[32,33] Relative to traditional NPEs, these instruments have the advantage of being automated and relatively brief. In addition, NCATs are designed to be repeatedly administered and thus have established reliable change indices to better quantify change in functioning.

Despite the popularity of NCATs, weaknesses have been identified. These include somewhat limited reliabilities across 4 different NCATs (ANAM4, CNS-Vital Signs, Cogstate, and ImPACT).[34] In a latter publication, Cole and colleagues compared these same 4 NCATs to traditional NPEs.[35] The results indicated rather small correlations and small effect sizes between NCAT and traditional NPE. Finally, studies have found these measures to have limited ability to identify individuals who intentionally underperform.[36,37] As such, while NCATs certainly have utility in the evaluation and management of acute and postacute concussion, continued development to assure optimized psychometric properties is warranted.

Various Contexts

Several special subpopulations are worth noting related to the NPE of TBI. First, as already noted, mild TBI tends to be seen quite commonly in civil forensic contexts, along with an associated higher rate of invalid performance. On the other end of the spectrum, there is TBI in sports. Many teams in sports whereby TBI is common (eg, football, soccer) have neuropsychologists on staff, who are tasked with making return to play decisions. NPE of TBI in sports is unique for 2 reasons: first, a heavy reliance on NCATs, and second, the issue of sandbagging, which is when an athlete underperforms at baseline. Then, if a head injury occurs, there appears to be no decline, and the athlete can return to play.[38] In other words, in forensic settings, there is an incentive to appear worse after an injury whereas in sports, the incentive is to avoid sitting out play time thus the need to appear worse prior to an injury.

A third unique context is that of military and Veterans Affairs. In the military, blast injury as a mechanism stands out as unique relative to civilian populations. Neuropathological effects of blast exposure is an ongoing area of research, given the primary blast wave interacts with fluid and air-fill spaces differently than blunt-force trauma;

however, cognitive outcomes do not appear significantly different from non-blast injuries.[39,40] After military service, many veterans elect to receive medical care within the VA system. As part of the VA, veterans may also pursue service-connected disability, a set of monetary entitlements for injuries incurred during service, including TBI. The problem is that the lines between clinical and disability can be blurred, given that examiners have access to clinical charts and exams may be completed within VA medical centers. Some have suggested that the system incentives veterans to be sick or preclude recovery.[41]

Return to Activity

Neuropsychologists are often asked to determine a person's ability to return to a specific activity, including work, sport, and driving, following TBI. In addition to determining if a person can return to an activity, neuropsychologists may be tasked with identifying accommodations that would make it possible for an individual to return to a given activity. These assessments are more likely to occur at the moderate and severe level of TBI, as individuals with mild TBI typically recover and return to activity without significant complication.[42] Unfortunately, neuropsychological tests do not perfectly overlap with many real-world tasks, and the predictive ability of specific tests to determine success is generally limited. In answering such questions, providers must consider the cognitive abilities that are necessary to successfully complete the task. Regarding the return to work, comparing the individual's cognitive abilities to those of a successful worker in their field plays an important role in determining if an individual is able to return to work. Regarding return to driving, processing speed and executive functioning are particularly relevant. Some suggest the use of trail making tests in predicting return to driving,[43] however others raise important questions regarding the methodological limitations of such assessment.[44]

SUMMARY

In summary, NPE can be helpful in informing care and functioning following TBI. NPEs will vary based on context, purpose, and the severity of TBI, but all will involve validated measures of cognitive functioning, with scores being converted to standardized scores based on normative samples.

CLINICS CARE POINTS

- When requesting a neuropsychological evaluation for a patient post-TBI, one should provide a specific, detailed referral question identifying the purpose of the requested examination.
- There are numerous nonneurological factors that are associated with recovery following TBI, particularly at mild injury severity.
- The standard of care for NPE is to assess performance and symptoms validity, regardless of context.

DISCLOSURE

This work was supported by the Salisbury VA Health Care System, VA Mid-Atlantic (VISN 6) Mental Illness Research, Education, and Clinical Center (MIRECC), and the Department of Veterans Affairs Office of Academic Affiliations Advanced Program in Mental Illness, Research, and Treatment. The authors declare that the research was conducted in the absence of any commercial or financial relationships that could be construed as a potential conflict of interest. The views, opinions, and/or findings contained in this article are those of the authors and should not be construed as an official Veterans Affairs, Department of Defense, or Defense Health Agency position, policy, or decision, unless so designated by other official documentation.

REFERENCES

1. Maas AIR, Harrison-Felix CL, Menon D, et al. Standardizing Data Collection in Traumatic Brain Injury. J Neurotrauma 2011;28(2):177–87.
2. Whyte J, Vasterling J, Manley GT. Common Data Elements for Research on Traumatic Brain Injury and Psychological Health: Current Status and Future Development. Arch Phys Med Rehabil 2010;91(11):1692–6.
3. McCrea M, Pliskin N, Barth J, et al. Official Position of the Military TBI Task Force on the Role of Neuropsychology and Rehabilitation Psychology in the Evaluation, Management, and Research of Military Veterans with Traumatic Brain Injury. Clin Neuropsychol 2008;22(1):10–26.
4. Novack TA, Dowler RN, Bush BA, et al. Validity of the orientation log, relative to the Galveston Orientation and Amnesia Test. J Head Trauma Rehabil 2000; 15(3):957–61.
5. Levin HS, O'Donnell VM, Grossman RG. The Galveston Orientation and Amnesia Test. A practical scale to assess cognition after head injury. J Nerv Ment Dis 1979; 167(11):675–84.
6. Bonfield CM, Lam S, Lin Y, et al. The impact of attention deficit hyperactivity disorder on recovery from mild traumatic brain injury. J Neurosurg Pediatr 2013; 12(2):97–102.
7. Iverson GL, Gardner AJ, Terry DP, et al. Predictors of clinical recovery from concussion: a systematic review. Br J Sports Med 2017;51(12):941–8.
8. Bayen E, Jourdan C, Ghout I, et al. Negative impact of litigation procedures on patient outcomes four years after severe traumatic brain injury: results from the PariS-traumatic brain injury study. Disabil Rehabil 2018;40(17):2040–7.
9. Denning JH, Shura RD. Cost of malingering mild traumatic brain injury-related cognitive deficits during compensation and pension evaluations in the veterans benefits administration. Appl Neuropsychol Adult 2019;26(1):1–16.
10. Iverson GL, Lange RT, Brooks BL, et al. "Good old days" bias following mild traumatic brain injury. Clin Neuropsychol 2010;24(1):17–37.
11. Gardner RC, Bahorik A, Kornblith ES, et al. Systematic review, meta-analysis, and population attributable risk of dementia associated with traumatic brain injury in civilians and veterans. J Neurotrauma 2023;40(7–8):620–34.
12. Schaffert J, Chiang HS, Fatima H, et al. History of traumatic brain injury does not alter course of neurocognitive decline in older adults with and without cognitive impairment. Neuropsychology 2023. https://doi.org/10.1037/neu0000892.
13. Godbolt AK, Cancelliere C, Hincapié CA, et al. Systematic review of the risk of dementia and chronic cognitive impairment after mild traumatic brain injury: results of the International Collaboration on Mild Traumatic Brain Injury Prognosis. Arch Phys Med Rehabil 2014;95(3 Suppl):S245–56.
14. Barnes DE, Byers AL, Gardner RC, et al. Association of mild traumatic brain injury with and without loss of consciousness with dementia in US military veterans. JAMA Neurol 2018;75(9):1055–61.
15. Iverson GL, Karr JE, Gardner AJ, et al. Results of scoping review do not support mild traumatic brain injury being associated with a high incidence of chronic cognitive impairment: Commentary on McInnes et al 2017. PLoS One 2019;14(9).

16. Lennon MJ, Brooker H, Creese B, et al. Lifetime traumatic brain injury and cognitive domain deficits in late life: The protect-tbi cohort study. J Neurotrauma 2023. https://doi.org/10.1089/neu.2022.0360.

17. McInnes K, Friesen CL, MacKenzie DE, et al. Mild Traumatic Brain Injury (mTBI) and chronic cognitive impairment: A scoping review. PLoS One 2017;12(4): e0174847.

18. Srinivasan G, Brafman DA. The emergence of model systems to investigate the link between traumatic brain injury and Alzheimer's disease. Front Aging Neurosci 2022;13:813544.

19. Martland HS. Punch drunk. J Am Med Assoc 1928;91(15):1103–7.

20. Miller H. Mental after-effects of head injury. Proc R Soc Med 1966;59(3):257–61.

21. Randolph C. Chronic traumatic encephalopathy is not a real disease. Arch Clin Neuropsychol 2018;33(5):644–8.

22. Iverson GL, Gardner AJ, McCrory P, et al. A critical review of chronic traumatic encephalopathy. Neurosci Biobehav Rev 2015;56:276–93.

23. Smith DH, Johnson VE, Trojanowski JQ, et al. Chronic traumatic encephalopathy - confusion and controversies. Nat Rev Neurol 2019;15(3):179–83.

24. Filley CM, Arciniegas DB, Brenner LA, et al. Chronic traumatic encephalopathy: A clinical perspective. J Neuropsychiatry Clin Neurosci 2019;31(2):170–2.

25. Laffey M, Darby AJ, Cline MG, et al. The utility of clinical criteria in patients with chronic traumatic encephalopathy. NeuroRehabilitation 2018;43(4):431–41.

26. Duff K. Evidence-based indicators of neuropsychological change in the individual patient: relevant concepts and methods. Arch Clin Neuropsychol 2012; 27(3):248–61.

27. Bush SS, Ruff RM, Tröster AI, et al. Symptom validity assessment: Practice issues and medical necessity: NAN Policy & Planning Committee. Arch Clin Neuropsychol 2005;20(4):419–26.

28. Heilbronner RL, Sweet JJ, Morgan JE, et al. American Academy of Clinical Neuropsychology consensus conference statement on the neuropsychological assessment of effort, response bias, and malingering. Clin Neuropsychol 2009;23(7): 1093–129.

29. Sweet JJ, Heilbronner RL, Morgan JE, et al. American Academy of Clinical Neuropsychology (AACN) 2021 consensus statement on validity assessment: Update of the 2009 AACN consensus conference statement on neuropsychological assessment of effort, response bias, and malingering. Clin Neuropsychol 2021; 35(6):1053–106.

30. Larrabee GJ, Millis SR, Meyers JE. 40 plus or minus 10, a new magical number: Reply to Russell. Clin Neuropsychol 2009;23(5):841–9.

31. LaDuke C, Barr W, Brodale DL, et al. Toward generally accepted forensic assessment practices among clinical neuropsychologists: A survey of professional practice and common test use. Clin Neuropsychol 2018;32(1):145–64.

32. Caccese JB, Eckner JT, Franco-MacKendrick L, et al. Interpreting clinical reaction time change and recovery after concussion: a baseline versus norm-based cutoff score comparison. J Athl Train 2021;56(8):851–9.

33. Schmidt JD, Register-Mihalik JK, Mihalik JP, et al. Identifying Impairments after concussion: normative data versus individualized baselines. Med Sci Sports Exerc 2012;44(9):1621–8.

34. Cole WR, Arrieux JP, Schwab K, et al. Test–retest reliability of four computerized neurocognitive assessment tools in an active duty military population. Arch Clin Neuropsychol 2013;28(7):732–42.

35. Cole WR, Arrieux JP, Ivins BJ, et al. A comparison of four computerized neurocognitive assessment tools to a traditional neuropsychological test battery in service members with and without mild traumatic brain injury. Arch Clin Neuropsychol 2018;33(1):102–19.

36. Manderino LM, Gunstad J. Improved post-injury cognitive test results: examining invalid baseline ImPACT testing. Brain Inj 2022;36(4):572–8.

37. Messa I, Korcsog K, Abeare C. An updated review of the prevalence of invalid performance on the Immediate Post-Concussion and Cognitive Testing (ImPACT). Clin Neuropsychol 2022;36(7):1613–36.

38. Schatz P, Elbin RJ, Anderson MN, et al. Exploring sandbagging behaviors, effort, and perceived utility of the ImPACT Baseline Assessment in college athletes. Sport Exerc Perform Psychol 2017;6(3):243–51.

39. Belanger HG, Proctor-Weber Z, Kretzmer T, et al. Symptom complaints following reports of blast versus non-blast mild TBI: Does mechanism of injury matter? Clin Neuropsychol 2011;25(5):702–15.

40. Greer N, Sayer N, Koeller E, et al. Outcomes associated with blast versus nonblast-related traumatic brain injury in US military service members and veterans: A systematic review. J Head Trauma Rehabil 2018;33(2):E16–29.

41. McNally RJ, Frueh BC. Why we should worry about malingering in the VA system: Comment on Jackson et al (2011). J Trauma Stress 2012;25(4):454–6.

42. Cancelliere C, Cassidy JD, Li A, et al. Systematic search and review procedures: results of the International Collaboration on Mild Traumatic Brain Injury Prognosis. Arch Phys Med Rehabil 2014;95(3 Suppl):S101–31.

43. Cullen N, Krakowski A, Taggart C. Early neuropsychological tests as correlates of return to driving after traumatic brain injury. Brain Inj 2014;28(1):38–43.

44. Ortoleva C, Brugger C, Van der Linden M, et al. Prediction of driving capacity after traumatic brain injury: a systematic review. J Head Trauma Rehabil 2012; 27(4):302–13.

45. Cappa KA, Conger JC, Conger AJ. Injury severity and outcome: A meta-analysis of prospective studies on TBI outcome. Health Psychol 2011;30(5):542–60.

46. Dikmen SS, Corrigan JD, Levin HS, et al. Cognitive outcome following traumatic brain injury. J Head Trauma Rehabil 2009;24(6):430–8.

47. Levine B, Kovacevic N, Nica EI, et al. The Toronto traumatic brain injury study: Injury severity and quantified MRI. Neurology 2008;70(10):771–8.

48. Moro F, Pischiutta F, Portet A, et al. Ageing is associated with maladaptive immune response and worse outcome after traumatic brain injury. Brain Commun 2022;4(2):fcac036.

49. Rabinowitz AR, Li X, McCauley SR, et al. Prevalence and predictors of poor recovery from mild traumatic brain injury. J Neurotrauma 2015;32(19):1488–96.

50. Donders J, Stout J. The Influence of Cognitive Reserve on Recovery from Traumatic Brain Injury. Arch Clin Neuropsychol Off J Natl Acad Neuropsychol 2019; 34(2):206–13.

51. McCrimmon S, Oddy M. Return to work following moderate-to-severe traumatic brain injury. Brain Inj 2006;20(10):1037–46.

52. Carroll LJ, Cassidy JD, Cancelliere C, et al. Systematic review of the prognosis after mild traumatic brain injury in adults: cognitive, psychiatric, and mortality outcomes: results of the International Collaboration on Mild Traumatic Brain Injury Prognosis. Arch Phys Med Rehabil 2014;95(3 Suppl):S152–73.

53. Eapen B, Cifu DX. Concussion E-Book: assessment, management and rehabilitation. Elsevier Health Sciences; 2019.

54. Larson EB, Kondiles BR, Starr CR, et al. Postconcussive complaints, cognition, symptom attribution and effort among veterans. J Int Neuropsychol Soc 2013; 19(1):88–95.
55. Lew HL, Otis JD, Tun C, et al. Prevalence of chronic pain, posttraumatic stress disorder, and persistent postconcussive symptoms in OIF/OEF veterans: polytrauma clinical triad. J Rehabil Res Dev 2009;46(6):697–702.
56. Mooney G, Speed J, Sheppard S. Factors related to recovery after mild traumatic brain injury. Brain Inj 2005;19(12):975–87.
57. Picon EL, Perez DL, Burke MJ, et al. Unexpected symptoms after concussion: Potential links to functional neurological and somatic symptom disorders. J Psychosom Res 2021;151:110661.
58. Kalmbach DA, Conroy DA, Falk H, et al. Poor sleep is linked to impeded recovery from traumatic brain injury. Sleep 2018;41(10):zsy147.
59. Saksvik SB, Smevik H, Stenberg J, et al. Poor sleep quality is associated with greater negative consequences for cognitive control function and psychological health after mild traumatic brain injury than after orthopedic injury. Neuropsychology 2021. https://doi.org/10.1037/neu0000751.
60. Sanchez E, Blais H, Duclos C, et al. Sleep from acute to chronic traumatic brain injury and cognitive outcomes. Sleep 2022;45(8):zsac123.

Chronic Traumatic Encephalopathy

Allison Wallingford, MD[a], Cherry Junn, MD[b],*

KEYWORDS

- Chronic traumatic encephalopathy • Neurodegenerative disease • Tau
- Traumatic brain injury • Tau protein

KEY POINTS

- Chronic traumatic encephalopathy (CTE) is a tauopathy characterized by neurofibrillary tangles and disordered neurites in the presence or absence of hyperphosphorylated tau (p-tau) immunoreactive astrocytes in surrounding small blood vessels, most prominently at the depts of the cortical sulci and in an irregular pattern.
- CTE is a neurodegenerative disease associated with repetitive head impacts (RHIs) and is diagnosed conclusively through neuropathological examination.
- The clinical presentation of CTE is unclear, but behavioral, mood, cognitive, and motor changes may be associated with CTE.
- Traumatic encephalopathy syndrome (TES) criteria of research diagnosis include 1) repetitive head trauma, 2) cognitive impairment and/or neurobehavioral dysregulation, 3) progressive course, and 4) not accounted for by another condition.
- TES is a research diagnostic term and should not be used in clinical settings.

INTRODUCTION

Chronic Traumatic Encephalopathy (CTE) is a tauopathy associated with repetitive head impacts (RHIs). This progressive neurodegenerative disease is diagnosed conclusively on neuropathological examination, based on the diagnosis for criteria established by the National Institute on Neurologic Disorders and Stroke and the National Institute of Biomedical Imaging and Bioengineering.[1]

Since CTE is a postmortem diagnosis, potential clinical symptoms of CTE have been gathered through retrospective reports about the deceased individual. Consequently, it has been challenging to determine a specific, identifiable clinical disorder or constellations of symptoms associated with CTE pathology. Additionally, while

[a] Department of Rehabilitation Medicine, University of Washington, Seattle, Washington, USA; [b] Department of Rehabilitation Medicine, University of Washington, 325 Ninth Avenue Box 359740, Seattle, WA 98104, USA
* Corresponding author. Harbroview Medical Center, 325 Ninth Avenue, Box 359740, Seattle, WA 98104.
E-mail address: cjp42@uw.edu

Phys Med Rehabil Clin N Am 35 (2024) 607–618
https://doi.org/10.1016/j.pmr.2024.02.011
pmr.theclinics.com

p-tau pathology, inflammation, white matter rarefaction, and arteriolosclerosis contribute to dementia in CTE, whether they also influence the behavioral and mood symptoms in CTE has yet to be determined.[2] Thus, there is a need to identify the presence of CTE during life to enable clinical trials for treatment and prevention. This need prompted the development of diagnostic criteria for Traumatic Encephalopathy Syndrome (TES) for research. Still, more research is needed to determine the clinical presentation of CTE and if TES represents it.

The past couple of decades have seen a dramatic increase in studies characterizing CTE neuropathology and symptoms as well as helping to establish the incidence and risk among populations with RHIs. These studies helped to associate CTE diagnosis risk with repetitive concussive and asymptomatic subconcussive impacts in multiple sports, military veterans, and potentially victims of domestic violence.

Research into both CTE and TES is in its early stages. Both diagnoses are a significant concern for patients and their families. Therefore, there is a significant need to elucidate the clinical implications of CTE, which can then help determine treatment and prevention. This article describes the current growing knowledge of CTE and its limitations.

HISTORY

The first description of CTE is thought to be by Martland in 1928, whereby cognitive deterioration, emotional lability, and parkinsonism were coined as "punch-drunk" among professional boxers.[3] This constellation of impairments appeared throughout the medical literature in the 30s, 40s, and 50s by many different names, including "dementia pugilista," "traumatic encephalopathy of pugilists," and "chronic boxer's encephalopathy," among others.[4,5] Other studies have noted psychotic states in those who sustained head and brain injuries.[5] This cognitive, behavioral, mood, and motor deterioration then continued to be noted in the literature, and Critchley used the term chronic traumatic encephalopathy to describe this constellation of symptoms among sailors who were former boxers.[6]

Autopsy studies of boxers in the 70s started to note many of the pathologic features that are now recognized as characteristic of CTE, including cortical atrophy, ventricular enlargement, cavum and fenestrated septum pellucidum, thinking of the corpus callosum, substantia nigra depigmentation, cerebellar scarring, neuronal loss, gliosis, and argyrophilic neurofibrillary tangles (NFTs) in neurons of the medial temporal lobe, cortex, and brainstem.[1,7–11]

The first detailed pathology reports were published in the 1990s, noting perivascular clusters of thioflavin, NFTs, and p-tau in the depths of the cortical sulci.[2] These studies also pointed out that these argyrophilic, p-tau positive cortical NFTs were mostly notably seen around small cortical blood vessels and noted diffuse granular neuronal cytoplasmic p-tau immunopositivity.[12]

Interest in CTE among professional athletes surged after the death of Mike Webster in 2005 at the age of 50 from a myocardial infarction. Before his death, Webster had experienced a decline in memory and judgment as well as depression, parkinsonism, and dementia. Webster's diagnosis of CTE on brain autopsy[13] raised public interest in CTE. It spurred donation and examination of many more brains of deceased athletes, accelerating research and understanding of the neuropathology, mechanism, and clinical characteristics of CTE. In 2009, McKee et al. described extensive p-tau deposits in 2 former boxers and one National Football League player and compared them to other reported cases of CTE.[14] These studies helped to establish the first criteria for neuropathology of chronic traumatic encephalopathy, which were described in the preliminary

National Institute of Neurologic Disorders and Stroke and National Institute of Biomedical Imaging and Bioengineering (NINDS/NIBIB) criteria.[15]

Since then, many other sports and conditions have been associated with CTE. CTE diagnosis had been made in the cases of repetitive concussive and asymptomatic subconcussive impacts in boxing,[16] bull rider,[17] wrestling,[18] mixed martial arts, American football,[13,19] soccer,[20–22] ice-hockey,[18] rugby,[23] "head-banging" behavior,[24] and seizures.[12] More recently, CTE has also been potentially identified in military veterans exposed to blast,[25,26] victims of domestic violence,[27,28] and a female professional athlete for the first time.[29]

DEFINITION

McKee et al. in 2009 noted the irregular distribution of the NFTs along the perivascular region was noted along the depth of the sulci.[14] The authors noted that these findings were different from those of other neurodegenerative diseases such as Alzheimer's disease (AD), progressive supranuclear palsy (PSP), corticobasal degeneration (CBD), primary age-related tauopathy (PART), and argyrophilic grain disease (AGD).

Subsequently, neuropathologic criteria for diagnosing and staging CTE have evolved over the past several years to establish CTE as a unique tauopathy with similar but distinct features from other neurodegenerative tauopathies, such as Alzheimer's disease (AD). Although other neurodegenerative diseases may be present alongside CTE, it is now recognized that CTE has a distinguishable phosphorylated tau (p-tau) deposition pattern. Neuropathologic criteria have generally focused on the presence of perivascular p-tau, neuritic rather than astrocytic plaques, and NFTs in the cortical sulci.

In 2011, Omalu and colleagues broadly defined CTE criteria as 4 phenotypes based on the general frequency and distribution of NFTs and NTs.[13,19,25] Shortly after, The McKee Criteria[18] was published in 2013, defining stricter pathologic criteria for CTE based on findings of perivascular p-tau and NFTs in a cortical distribution and establishing stages of severity (**Fig. 1**). This original criterion included the presence of p-tau immunoreactive astrocytes. This criterion was later removed as age-related p-tau immunoreactive astrocytic pathology of (ARTAG) was noted.[30,31]

McKee et al. also proposed 4 pathologic stages (stages I-IV): stages I and II being milder with a few smaller NFT legions, and stages III and IV being more severe, including larger, diffuse CTE lesions and NFTs, as well as macroscopic changes.[18]

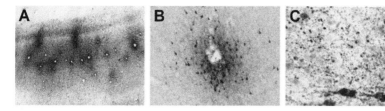

Fig. 1. The Pathognomonic lesions of CTE. The pathognomonic lesions of CTE consists of an accumulation of abnormally phosphorylated tau in neurons and astroglia distributed around small blood vessels at the depth of cortical sulci and in an irregular pattern. There are typically neurofibrillary tangles, p-tau inclusions in thorned astrocytes as well as dot-like structures in the neutropil. (*A*) Magnification X40, (*B*). Magnification X200, (*C*) Magnification X600; all images, CP-13 immunostained 50 μ tissue sections. C, counterstained with cresyl violet. (McKee AC, Alosco ML, Huber BR. Repetitive Head Impacts and Chronic Traumatic Encephalopathy. Neurosurg Clin N Am. 2016;27(4):529-535. https://doi.org/10.1016/j.nec.2016.05.009.)

The NINDS/NIBIB convened pathologists in 2015 to evaluate various cases of tauo-pathies and define preliminary consensus neuropathological criteria for CTE.[15] It was concluded that the pathognomonic lesion of CTE was "an accumulation of abnormal hyperphosphorylated tau (p-tau) in neurons and astroglia distributed around small blood vessels at the depths of cortical sulci and in an irregular pattern." This group also defined supportive that's non-p-tau related features such as disproportionate dilatation of the third ventricle, septal abnormalities, mammillary body atrophy, and contusions or other signs of previous traumatic injury (**Fig. 2**).

The second consensus panel convened in 2016 and refined the neuropathologic criteria for CTE to be that "the perivascular p-tau aggregates should include neurofi-brillary tangles, with or without astrocytes, and that the focus had to be in deeper cortical layers not restricted to subpial and superficial regions."[1] The group also sought to determine a minimum threshold for diagnosis based on a blinded review of cases of tauopathies by pathologists. Because staging by the McKee criteria proved inconsistent, this group proposed establishing a minimum threshold for CTE diagnosis based on a pathognomonic lesion and then using an algorithm for CTE severity as "low CTE" or "high CTE" based on points for NFT presence in each desig-nated region. The group asserts that this scoring system better accounts for variability in neuroanatomic patterns of CTE than the previously recommended stages.[1]

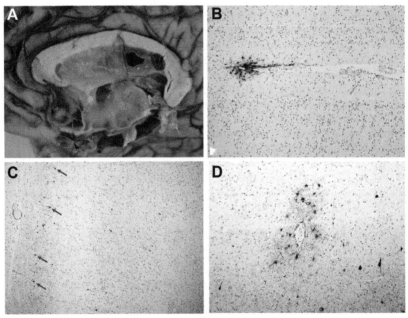

Fig. 2. Selected neuropathological features of CTE. (*A*) Mid-sagittal section of gross brain showing fenestrations in septum pellucidum. (*B*) P-tau immunoreactivity in neocortical brain tissue sample showing CTE pathognomonic lesion, defined as p-tau accumulations in neu-rons, astrocytes and cell processes distributed around small blood vessels at sulcal depths. (*C*) P-tau immunoreactivity in neocortical brain tissue sample showing NFTs (*arrows*) prefer-entially accumulating in superficial layers II-III. (*D*) Neocortical brain tissue sample showing perivascular p-tau immunoreactive neurons, astrocytes and cell processes. (Shively SB, Priemer DS, Stein MB, Perl DP. Pathophysiology of Traumatic Brain Injury, Chronic Traumatic Encephalopathy, and Neuropsychiatric Clinical Expression. Psychiatric Clinics of North Amer-ica. 2021;44(3):443-458. https://doi.org/10.1016/j.psc.2021.04.003.)

Neuropathologic descriptions of CTE have highlighted important differences between CTE and other tauopathies, including Alzheimer's Disease (AD), age-related tau astrogliopathy (ARTAG), primary age-related tauopathy (PART), supranuclear palsy (PSP), corticobasal degeneration (CBD), Guamanian parkinsonism dementia complex (GPDC), and argyrophilic grain disease (AGD). CTE is a primary tauopathy with a unique and defined pattern of p-tau pathology, characterized by the highest depositions of p-tau in the dorsolateral frontal cortex (DLF), superior temporal cortex, entorhinal cortex, amygdala, and locus coeruleus (LC).[32]

The data support CTE as a primary tauopathy. Amyloid beta (Aβ) deposition is neither a primary nor a consistent neuropathology in CTE. Nonetheless, Aβ deposition can occur with aging and is associated with the inheritance of the ApoE ε4 allele in those diagnosed with CTE.[18] Additionally, NFTs are distributed diffusely in the cortex in CTE, unlike the laminar distribution in AD.[2] Additionally, CTE can occur with comorbid neuropathologies. In one study, it was more common to have mixed or comorbid neuropathologies rather than one occurring in isolation.[33]

The other common comorbidity in older individuals is ARTAG.[2] Although initially, it was thought that p-tau immunopositive astrocytes in the subpial regions, temporal lobe white matter, and brainstem were characteristic of CTE, additional studies have demonstrated that these are part of the ARTAG instead. This clarification has been noted in the most recent NINDS criteria for CTE.[1]

Proving the existence of CTE as a distinct disease from other neurodegenerative conditions has been critical in showing CTE to be exclusively associated with a history of RHI.[2] Staging criteria for CTE have been helpful in studies demonstrating the dose-dependent relationship between RHI exposure and CTE severity.

Additional studies have examined new ways to determine the link between RHI and CTE, including the medical literature review through Bradford Hill criteria[34] and a reviews of the biomechanical properties.[35] These new studies and review of the biomechanical properties suggest potential mechanisms for tau deposition in CTE. Initial axonal injury may be a potential source of p-tau; the mechanical disruption of the axonal cytoskeleton may lead to microtubule accumulation at the site of injury leading to tau dissociation and hyperphosphorylation (**Fig. 3**).[36] These repetitive injuries lead to blood-brain barrier disruption, reduced glymphatic clearance, neuroinflammation, and neurovascular impairment, contributing to disease initiation and progression. Research into these processes and tauopathy will help elucidate the spread and propagation of the p-tau pathology in CTE.

CLINICAL SYNDROME

There has been a need to identify the presence of CTE during life. First, neuropsychological and cognitive features of CTE have been characterized based on behavior reports from family members of patients who were eventually diagnosed with CTE on autopsy. One review of the clinical presentation from family members by McKee et al.[18] described 4 progressively worsening clinical symptoms, ranging from stage I symptoms of headaches to stage IV symptoms of aggression and dementia.

Higher stages of CTE severity on the McKee criteria have been correlated with worse neurologic symptoms, higher odds of dementia, more years of football played,[37] and older age at death. The higher severity of CTE in patients with an older age of death and more years of retirement[38] has been noted and used as evidence of CTE as a progressive disease. On the other hand, CTE risk and severity have not been shown to correlate with the number of symptomatic concussions, years of education, steroid use, position played in American football, or age of first exposure to football.[2,18,39]

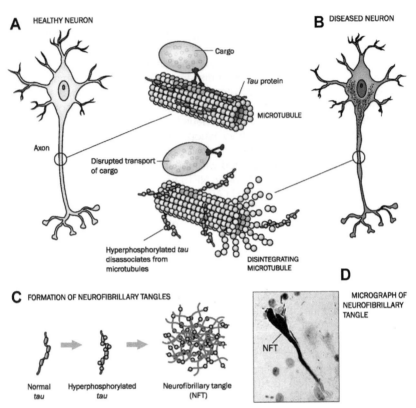

Fig. 3. (*A*) The endogenous brain protein tau normally binds microtubules within neuronal axons for stable transport of cargo with molecules necessary for cell viability and function. (*B*) In tauopathic disease (and axonal injury), tau gains phosphate groups and dissociates from microtubules, disrupting cargo transport and compromising cell function/viability. (*C*) Hyperphosphorylated tau (p-tau) forms insoluble aggregates within brain cells, including neurons (neurofibrillary tangles, NFTs). (*D*) Micrograph of p-tau immunoreactivity in a neuron (NFT). (Shively SB, Priemer DS, Stein MB, Perl DP. Pathophysiology of Traumatic Brain Injury, Chronic Traumatic Encephalopathy, and Neuropsychiatric Clinical Expression. Psychiatric Clinics of North America. 2021;44(3):443-458. https://doi.org/10.1016/j.psc.2021.04.003.)

Common clinical characteristics described in these clinical presentation studies include cognitive decline, especially decline in episodic memory and executive function, neuropsychologic symptoms, especially emotional explosivity, impulsivity, and lability.[40] Motor impairment, usually Parkinsonism,[11] is also described. Clinical presentation of CTE may have 2 different groups – younger age presenting with mood and behavior symptoms and older age with cognitive dysfunction.[40] Cognitive impairment was eventually noted in all the subjects.

A lack of accepted diagnostic and clinical criteria for CTE still needs to be addressed. In 2014, criteria were proposed for Traumatic Encephalopathy Syndrome (TES), a term used to describe the diagnosis of CTE manifestations during life for research purposes.[41] When the validity of this 2014 TES criteria for CTE pathology was conducted, it demonstrated sensitivity and specificity of 0.97 and 0.21[42] and was criticized for their lack of specificity and the need to separate neuropathology of CTE from the possible clinical features.[43]

Table 1
Neuropathologic criteria for CTE since 2011

Publication	Criteria for Diagnosis	Classification
Omalu et al,[44] 2011	The presence of sparse, moderate, or frequent band-shaped, flame-shaped, small globose, and large globose NFTs in the brain accompanied by sparse, moderate, or frequent NTs.	Four histologic phenotypes: 1. Sparse to frequent NFTs and NTs in the cerebral cortex and brainstem, ± NFTs and NTs in the subcortical nuclei/basal ganglia, no NFTs and NTs in the cerebellum, no diffuse amyloid plaques in the cerebral cortex. 2. Sparse to frequent NFTs and NTs in the cerebral cortex and brainstem, ± NFTs and NTs in the subcortical nuclei/basal ganglia, no NFTs and NTs in the cerebellum, sparse to frequent diffuse amyloid plaques in the cerebral cortex. 3. Moderate to frequent NFTs and NTs in the brainstem nuclei, none to sparse NFTs and NTs in the cerebral cortex and subcortical nuclei/brainstem nucelei, no NFTs and NTs in the cerebellum, no diffuse amyloid plaques in the cerebral cortex. 4. None to sparse NFTs and NTs in the cerebral cortex, brainstem, subcortical nuclei/basal ganglia, no NFTs and NTs in the cerebellum, no diffuse amyloid plaques in the cerebral cortex. Each phenotype may have none to sparse or moderate to frequent NFTs and NTs ± diffuse amyloid plaques in the hippocampus.
McKee et al,[18] 2013	(1) the presence of perivascular foci of p-tau NFTs and astrocytic tangles; (2) an irregular cortical distribution of p-tau NFTs and astrocytic tangles with a predilection for the depth of cerebral sulci; (3) clusters of subpial and periventricular astrocytic tangles in the cerebral cortex, diencephalon, basal ganglia, and brainstem; and (4) NFTs in the cerebral cortex located preferentially in the superficial layers	Four stages of increasing severity: Stage I – One or two isolated epicenters of NFTs and dotlike neurites arranged around small blood vessels at the depths of the sulci in the frontal, temporal, or parietal cortices. Stage II – three or more larger CTE lesions in multiple cortical regions, superficial NFTs along the sulcal wall and at gyral crests of the adjacent cortices, and more neurofibrillary pathology in the locus coeruleus and nucleus basalis of Meynert

(continued on next page)

Table 1
(continued)

Publication	Criteria for Diagnosis	Classification
NINDS/NIBIB 2015[1]	The presence of a single pathognomonic lesion, defined as "an accumulation of abnormal p-tau in neurons, astrocytes, and cell processes around small vessels in an irregular pattern at the depths of the cortical sulci," is required. Supportive neuropathologic features are also listed, such as NFTs preferentially affecting the superficial layers and p-tau pretangles and NFTs affective CA2 and CA4 of the hippocampus.	Stage III – confluent perivascular patches of p-tau immunoreactive NFTs and dotlike and threadlike neurites in the sulcal depths, NFTs in the superficial cortical laminae, and NFTs diffusely distributed in medial temporal lobe structures. Neurofibrillary degeneration of CA1, CA4 and CA2 of the hippocampus Stage IV - CTE lesions and NFTs are densely distributed throughout the cerebral cortex, diencephalon, brainstem, cerebellar dentate nucleus, and spinal cord, with neuronal loss and gliosis in the frontal and temporal cortices and astrocytic p-tau pathology
NINDS/NIBIB 2021[1]	A pathognomonic lesion consists of p-tau aggregates in neurons, with or without glial tau in TSA, at the depth of a cortical sulcus around a small blood vessel, in deeper cortical layers not restricted to subpial and superficial region of the sulcus.	Staging the level of severity is based on a points system (out of 10 points max): 1 point is given for the presence of NFTs in the bank or crest of the gyrus each count. NFTs in the superficial cortical laminae (often most prominent in the temporal lobe) also count as 1 point. 1 point is given for the presence of NFTs in CA1 and CA4 of the hippocampus, entorhinal cortex, amygdala, thalamus, mamillary body, and cerebellar dentate nucleus. Cases with < 5 points are designated as "low" CTE and cases with ≥ 5 points are designated as "high" CTE.

Detailed pathologic criteria for CTE published by different research groups. Omalu et al characterized histologic phenotypes but did not identify different levels of severity correlating to different patterns. Later criteria by the McKee group and NINDS created systems of grading severity based on pathologic findings.

Abbreviations: CTE, chronic traumatic encephalopathy; NFT, neurofibrillary tangles; NT, neuropil threads; TSA, throne-shaped astrocytes.

Subsequently, the National Institute of Neurologic Disorders and Stroke (NINDS) proposed new criteria in 2019 for TES, requiring (1) substantial exposure to RHIs, (2) core clinical features of cognitive impairment (in episodic memory and/or executive functioning) and/or neurobehavioral dysregulation, (3) progressive course; and (4) presentation not fully accounted for by other disorders (**Table 1**).[45] Once these criteria are met for TES, then the level of functional dependence is graded on 5 levels, ranging from independent to dementia. Lastly, a provisional level of certainty for CTE pathology is determined based on specific RHI exposure thresholds, core clinical features, functional status, and additional supportive features, including delayed onset, motor signs, and psychiatric features. TES remains a separate diagnosis from CTE, and the hope is that biomarkers will be identified to aid the diagnosis of CTE during life.

This updated NINDS criteria attempted to improve the previous criteria's specificity by excluding some nonspecific features of TES, such as depression, anxiety, and headache. However, it continues to have limitations in the definition of "substantial repetitive head trauma" and lacks objective diagnostic criteria for "neurobehavioral dysregulation."[46] As updated clinical and pathologic information and in vivo biomarkers become available, these criteria will be revised.

DISCUSSION

CTE is a unique neurodegenerative disease that is progressive and associated with RHIs; definitive diagnosis is made only through autopsy. TES has been defined to help with CTE research and will need continued research to determine the specific clinical presentation and course of CTE. Understanding risk factors that affect CTE's clinical and pathologic development is needed to provide targeted treatment for this population.

SUMMARY

CTE is a neurodegenerative disease characterized by primary tauopathy with a pathognomonic deposit pattern in neurofibrillary tangles, neurites, and astrocytes surrounding small blood vessels at the sulcal depths of the cerebral cortex. It is only diagnosed conclusively by a neuropathological examination of brain tissue, creating a need to determine clinical symptoms to help with research and treatment. TES is a diagnostic term to help guide current CTE research. CTE neuropathology and neurobehavioral symptoms need additional research to determine whether TES represents a unique clinical syndrome of CTE to identify CTE in life for prevention and treatment.

CLINICS CARE POINTS

- CTE is diagnosed conclusively by a neuropathological examination and should not be given as a diagnosis to a patient without one. Thus, it is not possible to diagnose CTE during life.
- TES is for research purposes and should not be used in clinical settings.
- Patients should be evaluated and treated for relevant and/or treatable conditions such as sleep disorders or cardiovascular diseases.
- Patients should be evaluated and treated for neurobehavioral dysregulation and other symptoms associated with CTE.
- Emphasis should be placed on improving quality of life, providing appropriate treatment for symptoms, and counseling on appropriate lifestyle changes that are helpful in other neurodegenerative diseases.

DISCLOSURE

None.

REFERENCES

1. Bieniek KF, Cairns NJ, Crary JF, et al. The Second NINDS/NIBIB Consensus Meeting to Define Neuropathological Criteria for the Diagnosis of Chronic Traumatic Encephalopathy. J Neuropathol Exp Neurol 2021;80(3):210–9.
2. McKee AC. The Neuropathology of Chronic Traumatic Encephalopathy: The Status of the Literature. Semin Neurol 2020;40(4):359–69.
3. Martland HS. Punch drunk. J Am Med Assoc 1928;91(15):1103.
4. Montenigro PH, Corp DT, Stein TD, et al. Chronic traumatic encephalopathy: historical origins and current perspective. Annu Rev Clin Psychol 2015;11(1): 309–30.
5. Bowman KM, Blau A. Psychotic states following head and brain injury in adults and children. In: Brock S, editor. Injuries of the skull, brain and spinal cord: neuro-psychiatric, surgical, and medico-legal aspects. Washington, DC: Williams & Wilkins Co; 1940. p. 309–60.
6. Critchley M. Medical aspects of boxing, particularly from a neurological standpoint. BMJ 1957;1(5015):357–62.
7. Payne E. Brains of boxers. Minim Invasive Neurosurg 1968;11(05):173–88.
8. Mawdsley C, Ferguson FR. Neurological disease in boxers. Lancet 1963; 282(7312):795–801.
9. Spillane JD. Five Boxers. BMJ 1962;2(5314):1205–12.
10. Neubuerger KT, Sinton D, Denst J. Cerebral atrophy associated with boxing. Arch Neurol Psychiatr 1959;81(4):403.
11. Corsellis JAN, Bruton CJ, Freeman-Browne D. The aftermath of boxing. Psychol Med 1973;3(3):270–303.
12. Geddes JF, Vowles GH, Nicoll JAR, et al. Neuronal cytoskeletal changes are an early consequence of repetitive head injury. Acta Neuropathol 1999;98(2):171–8.
13. Omalu BI, DeKosky ST, Minster RL, et al. Chronic Traumatic Encephalopathy in a National Football League Player. Neurosurgery 2005;57(1):128–34.
14. McKee AC, Cantu RC, Nowinski CJ, et al. Chronic traumatic encephalopathy in athletes: progressive tauopathy after repetitive head injury. J Neuropathol Exp Neurol 2009;68(7):709–35.
15. McKee AC, Cairns NJ, Dickson DW, et al. The first NINDS/NIBIB consensus meeting to define neuropathological criteria for the diagnosis of chronic traumatic encephalopathy. Acta Neuropathol 2016;131(1):75–86.
16. Goldfinger MH, Ling H, Tilley BS, et al. The aftermath of boxing revisited: identifying chronic traumatic encephalopathy pathology in the original Corsellis boxer series. Acta Neuropathol 2018;136(6):973–4.
17. Keene CD, Latimer CS, Steele LM, et al. First confirmed case of chronic traumatic encephalopathy in a professional bull rider. Acta Neuropathol 2018;135(2):303–5.
18. McKee AC, Stein TD, Nowinski CJ, et al. The spectrum of disease in chronic traumatic encephalopathy. Brain 2013;136(1):43–64.
19. Omalu BI, DeKosky ST, Hamilton RL, et al. Chronic Traumatic Encephalopathy in a National Football League Player: part II. Neurosurgery 2006;59(5):1086–93.
20. Ling H, Morris HR, Neal JW, et al. Mixed pathologies including chronic traumatic encephalopathy account for dementia in retired association football (soccer) players. Acta Neuropathol 2017;133(3):337–52.

21. Lee EB, Kinch K, Johnson VE, et al. Chronic traumatic encephalopathy is a common co-morbidity, but less frequent primary dementia in former soccer and rugby players. Acta Neuropathol 2019;138(3):389–99.
22. McKee AC, Daneshvar DH, Alvarez VE, et al. The neuropathology of sport. Acta Neuropathol 2014;127(1):29–51.
23. Buckland ME, Sy J, Szentmariay I, et al. Correction to: Chronic traumatic encephalopathy in two former Australian National Rugby League players. Acta Neuropathol Commun 2019;7(1):122.
24. Hof PR, Knabe R, Bovier P, et al. Neuropathological observations in a case of autism presenting with self-injury behavior. Acta Neuropathol 1991;82(4):321–6.
25. Omalu B, Hammers JL, Bailes J, et al. Chronic traumatic encephalopathy in an Iraqi war veteran with posttraumatic stress disorder who committed suicide. Neurosurg Focus 2011;31(5):E3.
26. Goldstein LE, Fisher AM, Tagge CA, et al. Chronic traumatic encephalopathy in blast-exposed military veterans and a blast neurotrauma mouse model. Sci Transl Med 2012;4(134).
27. Costello K, Greenwald BD. Update on domestic violence and traumatic brain injury: a narrative review. Brain Sci 2022;12(1).
28. Danielsen T, Hauch C, Kelly L, et al. Chronic Traumatic Encephalopathy (CTE)-Type Neuropathology in a Young Victim of Domestic Abuse. J Neuropathol Exp Neurol 2021;80(6):624–7.
29. Suter CM, Affleck AJ, Pearce AJ, et al. Chronic traumatic encephalopathy in a female ex-professional Australian rules footballer. Acta Neuropathol 2023;146(3):547–9.
30. Kovacs GG, Milenkovic I, Wöhrer A, et al. Non-Alzheimer neurodegenerative pathologies and their combinations are more frequent than commonly believed in the elderly brain: a community-based autopsy series. Acta Neuropathol 2013;126(3):365–84.
31. Kovacs GG, Molnár K, László L, et al. A peculiar constellation of tau pathology defines a subset of dementia in the elderly. Acta Neuropathol 2011;122(2):205–22.
32. Alosco ML, Cherry JD, Huber BR, et al. Characterizing tau deposition in chronic traumatic encephalopathy (CTE): utility of the McKee CTE staging scheme. Acta Neuropathol 2020;140(4):495–512.
33. Boyle PA, Yu L, Wilson RS, et al. Person-specific contribution of neuropathologies to cognitive loss in old age. Ann Neurol 2018;83(1):74–83.
34. Nowinski CJ, Bureau SC, Buckland ME, et al. Applying the Bradford Hill Criteria for Causation to Repetitive Head Impacts and Chronic Traumatic Encephalopathy. Front Neurol 2022;13. https://doi.org/10.3389/fneur.2022.938163.
35. Cherry JD, Babcock KJ, Goldstein LE. Repetitive Head Trauma Induces Chronic Traumatic Encephalopathy by Multiple Mechanisms. Semin Neurol 2020;40(4):430–8.
36. Shively SB, Priemer DS, Stein MB, et al. Pathophysiology of Traumatic Brain Injury, Chronic Traumatic Encephalopathy, and Neuropsychiatric Clinical Expression. Psychiatr Clin 2021;44(3):443–58.
37. Mez J, Daneshvar DH, Abdolmohammadi B, et al. Duration of American Football Play and Chronic Traumatic Encephalopathy. Ann Neurol 2020;87(1):116–31.
38. Mez J, Daneshvar DH, Kiernan PT, et al. Clinicopathological Evaluation of Chronic Traumatic Encephalopathy in Players of American Football. JAMA 2017;318(4):360.
39. Alosco ML, Mez J, Tripodis Y, et al. Age of first exposure to tackle football and chronic traumatic encephalopathy. Ann Neurol 2018;83(5):886–901.

40. Stern RA, Daneshvar DH, Baugh CM, et al. Clinical presentation of chronic traumatic encephalopathy. Neurology 2013;81(13):1122–9.
41. Montenigro PH, Baugh CM, Daneshvar DH, et al. Clinical subtypes of chronic traumatic encephalopathy: Literature review and proposed research diagnostic criteria for traumatic encephalopathy syndrome. Alzheimer's Res Ther 2014;6(5–8).
42. Mez J, Alosco ML, Daneshvar DH, et al. Validity of the 2014 traumatic encephalopathy syndrome criteria for CTE pathology. Alzheimer's Dementia 2021;17(10):1709–24.
43. Iverson GL, Keene CD, Perry G, et al. The Need to Separate Chronic Traumatic Encephalopathy Neuropathology from Clinical Features. J Alzheim Dis 2017;61(1):17–28.
44. Omalu B, Bailes J, Hamilton RL, et al. Emerging Histomorphologic Phenotypes of Chronic Traumatic Encephalopathy in American Athletes. Neurosurgery 2011;69(1):173–83.
45. Katz DI, Bernick C, Dodick DW, et al. National Institute of Neurological Disorders and Stroke Consensus Diagnostic Criteria for Traumatic Encephalopathy Syndrome. Neurology 2021;96(18):848–63.
46. Cullum CM, LoBue C. Defining traumatic encephalopathy syndrome — advances and challenges. Nat Rev Neurol 2021;17(6):331–2.

Neuropharmacology in Traumatic Brain Injury

Gabriel Sanchez, DO[a], Merideth Byl, DO, MBA[a],
Quynh Giao Pham, MD[b,c], Blessen C. Eapen, MD[d,e],*

KEYWORDS

- Traumatic injury • TBI • Head injury • Drug therapy • Medication • Pharmacology

KEY POINTS

- Evidence supporting pharmacologic management for post-traumatic agitation is limited but consensus recommendations do exist and are often geared toward targeting symptoms.
- The primary goals in TBI treatment is to minimize secondary brain damage and promote neuroprotection but many pharmacological treatments for related symptoms have adverse side effects, potentially delaying recovery.
- Post-traumatic headache (PTH) is one of the most common complaints following TBI of any severity ,Headache subtypes are not always clear-cut and treatment should be multi-disciplinary with pharmacologic management dictated by the closest clinical phenotype that the patient's clinical features.

INTRODUCTION

Traumatic brain injury (TBI) is a complex condition that occurs when an external force disrupts the normal functioning of the brain. It is a major source of disability worldwide, with a staggering incidence estimated at 27 to 69 million and prevalence estimated at 55.5 million annually.[1] In the United States, the Global Burden of Disease study estimates a TBI incidence of 1.1 million and prevalence of 2.3 million in 2016.[2] However, these figures likely underestimate the occurrence of TBIs as they do not account for those persons who did not receive medical care, had outpatient visits, or those who received care at a federal facility (ie, active US military or veterans).

TBI is a serious injury that can have a devastating and lasting impact on individuals and their families. Some studies have estimated that 3.2 to 5.3 million persons in the

[a] Physical Medicine & Rehabilitation Residency Program, Greater Los Angeles VA Healthcare System, 11301 Wilshire Boulevard, Los Angeles, CA 90073, USA; [b] Division of Physical Medicine and Rehabilitation, Department of Medicine, David Geffen School of Medicine at UCLA; [c] Physical Medicine & Rehabilitation Residency Program, Greater Los Angeles VA Healthcare System, David Geffen School of Medicine at UCLA; [d] Division of Physical Medicine and Rehabilitation, University of California, Los Angeles (UCLA); [e] Physical Medicine and Rehabilitation Service, VA Greater Los Angeles Healthcare System; David Geffen School of Medicine at UCLA
* Corresponding author.
E-mail address: Blessen.Eapen2@va.gov

Phys Med Rehabil Clin N Am 35 (2024) 619–636
https://doi.org/10.1016/j.pmr.2024.02.001
1047-9651/24/© 2024 Elsevier Inc. All rights reserved.

United States are living with a TBI-related disability[3,4] and globally some staggering 8.1 million years of living with disability.[1] Common symptoms of TBI include cognitive difficulties, headaches, dizziness, memory problems, fatigue and sleep disturbances, mood disturbances, seizures, and sensory disturbances. In this article, we review the latest research and guidelines in pharmacologic management of TBI-related seque-lae.(**Table 1**)

DISORDERS OF CONSCIOUSNESS: HYPOAROUSAL STATE

Disorders of consciousness (DoCs) are characterized by changes in arousal and awareness commonly due to TBI, cardiac arrest, intracerebral hemorrhage, and ischemic stroke. DoCs are caused by direct damage to the neural systems that control arousal and awareness or by indirect damage to connections between these systems. Arousal refers to a state of wakefulness that can range from extreme hypoarousal (ie, coma) to hyperarousal (ie, manic excitement). This section focuses on discussing hypoarousal with respect to DoC, whereas hyperarousal or agitation will be discussed in later section.

Our current understanding of the neurochemistry of arousal systems suggests that glutamate-modulating, catecholamine-augmenting, and/or procholinergic agents may be useful treatments for hypoarousal disorders.[5] Currently, amantadine—a noncompetitive N-methyl-D-aspartate (NMDA) antagonist that also indirectly facilitates dopaminergic function—is regarded as the first-line treatment of DoC after TBI.[6] A placebo-controlled study of 184 inpatient rehabilitation patients who were in a vegetative or minimally conscious state 4 to 6 weeks after TBI found that recovery was significantly faster in the amantadine group compared to placebo.[7] Thus, it was concluded that amantadine sped up the rate of functional improvement during active treatment in patients with post-traumatic DoC.[7] Other studies have shown amantadine to improve cognition, specifically with respect to attention, concentration, processing time, initiation, orientation, sequencing, verbalization, and participation.[8]

There are also few reports describing improvements in patients with DoC in response to other neurochemistry-altering agents including bromocriptine,[9] levodopa,[10] pramipexole,[10] methylphenidate,[11] lamotrigine,[12] modafinil,[13] and zolpidem.[14] Although the evidence supporting the use of these other agents remains limited, the improvements in patients with DoC warrant further research into the application of these medications. Regardless, these medications can be considered as treatment options in case amantadine is ineffective or when side-effects are intolerable.

AGITATION: HYPERAROUSAL STATE

The TRIUMPH TBI guidelines define agitation as a subtype of delirium which occurs during a period of post-traumatic amnesia characterized by excess of behavior that includes some combination of aggression, disinhibition, akathisia, and emotional lability.[15] Evidence supporting pharmacologic management for post-traumatic agitation is limited as most studies lack the methodological rigor necessary to support standardized treatment. However, consensus recommendations do exist and are often geared toward targeting symptoms.

For treatment of acute agitation, antipsychotics can also be considered, although certain antipsychotics are more favorable than others in the TBI population. The first-generation antipsychotics have been shown to slow cognitive recovery and slow motor recovery[16] and are associated with a longer period of post-traumatic amnesia.[17] As such, these typical antipsychotics should generally be avoided in the TBI population. The second-generation or atypical antipsychotics are better tolerated

Table 1
Medications in traumatic brain injury[15,36,69-71]

Disorders	Drugs	Classification	Dosing (Parenteral Route Unless Noted)	Comments
Disorders of consciousness: hypoarousal state	Amantadine	Noncompetitive NMDA antagonist; dopaminergic stimulant	50–400 mg/day in divided doses	Positive effect on cognition; can lower seizure threshold. Avoid during nighttime due to insomnia risk
	Bromocriptine	Dopamine D2 agonist	1.25–2.25 mg bid	Second line— limited evidence of efficacy
	Levodopa	Dopamine precursor	100–200 mg daily	
	Pramipexole	Dopaminergic agent	0.375 mg daily to max 4.5 mg daily	
	Methylphenidate	Norepinephrine and dopamine reuptake inhibitor	5–20 mg tid/bid	
	Lamotrigine	Anticonvulsant	60 mg/day max	
	Modafinil	CNS stimulant	100–400 mg daily	
	Zolpidem	Sedative hypnotics	5–12.5 mg daily	
Disorders of consciousness: agitation	Propranolol	Nonselective beta-blockers	40–60 mg/day divided dose (bid/qid)	Preventive treatment; highly lipophilic; may cause hypotension and bradycardia
	Amantadine	Noncompetitive NMDA antagonist	100 mg bid (daytime)	Used in acute or chronic TBI agitation by improving cognition. Can lower seizure threshold
	Valproic acid	Anticonvulsant	250 mg tid with target of 1000–2500 mg daily	First-line preventive treatment; limited by gradual titration
	Carbamazepine	Anticonvulsant	300–400 mg/day	Rapid onset but high side effects limited its use

(continued on next page)

Table 1
(continued)

Disorders	Drugs	Classification	Dosing (*Parenteral Route Unless Noted*)	Comments
	Levetiracetam	Anticonvulsant	500–1500 mg bid	Baseline prevention for agitated behavior and seizure prophylaxis
	Olanzapine	Atypical antipsychotic	10 mg IM once, then 2.5–10 mg q2h if needed	Control acute agitation; can cause QT prolongation
	Quetiapine	Atypical antipsychotic	25–300 mg divided dose	Control acute agitation; reduce irritability and aggression
	Lorazepam	Benzodiazepine	4 mg IV (2 mg/min); repeat q 10–15 min if needed max 8 mg	Rapid resolution of violent agitation: caution use of benzodiazepines due to paradoxic or rebound response
	Tizanidine	Central alpha-2-adrenergic receptor agonist	2 mg q6–8 h as needed; max 3 dose/24 h	Acute agitation and controlling spasticity.
Seizure	Phenytoin	Anticonvulsant	15–20 mg/kg IV load → 100 mg tid × 7d	Use for 7 d after TBI drug of choice due to minimal sedation
	Levetiracetam	Anticonvulsant	1000 mg IV load, then 500 mg iv/po × 7d	Use for 7 d after TBI
PSH	Propranolol	Noncardio selective beta-blocker	10 mg tid	Drug of choice; penetrate bb barrier due to High lipophilicity
	Gabapentin	Anticonvulsant (acts at α2δ subunit of voltage-gated Ca^{++}channel)	100–300 mg tid;	Preventive
	Clonidine	Antihypertensive (central α2-adrenergic receptor agonist)	0.1–0.3 mg tid	Abortive, may cause hypotension
	Bromocriptine	Dopamine agonist	5–10 mg bid to tid	May cause hypertension and dyskinesia

Dantrolene	Antispasmodic (sarcoplasmic reticulum Ca^{++} inhibitor)	25 mg daily po	Abortive; side effects of severe hepatotoxicity
Baclofen	Antispasmodic (gamma-aminobutyric Acid B [GABAB] agonist)	5 mg tid to max 80 mg/day	Preventive, can cause sedation
Morphine	Opiate	1–10 mg IV q3–6 h	May help in acute PSH episodes refractory to other meds
Post-traumatic headaches			
Aspirin/acetaminophen	Nonopioid analgesics	Standard dosing	For mild-to-moderate headache
Ibuprofen; diclofenac	NSAIDs	Standard dosing	Acute migraine; more effective when combined with acetaminophen and caffeine
Sumatriptan; almotriptan; eletriptan; frovatriptan; naratriptan; rizatriptan; zolmitriptan	Triptans	Standard dosing	Migraine abortive therapy; avoid in cardiovascular or cerebrovascular disease
Fremanezumab; galcanezumab; eptinezumab	CGRP antagonist	Standard dosing	Migraine abortive therapy for those whose triptans was ineffective or contraindicated.
Onabotulinum toxin A	Botulinum toxin	100–155 unit to muscles of the face and neck	Migraine prophylaxis
Topiramate	Anticonvulsant	25 mg once daily (qd) titrating to 50 mg twice daily (bid)	Migraine prophylaxis; may slow neurologic recovery
Carbamazepine	Anticonvulsant	200–400 mg in 2–4 divided doses	For trigeminal neuralgia caution in syndrome of inappropriate antidiuretic hormone (SIADH), monitor for Stevens–Johnson syndrome

(continued on next page)

Table 1
(continued)

Disorders	Drugs	Classification	Dosing (Parenteral Route Unless Noted)	Comments
Spasticity	Baclofen	Antispasmodic (GABAB agonist)	5–20 mg tid; max 80 mg/day	Intrathecal route is superior to oral route; sedative effect may affect cognitive function.
	Tizanidine	Antispasmodic (alpha-2 agonist)	5 mg tid to maximum (max) 80 mg/day	May have negative cognitive effect
	Botulinum toxin A	Botulinum toxin	Dose variable IM injection	Use for selected muscle group
Sleep–wake disturbance: hypersomnolence	Modafinil	CNS stimulant	100–400 mg daily	Promote wakefulness
	Methylphenidate	CNS stimulant (norepinephrine and dopamine reuptake inhibitor)	5–20 mg three times a day (tid)/bid	Caution of effect on sleep–wake cycle
Insomnia	Melatonin	Natural supplement	1 mg bedtime (qhs) (max 10 mg)	Effect on circadian rhythm
	Quetiapine	Atypical antipsychotic	25–200 mg/day	Sedating effect; limited study for treatment of insomnia.
	Trazadone	Antidepressant SSRI	50–100 mg qhs	Help regulate sleep–wake cycle; sedating effect
Post-TBI fatigue	Methylphenidate	Neurostimulant (mixed dopamine and noradrenergic reuptake inhibitor)	5–20 mg tid/bid	Avoid evening dosing.
	Melatonin	Natural supplement	1 mg qhs (max 10 mg)	May improve sleep-related fatigue

Category	Drug	Class	Dosing	Comments
Memory and cognitive slowing	Methylphenidate	Neurostimulant	5–20 mg tid/bid	Improve attention and processing speeds.
	Amantadine	Noncompetitive NMDA antagonist; dopaminergic stimulant	50–400 mg/day in divided doses	Stimulate dopamine release; some efficacies in treating TBI cognitive symptoms; caution use in agitated patients
	Donepezil	Cholinesterase inhibitor	5–10 mg/day	May improve cognitive function; limited evidence.
	Rivastigmine; galantamine; physostigmine	Cholinesterase inhibitor	Standard dosing	Generally well tolerated
Anxiety and/depression	Sertraline Venlafaxine	SSRI	100 mg qd 37.5–75 mg bid to tid (max 225 mg/day)	First-line therapy; watch for serotonin syndrome, QTc prolongation
	Duloxetine		40–60 mg bid to qid (max 420 mg/day)	
	Citalopram		40 mg/day	Less activating
	Buspirone	Antianxiety	5–20 mg TID	Preferred anxiolytic; no significant adverse cognitive effect; delayed therapeutic action

and can be considered as practical alternatives for as-needed management of TBI agitation. Olanzapine has been shown to be effective in treating acute agitation.[18] Low doses can be given at frequent intervals until the agitated behavior abates, and repeated dosing to the point of sedation may be required. Additionally, the administration of quetiapine has been shown effective in reducing irritability and aggression resulting from TBI.[19] Quetiapine can be timed for when the patient is known to be agitated. Use caution in patients with cardiac comorbidities as atypical antipsychotics are associated with QT prolongation.

For baseline agitation prevention, evidence suggests that beta-blockers are the most effective.[20] Propranolol, a lipho-philic beta-blocker, has been studied most extensively based on the theory that higher lipophilicity permits greater central nervous system effects. One randomized control trial that compared propranolol to placebo showed that propranolol had a significant effect in reducing the intensity of agitation and reducing the need for physical restraints.[21] Other studies showed that propranolol improved restlessness and disinhibition without adverse effect on motor recovery.[22] The most common adverse effects are hypotension and bradycardia, whereas some experience lethargy and depression.

Anticonvulsants have also been shown to reduce TBI-related agitation with minimal sedative effect. These may be a good choice in patients who have additional indications such as post-traumatic epilepsy. Expert consensus recommends valproic acid and carbamazepine as the first-line agents to treat agitation, aggressiveness, anger, and irritability after TBI.[23,24] Valproic acid has the most evidence in TBI populations supporting a rapid onset of effect on target symptoms with few adverse effects on cognition.[25] Carbamazepine has also been shown to be efficacious, but its extensive side effect profile and risk for toxicity complicate its use.

Amantadine was discussed previously in the treatment of hypoarousal disorders as it can be used as a wakefulness-promoting agent for having a positive effect on cognition. Some studies have also shown amantadine is effective in treatment of acute or chronic TBI agitation through improving cognition. Amantadine can be considered for treatment in TBI agitation, especially in the presence of additional target symptoms such as cognitive deficits or reduced alertness. Nighttime dosing should generally be avoided due to potential risk for insomnia. Caution use in those with seizure history or at risk for increased intracranial pressure as the medication can potentially lower seizure threshold.

Other medications that are not only effective in treating agitation but also target separate indications in the TBI population include selective serotonin reuptake inhibitors (SSRIs), tizanidine, and levetiracetam. Specific SSRIs which have a favorable effect on behavior and anger are citalopram, escitalopram, and fluoxetine.[26] SSRIs are often used concurrently after TBI for adjustment or organic depression. Tizanidine, a central alpha-2-adrenergic receptor agonist, can be effective for as-needed medication to treat acute agitation and also useful for concurrent spasticity. Levetiracetam commonly used in the TBI population for seizure prophylaxis or control can also be effective in providing baseline prevention for agitated behaviors.

SEIZURES

Several potential mechanisms for TBI etiologies have been identified, including axonal injury, apoptosis, microhemorrhage, demyelination, microgliosis, generalized inflammation, and oxidative stress. These early phases of injury lead to various types of remodeling and potential neurocircuitry changes that can ultimately cause epilepsy. Prophylactic treatment remains challenging. While certain antiepileptic drugs (AEDs) show promise in reducing early seizures after TBI, they have limited efficacy in preventing late seizures or reducing mortality.

Currently, AEDs are approved for use during the first 7 days after TBI. Phenytoin is the anticonvulsant of choice for its minimal sedation effect and availability in intravenous (IV) formulation.[27] Levetiracetam is also a reasonable alternative. Studies have shown beneficial treatment effects of phenytoin and levetiracetam in reducing early seizure incidence.[28,29] After the initial 7 days, these medications should be discontinued due to potential side effects and the lack of evidence supporting prolonged use. No significant benefit has been found for antiepileptic prophylaxis for late seizures.[28,29]

PAROXYSMAL SYMPATHETIC HYPERACTIVITY

Paroxysmal sympathetic hyperactivity (PSH) is a phenomenon that can occur after any brain lesion, but most notably reported as high as 80% of cases following TBI.[30] Common associated symptoms include hyperthermia, hypertension, tachycardia, tachypnea, diaphoresis, dystonia, and even motor symptoms such as posturing. Although the pathophysiology is not yet completely understood, most researchers agree that PSH is driven by a loss of inhibition on the sympathetic nervous system after TBI. The severity of TBI seems to have a direct correlation with the likelihood of developing PSH. Additionally, PSH tends to be more prevalent in younger male patients who sustain more severe TBI. Researchers have found a specific association between PSH and direct injury in the splenium of the corpus callosum and posterior limb of the internal capsule.[30]

When managing PSH, the primary goal is symptomatic management.[31] This often includes reducing fevers, managing cardiovascular symptoms such as tachycardia and hypertension, and treating spasticity.[31] The drug of choice for prevention of PSH is propranolol, which is known for its higher lipophilicity and better penetration of the blood–brain barrier. However, adrenergic drugs should be avoided in the presence of hypotension for their effect on lowering blood pressure. These drugs may also lead to decreased alertness, cognition, and have been linked to the development of depression.[32] Other medications that are helpful in management include gabapentin, clonidine, bromocriptine, dantrolene, baclofen, and morphine.[30] Careful monitoring and consideration of various medication side effects are necessary to ensure optimal management and minimize potential adverse effects on cognition and mental function.

PAIN

Acute and chronic pain are prevalent in the TBI population with headaches being one of the most common complaints after TBI.[33] The pain can either be a direct consequence of TBI or secondary to other physical injuries sustained during the traumatic event. As such, pain medications are commonly prescribed to TBI patients, with opioids having the highest odds for new prescription after hospitalization for TBI.[34] Premorbid substance abuse is a significant risk factor for TBI. Thus, practitioners must weigh the risks of potential medication misuse from the benefit of pain relief. Research has estimated that 10% to 20% of people with TBI develop new-onset substance use after injury.[35] Practitioners must also consider concurrent prescriptions with other psychotropic medications and how they interact with opioids. Medications that potentially alter cognition or any other aspect of neurologic status should be used with caution.

Currently, there are no standard guidelines for treatment of pain specific to the TBI population. Good clinical practice includes identifying and treating the primary pain generators, rather than treating the symptom of pain alone. In acute TBI pain, the primary pain generators more likely involve fractures, visceral injuries, peripheral nerve injuries, and postsurgical pain.[36] On the other hand, common chronic pain generators include spasticity, hypertonicity, contracture, myofascial pain, fibromyalgia, complex regional pain syndrome, dystonia, central pain, central sensitization, chronic fracture pain, and craniofacial neuralgias.[36]

Pain medicines to consider in post-TBI pain syndromes can be categorized depending on the levels of severity. Mild pain medicines to consider include aspirin, acetaminophen, and nonsteroidal anti-inflammatory drugs (NSAIDs). Moderate pain may require stronger prescriptions with consideration for high-dose aspirin or acetaminophen, oral or injectable NSAIDs, mixed opiate analgesics with aspirin or acetaminophen, and tramadol. For severe pain, medications to consider include parenteral opioids, partial agonist opioids, antidepressants, and anticonvulsants.

POST-TRAUMATIC HEADACHE

Post-traumatic headache (PTH) is one of the most common complaints following TBI of any severity with rates ranging from 57% to 80%.[37] The most common clinical presentations of PTH are migraine-like or tension-type headaches.[36] PTH can be especially difficult to treat given concomitant cognitive, physical, and emotional problems often present after TBI. Headache subtypes are not always clear-cut, and it is not uncommon for characteristics to overlap. Thus, pharmacologic management should be dictated by the closest clinical phenotype that the patient's clinical features resemble most, and treatment should incorporate multiple modalities.

For PTH with migraine characteristics, the treatment plan can include abortive and prophylactic therapies. Some abortive medications to consider include NSAIDs, selective serotonin receptor agonists (-triptans), and calcitonin gene-related peptide (CGRP) antagonists (-gepants). The US Headache Consortium recommends aspirin, naproxen, ibuprofen, and diclofenac-K for oral treatment of migraines.[36] NSAIDs are shown to be more effective than placebo for acute migraines, but not more effective than combination aspirin, acetaminophen, and caffeine.[38,39] Combination aspirin, acetaminophen, and caffeine are preferred over ibuprofen in acute migraines. Intramuscular ketorolac can also be considered if parenteral administration is required.

The US Headache Consortium also recommends several triptans for abortive treatment of acute migraines.[40] Triptans are selective serotonin agonists at 5-hydroxytryltmine 1B/1D (5-HT 1D/1B) receptors. These serotonin receptors are found on intracranial blood vessels and sensory nerves of the trigeminal system. Activation at these receptors causes vasoconstriction and reduces inflammation.[36] Given vasoconstrictive effects, triptans are contraindicated in those with a significant history of coronary or cerebrovascular disease. Prescribe cautiously in the TBI population for greater risk of stroke, especially in the presence of vascular injuries.

A landmark study in 2004 using CGRP antagonist for migraine abortion launched CGRP into prominence as a causative factor in migraine pathophysiology.[41] CGRP has been implicated in the pathophysiology of headache through meningeal vasodilation. CGRP antagonists (-gepants) inhibit this pathway without producing vasoconstrictive effects. Thus, they may be beneficial for those who failed triptans or those in whom triptans are contraindicated. Botulinum toxin injections have also become increasingly popular as treatment of migraine prophylaxis. Phase III PREEMPT trial showed that onabotulinum toxin A is an effective prophylactic treatment against migraine and even in treatment of chronic tension-type headaches.[42]

Certain prophylactic agents are associated with side effects that can be problematic in TBI patients. For example, tricyclic Antidepressant (TCAs) have historically been used first-line as prophylaxis for chronic tension-type headaches. However, TCAs have also been shown to lower seizure threshold which can be catastrophic in this high-risk population. Additionally, anticonvulsants such as topiramate have shown efficacy in preventing migraines. However, topiramate has also been shown to produce significant cognitive impairments which could theoretically slow neurologic recovery in patients healing from TBI.

In craniofacial neuralgias, TCAs, SSRIs, serotonin-norepinephrine reuptake inhibitors (SNRIs), and anticonvulsants have been found useful. TCAs should generally be used with caution as described earlier. Carbamazepine is an anticonvulsant that has historically been considered first-line treatment of trigeminal neuralgia. Caution carbamazepine use in TBI patients with inappropriate antidiuretic hormone (ADH) secretion for concerns of worsening of hyponatremia and closely monitor for potentially life-threatening Stevens–Johnson syndrome or toxic epidermal necrolysis.

SPASTICITY

Spasticity is a common consequence of moderate and severe TBI and can significantly impact a patient's quality of life. Various oral muscle relaxants have shown promise in alleviating spasticity, with good evidence for use of oral baclofen or tizanidine. Oral baclofen has been shown to improve the lower extremity modified Ashworth scale (MAS).[43] Oral tizanidine has been shown to reduce the MAS, enhance motor strength, and reduce muscle tone.[44] Intrathecal baclofen has shown promise as a potential superior option to oral baclofen in reducing muscle spasms, especially in the lower extremities.[26] Caution, however, as sedating side effects of many spasticity-managing medications can be counterproductive in TBI. In TBI patients, prioritizing cognitive function to achieve rehabilitation goals is crucial, requiring a careful balance of medication dosing.[45]

Certain medications such as benzodiazepines are effective in treating spasticity and dystonia in the non-TBI population; however, these should be avoided in TBI for their negative effects on neuroplasticity and other adverse effects such as somnolence, memory impairment, depression, and respiratory depression.[32]

Botulinum toxin injection has also emerged as a modality to treat spasticity in TBI patients.[26] While it may offer some relief, studies comparing placebo and botulinum toxin A injection in TBI survivors have yielded limited results regarding sustained improvement of spasticity.[28]

SLEEP–WAKE DISTURBANCES

The link between sleep–wake disturbances (SWDs) and TBI remains intricate and not fully understood. Research has shed light on the prevalence of SWD in TBI patients, with rates ranging from 30% to 84%.[46] Hypersomnolence emerges as the most common SWD in patients with moderate and severe TBI, while those with mild TBI are more prone to circadian rhythm disturbance and insomnia.[46]

For treatment of hypersomnolence or excess fatigue, wakefulness-promoting agents such as modafinil[47] and stimulants such as methylphenidate have been shown effective.[48] While stimulants can offer benefits, their impact on sleep and wakefulness must be taken into account to avoid further exacerbating SWD.[49]

For all medications to treat insomnia, patients should be treated with the lowest effective dose and the shortest time period possible. Melatonin can be considered for its effects on circadian rhythm and overall safety. For TBI patients with insomnia and concomitant behavioral or cognitive indications, medications such as quetiapine or trazodone can be useful with regard to their sedating side effects.

POST-TRAUMATIC BRAIN INJURY FATIGUE

Post-TBI fatigue (PTBIF) is one of the most common disabling symptoms following TBI of any severity. Fatigue and concentration deficits are acknowledged as some of the most distressing and long-lasting symptoms with a significant negative impact on well-being and quality of life.[50] Fatigue in general is a broad symptom with many possible etiologies to consider. As such, providers must rule out secondary causes of fatigue and correct what may be correctable before making a PTBIF diagnosis. There are currently no standard treatments, although the most widely used medication for cognitive impairments after TBI is methylphenidate. Methylphenidate is a mixed dopaminergic and noradrenergic neurostimulant medication that is usually prescribed for attention-deficit disorder. Studies have revealed that persons with TBI treated with methylphenidate had reduced mental fatigue and improved cognitive function.[51] Avoid dosing in the evening time to prevent stimulation-induced insomnia. Use cautiously in individuals with pre-existing cardiovascular disease as common side effects include increased blood pressure and heart rate. Melatonin has also been shown to reduce post-TBI fatigue in randomly controlled trials, although the benefits may be related to sleep-related fatigue Agents that affect the dopamine and norepinephrine pathways such as amphetamines, amantadine, bromocriptine, and atomoxetine have also been studied with limited benefits.

MEMORY AND COGNITIVE SLOWING

Cognitive and neuropsychiatric symptoms can be present after TBI, thought to arise from direct disruption to the neural circuits that underlie cognitive function and neuropsychiatric regulation.[36] Thus, most pharmacologic interventions to address these complications will target neurotransmitter systems that may be disrupted by brain injury. The systems that are typically targeted include the dopaminergic, cholinergic, serotonergic, and noradrenergic pathways.

Dopamine is a neurotransmitter that has important roles in motor and cognitive function. Problems with memory and other neuropsychiatric symptoms can be seen when dopaminergic pathways are damaged. Dopamine levels have been directly correlated to arousal.[52] Medications that stimulate dopamine release and/or reduce uptake have shown efficacy in treating cognitive symptoms following TBI. Methylphenidate, as previously discussed, has also been shown to improve attention and processing speeds.[53] Amantadine directly stimulates dopamine release and reduces uptake has also shown some efficacy in treating cognitive symptoms following TBI. Caution in severely agitated patients as dopamine excess can lead to neuropsychiatric problems such as psychosis, anxiety, and impulsivity.

Some studies suggest the benefit of stimulants on improving memory, thought to work by augmentation of attention and processing speeds. Methylphenidate and other neurostimulants can be considered as adjunctive treatment to improve memory and concentration. The cholinergic system is best known for its role in memory, especially as it relates to Alzheimer's disease. This pathway has also been found to be important in attention, arousal, and executive function.[54] Thus, there is literature that supports typical Alzheimer's disease treatments such as donepezil and acetylcholinesterase inhibitors as treatment consideration to improve memory after TBI.[55] Physostigmine, rivastigmine, and galantamine have been shown superior to placebo in a few small studies.[56]

ANXIETY AND DEPRESSION

Treating depression and other neuropsychiatric symptoms after TBI is important, as successful treatment may influence improvements in other symptom domains. One study highlighted additional benefits to antidepressant treatment including reduced concurrent irritability, reduced aggression, and improved cognitive functioning.[57] Overall, the current literature on pharmacologic treatment of depression post-TBI lacks methodological rigor. Current treatment approaches rely on evidence based on anxiety or depression treatment in the non-TBI population.

SSRIs have received the most attention in research literature. They are considered first-line treatment of depression post-TBI, likely attributed to their evidence base regarding their use in major depressive disorder. Randomized controlled trials evaluating sertraline to treat depression in the context of TBI have demonstrated some benefits over placebo. Activating antidepressants such as fluoxetine, sertraline, venlafaxine, and duloxetine can be considered when treating depression associated with a component of fatigue. Citalopram is not as activating but may be helpful in depression associated with anxiety.

The efficacy and tolerability of other antidepressants such as SNRI, bupropion, and the monoamine oxidase inhibitors (MAOIs) in TBI are not well established. MAOIs should be avoided in TBI patients with severe cognitive or behavioral impairments as these individuals may have difficulty following the strict dietary restrictions necessary for safe MAOI use. Bupropion should also be avoided in this population as it can potentially lower seizure thresholds. TCAs, often used for treatment of depression in the general population, should be avoided in the depressed TBI population due to greater risk for complications as mentioned earlier.[58]

Literature regarding pharmacologic therapy for anxiety post-TBI is lacking, and no controlled trials have studied efficacy specific to the TBI population. Here, we again rely on the typical evidence-based treatments for anxiety in the general population. SSRIs and SNRIs are considered first-line for anxiety treatment in the TBI population, given their efficacy and tolerability in treatment of generalized anxiety and other similar psychiatric disorders.[59] Benzodiazepines should generally be avoided in this population for concern of sedating effects and addictive potential.

MEDICATIONS TO AVOID IN TRAUMATIC BRAIN INJURY

Neuroleptics commonly known as antipsychotics are the medication class with the greatest potential for negative outcomes in the TBI population. Most brain injury patients are already in a state of dopamine insufficiency following the traumatic event, and antipsychotics' primary mechanism involves interfering with dopamine function. Thus, antipsychotics may exacerbate the already dopamine-deficient state seen in TBI. The first-generation antipsychotics such as haloperidol have the strongest negative potential due to their high potency. Studies have shown that haloperidol adversely affects neurologic recovery when used after brain injury.[60] Aside from mechanistic effects that could negatively affect outcomes, TBI patients have a greater risk for developing neuroleptic malignant syndrome with use of first-generation antipsychotics.[61] If antipsychotic use is necessary for management of psychosis or severe agitation, then the second generation can be considered if other safer medications have failed.

Antihistamines are known to have negative consequences with significant impact on central nervous system (CNS) function, especially in older adults.[62] The effects of antihistamines on people with brain injury should be considered in the same way as they are for older adults. Newer antihistamines are thought to be safer and less sedating than older generations as their larger size limits permeation across the blood–brain barrier. However, people with brain injury have a disrupted blood–brain barrier and thus may still be susceptible to CNS effects of newer antihistamines.

AEDs generally work to suppress nerve cell firing. They can also have negative effects on neurologic recovery after brain injury and thus should be avoided when possible.[63] In healthy adults, AEDs have been shown to cause cognitive impairment particularly with respect to memory, attention, and psychomotor speed.[64] Clinicians must balance the potential hindrance of neurologic recovery with post-TBI increased risk for seizures. Phenytoin is often used because it does not cause significant sedation and can be loaded intravenously.[65] Levetiracetam is also a reasonable alternative.

Benzodiazepines can be effective in controlling spasticity and dystonia following TBI. However, regular use of these medications is not recommended as they can interfere with neurologic recovery. Like AEDs, benzodiazepines work by suppressing the activity of neurons. Furthermore, some studies have shown that they can inhibit sprouting of new dendrites[66] which are an important mechanism for learning and memory. Aside from their potential negative effects on neurologic recovery, benzodiazepines have a high abuse potential which could be problematic in this high-risk TBI population.

Anticholinergic medications are commonly prescribed to treat a variety of symptoms after brain injury, but they can also have negative effects on cognition. Cholinergic mechanisms are involved in cognitive function,[67] and anticholinergic medications work to inhibit these mechanisms. This can potentially lead to problems with memory, attention, and learning.[68] TCAs are commonly used to treat depression in the non-TBI population; however, there are non-TCA antidepressants that do not have anticholinergic side effects. As discussed earlier, SSRIs are preferred for treatment of depression in TBI as they are generally safer and more effective in this population.

Adrenergic blockers are a class of medications that can affect cognitive function, blood pressure, and mood. They can also potentially cause drowsiness, decreased alertness, and depression. In the rehabilitation setting, these medications can be dangerous as they can interfere with normal homeostatic mechanisms with positional changes. Interestingly, beta-blockers such as propranolol are considered effective in treating agitation following TBI and considered less offensive compared to other options such as antipsychotics or benzodiazepines.

CLINICS CARE POINTS

- The primary goals in TBI treatment is to minimize secondary brain damage and promote neuroprotection.
- Treatment for disorders of consciousness typically involves medications like amantadine, which facilitate dopamine function and improve cognitive parameters.Other pharmacological options include bromocriptine, levodopa, and methylphenidate, showing potential for enhancing cognition and arousal.
- Second-generation antipsychotics like olanzapine and quetiapine can be considered for managing acute agitation, with caution in patients with cardiac comorbidities.
- For paroxysmal sympathetic hyperactivity, propranolol is the preferred preventive agent, although caution is advised in patients with hypotension.
- Phenytoin and levetiracetam are commonly used within the first seven days post-TBI to reduce early seizure incidence.However, prolonged antiepileptic use lacks evidence beyond the initial period and may pose risks.
- Opioid prescription for pain management should be used cautiously due to the risk of misuse and potential interactions with psychotropic medications.
- For post TBI headaches, NSAIDs, triptans, and CGRP antagonists can be used for abortive therapy and antiepileptics and antidepressants can help with prevention.

ACKNOWLEDGMENTS

The authors would like to thank Vanessa Tran for her expertise and assistance throughout all aspects of our study and for her help in writing the article and creating the summary table.

DISCLOSURE

None.

REFERENCES

1. Centers for Disease Control and Prevention. Report to congress on traumatic brain injury in the United States: epidemiology and rehabilitation. Atlanta, GA: U.S, Department of Health and Human Services; 2015.
2. GBD 2016 Traumatic Brain Injury and Spinal Cord Injury Collaborators. Global, regional, and national burden of traumatic brain injury and spinal cord injury, 1990-2016: a systematic analysis for the Global Burden of Disease Study 2016. Lancet Neurol 2019 Jan;18(1):56–87.
3. Thurman DJ, Alverson C, Dunn KA, et al. Traumatic brain injury in the United States: A public health perspective. J Head Trauma Rehabil 1999 Dec;14(6): 602–15.
4. Zaloshnja E, Miller T, Langlois JA, et al. Prevalence of long-term disability from traumatic brain injury in the civilian population of the United States, 2005. J Head Trauma Rehabil 2008;23(6):394–400.
5. Arciniegas DB, Silver JM. Pharmacotherapy of posttraumatic cognitive impairments. Behav Neurol 2006;17(1):25–42.
6. Giacino JT, Katz DI, Schiff ND, et al. Comprehensive systematic review update summary: Disorders of consciousness. Neurology 2018;91(10):461–70.
7. Giacino JT, Whyte J, Bagiella E, et al. Placebo-Controlled Trial of Amantadine for Severe Traumatic Brain Injury. N Engl J Med 2012;366(9):819–26.
8. Nickels JL, Schneider WN, Dombovy ML, et al. Clinical use of amantadine in brain injury rehabilitation. Brain Inj 1994;8(8):709–18.
9. Passler MA, Riggs RV. Positive outcomes in traumatic brain injury–vegetative state: Patients treated with bromocriptine. Arch Phys Med Rehabil 2001;82(3): 311–5.
10. Patrick PD, Buck ML, Conaway MR, et al. The use of dopamine enhancing medications with children in low response states following brain injury. Brain Inj 2003; 17(6):497–506.
11. Hornyak JE, Nelson VS, Hurvitz EA. The use of methylphenidate in paediatric traumatic brain injury. Pediatr Rehabil 1997;1(1):15–7.
12. Peggy E, Chatham Showalter D. Stimulating consciousness and cognition following severe brain injury: a new potential clinical use for lamotrigine. Brain Inj 2000;14(11):997–1001.
13. Rivera VM. Modafinil for the treatment of diminished responsiveness in a patient recovering from brain surgery. Brain Inj 2005;19(9):725–7.
14. Whyte J, Myers R. Incidence of Clinically Significant Responses to Zolpidem Among Patients with Disorders of Consciousness. Am J Phys Med Rehabil 2009;88(5):410–8.
15. Rani Lindberg M. TRIUMPH Traumatic Brain Injury Guidelines: Management of Post Traumatic Brain Injury (TBI) Agitation. 2020 Aug.

16. Feeney DM, Gonzalez A, Law WA. Amphetamine, haloperidol, and experience interact to affect rate of recovery after motor cortex injury. Science 1982; 217(4562):855–7.

17. Rao N, Jellinek HM, Woolston DC. Agitation in closed head injury: haloperidol effects on rehabilitation outcome. Arch Phys Med Rehabil 1985;66(1):30–4.

18. Phyland RK, McKay A, Olver J, et al. Use of olanzapine to treat agitation in traumatic brain injury: study protocol for a randomised controlled trial. Trials 2020; 21(1):662.

19. Kim E, Bijlani M. A pilot study of quetiapine treatment of aggression due to traumatic brain injury. J Neuropsychiatry Clin Neurosci 2006;18(4):547–9.

20. Fleminger S, Greenwood RJ, Oliver DL. Pharmacological management for agitation and aggression in people with acquired brain injury. Cochrane Database Syst Rev 2006;(4):CD003299.

21. Brooke MM, Patterson DR, Questad KA, et al. The treatment of agitation during initial hospitalization after traumatic brain injury. Arch Phys Med Rehabil 1992; 73(10):917–21.

22. Mysiw WJ, Sandel ME. The agitated brain injured patient. Part 2: Pathophysiology and treatment. Arch Phys Med Rehabil 1997;78(2):213–20.

23. Chatham Showalter PE, Kimmel DN. Agitated symptom response to divalproex following acute brain injury. J Neuropsychiatry Clin Neurosci 2000;12(3):395–7.

24. Plantier D, Luauté J. Drugs for behavior disorders after traumatic brain injury: Systematic review and expert consensus leading to French recommendations for good practice. Ann Phys Rehabil Med [Internet 2016;59(1):42–57. Available at: https://www.sciencedirect.com/science/article/pii/S1877065715005540.

25. Hicks AJ, Clay FJ, Hopwood M, et al. The Efficacy and Harms of Pharmacological Interventions for Aggression After Traumatic Brain Injury-Systematic Review. Front Neurol 2019;10:1169.

26. Tani J, Wen YT, Hu CJ, et al. Current and Potential Pharmacologic Therapies for Traumatic Brain Injury. Pharmaceuticals 2022;15(7).

27. Ripley D. Neuropharmacology: a neurorehab perspective. In: Zasler ND, Katz DI, Zafonte RD, editors. *Brain injury medicine- principles and practice*. 3rd edition. New York: Springer Publishing Company, LLC; 2022. p. 1126–37.

28. Vasudevan V, Amatya B, Khan F. Overview of systematic reviews: Management of common Traumatic Brain Injury-related complications. PLoS One 2022;17(9): e0273998.

29. Fordington S, Manford M. A review of seizures and epilepsy following traumatic brain injury. J Neurol 2020;267(10):3105–11.

30. Perkes I, Baguley IJ, Nott MT, et al. A review of paroxysmal sympathetic hyperactivity after acquired brain injury. Ann Neurol 2010;68(2):126–35.

31. Samuel S, Allison TA, Lee K, et al. Pharmacologic Management of Paroxysmal Sympathetic Hyperactivity After Brain Injury. J Neurosci Nurs 2016 Apr; 48(2):82–9.

32. Ripley D, Driver S. Pharmacologic Management of the patient with traumatic brain injury. In: Eapen B, Cifu D, editors. Rehabilitation after traumatic brain injury. Amsterdam: Elsevier; 2018. p. 133–63.

33. Bhatnagar S, Iaccarino MA, Zafonte R. Pharmacotherapy in rehabilitation of post-acute traumatic brain injury. Brain Res 2016;1640(Pt A):164–79.

34. Molero Y, Sharp DJ, D'Onofrio BM, et al. Psychotropic and pain medication use in individuals with traumatic brain injury-a Swedish total population cohort study of 240 000 persons. J Neurol Neurosurg Psychiatry 2021;92(5):519–27.

35. Bjork JM, Grant SJ. Does traumatic brain injury increase risk for substance abuse? J Neurotrauma 2009;26(7):1077–82.

36. Zasler ND, Arciniegas DB, Katz DI, et al, editors. Brain injury medicine. New York, NY: Springer Publishing Company; 2021.

37. Nampiaparampil DE. Prevalence of chronic pain after traumatic brain injury: a systematic review. JAMA 2008;300(6):711–9.

38. Goldstein J, Silberstein SD, Saper JR, et al. Acetaminophen, Aspirin, and Caffeine in Combination Versus Ibuprofen for Acute Migraine: Results From a Multicenter, Double-Blind, Randomized, Parallel-Group, Single-Dose, Placebo-Controlled Study. Headache: The Journal of Head and Face Pain 2006;46(3):444–53.

39. Ramadan N, Silberstein S, Freitag F, et al. Evidence-Based Guidelines for Migraine Headache in the Primary Care Setting: Pharmacological Management for Prevention of Migraine. Neurology 2000 Jul;55.

40. Holland S, Silberstein SD, Freitag F, et al. Evidence-based guideline update: NSAIDs and other complementary treatments for episodic migraine prevention in adults: [RETIRED]. Neurology 2012;78(17):1346–53.

41. Olesen J, Diener HC, Husstedt IW, et al. Calcitonin Gene–Related Peptide Receptor Antagonist BIBN 4096 BS for the Acute Treatment of Migraine. N Engl J Med 2004;350(11):1104–10.

42. Silberstein SD, Stark SR, Lucas SM, et al. Botulinum toxin type A for the prophylactic treatment of chronic daily headache: a randomized, double-blind, placebo-controlled trial. Mayo Clin Proc 2005;80(9):1126–37.

43. Meythaler JM, Clayton W, Davis LK, et al. Orally Delivered Baclofen to Control Spastic Hypertonia in Acquired Brain Injury. J Head Trauma Rehabil 2004; 19(2):101–8.

44. Meythaler JM, Guin-Renfroe S, Johnson A, et al. Prospective assessment of tizanidine for spasticity due to acquired brain injury. Arch Phys Med Rehabil 2001; 82(9):1155–63.

45. Synnot A, Chau M, Pitt V, et al. Interventions for managing skeletal muscle spasticity following traumatic brain injury. Cochrane Database Syst Rev 2017;11(11): CD008929.

46. Paredes I, Navarro B, Lagares A. Sleep disorders in traumatic brain injury. Neurocirugia (English Edition) 2021;32(4):178–87.

47. Kaiser PR, Valko PO, Werth E, et al. Modafinil ameliorates excessive daytime sleepiness after traumatic brain injury. Neurology 2010;75(20):1780–5.

48. Francisco GE, Ivanhoe CB. Successful treatment of post-traumatic narcolepsy with methylphenidate: a case report. Am J Phys Med Rehabil 1996;75(1):63–5.

49. Wiseman-Hakes C, Murray B, Moineddin R, et al. Evaluating the impact of treatment for sleep/wake disorders on recovery of cognition and communication in adults with chronic TBI. Brain Inj 2013;27(12):1364–76.

50. Lannsjö M, Geijerstam JL af, Johansson U, et al. Prevalence and structure of symptoms at 3 months after mild traumatic brain injury in a national cohort. Brain Inj 2009;23(3):213–9.

51. Johansson B, Andréll P, Rönnbäck L, et al. Follow-up after 5.5 years of treatment with methylphenidate for mental fatigue and cognitive function after a mild traumatic brain injury. Brain Inj 2020;34(2):229–35.

52. Horvitz JC. Mesolimbocortical and nigrostriatal dopamine responses to salient non-reward events. Neuroscience 2000;96(4):651–6.

53. Zhang WT, Wang YF. Efficacy of methylphenidate for the treatment of mental sequelae after traumatic brain injury. Medicine 2017;96(25):e6960.

54. Arciniegas DB. Cholinergic dysfunction and cognitive impairment after traumatic brain injury. Part 2: evidence from basic and clinical investigations. J Head Trauma Rehabil 2011;26(4):319–23.
55. Zhang L, Plotkin RC, Wang G, et al. Cholinergic augmentation with donepezil enhances recovery in short-term memory and sustained attention after traumatic brain injury. Arch Phys Med Rehabil 2004;85(7):1050–5.
56. Cardenas DD, McLean A, Farrell-roberts L, et al. Oral physostigmine and impaired memory in adults with brain injury. Brain Inj 1994;8(7):579–87.
57. Kant R, Smith-seemiller L, zeiler D. Treatment of aggression and irritability after head injury. Brain Inj 1998;12(8):661–6.
58. Wroblewski BA, Mccolgan K, Smith K, et al. The Incidence of Seizures during Tricyclic Antidepressant Drug Treatment in a Brain-Injured Population. J Clin Psychopharmacol 1990;10(2):124–8.
59. Polich G, Iaccarino MA, Zafonte R. Psychopharmacology of traumatic brain injury. Handb Clin Neurol 2019;253–67.
60. Kline AE, Hoffman AN, Cheng JP, et al. Chronic administration of antipsychotics impede behavioral recovery after experimental traumatic brain injury. Neurosci Lett 2008;448(3):263–7.
61. Bellamy CJ, Kane-Gill SL, Falcione BA, et al. Neuroleptic Malignant Syndrome in Traumatic Brain Injury Patients Treated With Haloperidol. J Trauma Inj Infect Crit Care 2009;66(3):954–8.
62. Agostini JV, Leo-Summers LS, Inouye SK. Cognitive and Other Adverse Effects of Diphenhydramine Use in Hospitalized Older Patients. Arch Intern Med 2001; 161(17):2091.
63. Bhullar IS, Johnson D, Paul JP, et al. More harm than good. J Trauma Acute Care Surg 2014;76(1):54–61.
64. Meador KJ, Gilliam FG, Kanner AM, et al. Cognitive and Behavioral Effects of Antiepileptic Drugs. Epilepsy Behav 2001;2(4). SS1–17.
65. Temkin NR, Dikmen SS, Wilensky AJ, et al. A Randomized, Double-Blind Study of Phenytoin for the Prevention of Post-Traumatic Seizures. N Engl J Med 1990; 323(8):497–502.
66. Villasana LE, Peters A, McCallum R, et al. Diazepam Inhibits Post-Traumatic Neurogenesis and Blocks Aberrant Dendritic Development. J Neurotrauma 2019; 36(16):2454–67.
67. Arciniegas DB. The cholinergic hypothesis of cognitive impairment caused by traumatic brain injury. Curr Psychiatr Rep 2003;5(5):391–9.
68. Sakel M, Boukouvalas A, Buono R, et al. Does anticholinergics drug burden relate to global neuro-disability outcome measures and length of hospital stay? Brain Inj 2015;29(12):1426–30.
69. Talsky A, Pascione L, Shaw T, et al. Pharmacological interventions for traumatic brain injury. Br Columbia Med J 2011;53(1):26–31.
70. Ali A, Morfin J, Mills J, et al. Fatigue After Traumatic Brain Injury: A Systematic Review. J Head Trauma Rehabil 2022;37(4):E249–57.
71. Raithel DS, Ohler KH, Porto I, et al. Morphine: An Effective Abortive Therapy for Pediatric Paroxysmal Sympathetic Hyperactivity After Hypoxic Brain Injury. J Pediatr Pharmacol Therapeut 2015;20(4):335–40.

Community Reintegration After Traumatic Brain Injury

Brian D. Greenwald, MD[a,b,]*, Kristen A. Harris, MD[a,b],
Harsha Ayyala, MD[a,b], Dustin J. Gordon, PhD[c]

KEYWORDS

- Traumatic brain injury • Acquired brain injury • Community reintegration • Mobility
- Caregiver • Medical complications

KEY POINTS

Community reintegration is important to facilitate independence and social connectivity for patients with traumatic brain injury (TBI), while limiting caregiver burden and improving satisfaction with quality of life.

- Many medical complications common in patients with TBI may impact community reintegration, including pain, seizures, sleep, vision, fatigue, mood, loss of taste and smell, and balance.
- A number of environmental and social factors also impact effective community reintegration, including mobility, considerations for return to work or school, alcohol use, and sexuality.
- Inpatient/residential and outpatient programs should facilitate community reintegration for patients with TBI and should be staffed with a multidisciplinary rehabilitation team including neuropsychologists, physical, occupational and speech therapists, recreational therapists, and case managers.

INTRODUCTION

Maximizing community reintegration for persons with disabilities is a standard protected by the Americans with Disabilities Act and the United Nations Convention on the Rights of Persons with Disabilities. Community reintegration is important for independence, social connectivity, limiting caregiver burden, and improving both patient and caregiver satisfaction with quality of life. Achieving community reintegration can be complicated in patients with traumatic brain injury (TBI) due to a unique

[a] Department of Physical Medicine and Rehabilitation, Hackensack Meridian School of Medicine, JFK Johnson Rehabilitation Institute, 65 James Street, Edison, NJ 08820, USA; [b] Department of Physical Medicine & Rehabilitation, JFK Johnson Rehabilitation Institute, 65 James Street, Edison, NJ 08820, USA; [c] Rehabilitation Specialists, 18-01 Pollitt Drive Suite 1A, Fair Lawn, NJ 07410, USA
* Corresponding author.
E-mail address: brian.greenwald@hmhn.org

Phys Med Rehabil Clin N Am 35 (2024) 637–650
https://doi.org/10.1016/j.pmr.2024.02.012
pmr.theclinics.com

constellation of neurologic and behavioral symptoms. In this article we review the unique impact of medical complications common in patients with TBI; environmental and social factors relating to community reintegration; characteristics of inpatient/residential and outpatient community reintegration programs; and coordination of care, case management, and family involvement.

DISCUSSION
Medical Complications Impacting Community Reintegration

Many medical complications that are common after TBI can impact patients' community participation. Outpatient management of symptom burden by the rehabilitation physician is important to facilitate successful community reintegration. Readers should consider reviewing and sharing the patient fact sheets on these topics and other TBI-related topics on the TBI Model System Knowledge Translation Center (msktc.org/tbi/factsheets), which can be helpful for patients and caregivers. Specific medical complications impacting community reintegration are summarized in **Box 1** and discussed below.

Headaches and pain
Headaches are common after TBI and can occur after mild, moderate, or severe TBI. For many patients, headaches persist even for years after their injury.[1] Headaches can impede community reintegration by limiting patients' attention and impacting memory. Medication overuse headaches may occur in the community setting as patients begin utilizing over the counter medications to treat symptoms independently. There are numerous effective pharmacologic and non-pharmacologic treatments for post-traumatic headaches, and physicians can contribute to successful community reintegration by offering management options for headaches.[2,3] Pain issues beyond headaches are also common after TBI, either due to neuropathic or somatic causes as a result of the injury complex. Inadequate pain management can limit community reintegration due to the biopsychosocial nature of pain. Conversely, certain medications used for pain management may cause sedation limiting activity participation.

Seizures
Seizures are common after TBI. Although patients are at highest risk for seizures in the first week after injury, patients with TBI remain at increased risk for seizure even years after their injury. Cumulative incidence of late post-traumatic seizures at 5 years has been suggested to be as high as 20.5%, with certain risk factors such as bi-parietal contusions and dural penetration further increasing risk of seizures.[4,5] Post-

Box 1
Medical complications impacting community reintegration
Headaches and pain
Seizure
Sleep
Vision
Fatigue
Mood
Loss of smell/taste
Balance

traumatic seizures can limit patients' ability to participate in activities, including driving, climbing, and swimming. Patients with seizures may experience postictal symptoms including fatigue and further limiting participation in activities. Furthermore, many antiepileptic medications can also cause fatigue. Patients with post-traumatic seizures should be referred to neurology for management to maximize community participation.

Sleep
Traumatic brain injury increases patients' risk of sleep disturbance including insomnia, excessive daytime sleepiness, delayed sleep phase syndrome, and narcolepsy.[6,7] Sleep disorders can worsen symptoms of depression, anxiety, and fatigue which may impact work performance and place patients at risk of traffic accidents. Sleep disturbances can also impact relationships with friends and family, including bed partners. Review of medications, sleep habits, mood disturbances (ie, depression and anxiety), drug and alcohol use can be helpful as an initial evaluation of patients with sleep disorders after TBI.

Vision
Patients may develop disorders of vision after TBI, either due to direct injury to the eyes, visual pathways, extraocular muscles, or due to impaired ability to process visual information.[8] Symptoms may include blurred vision, diplopia, and decreased peripheral vision. Persistent visual symptoms after brain injury may impact patients after community discharge due to intolerance of glare or bright lights, impact on balance and depth perception, and intolerance of visual overload. Outpatient services such as evaluation by a neuro-ophthalmologist or neuro-optometrist can be helpful. Vision therapy and recommendations for optical devices and strategies to limit symptom burden may improve patients' ability to return to activities.

Fatigue
Fatigue is one of the most common problems people have after TBI. 70% of survivors of TBI complain of mental fatigue. It may present after TBI as physical, psychological, or mental fatigue. Fatigue can impact mood, physical function, and many aspects of cognitive function including attention, concentration, memory, and communication. Important ways to reduce fatigue include identifying triggers, encouraging proper sleep patterns and rest when needed, avoiding alcohol, recreational drug use, and improving time management. It is also recommended that patients exercise daily to improve mental function and alertness.[9] Many medications used in management of patients with TBI are associated with fatigue, these are outlined in **Table 1**.

Mood
Anxiety and depression may be prevalent in the general population and in people with moderate to severe TBI. This may be due to injury to areas of the brain that control emotions and chemical cascades. Anxiety and depression can also be due to compromised function with loss of function and independence. Grief reaction due to these losses should also be considered. Anxiety may lead to intense fear and worry leading to physical manifestations such as tachycardia, tachypnea, diaphoresis, or tremor. Depression may present as feelings of sadness, irritability, or worthlessness that could lead to changes in sleep or appetite. Uncontrolled depression can lead to thoughts of hurting oneself and loss of activities that were previously enjoyed. Different methods of addressing mood issues include psychotherapy, support groups, and pharmacotherapy from medical providers. In addition, reducing triggers by setting a regular

---

Table 1
Common drug classes with side effects of fatigue[37]

Drug Class	Common Medications
Antispasticity agents	Baclofen[a], Clonidine, Tizanidine, Dantrolene, Benzodiazepines[a]
Analgesics	Opioid/opiate medications[a], barbiturates[a], neuropathic medications
Anticonvulsants	Keppra (levetiracetam), Valproic Acid (Depakote), Phenytoin, Phenobarbital[a], Benzodiazepines[a]
Antihistamines	Benadryl[a], allergy medications (Zyrtec, Claritin), Vistaril
Anti-inflammatories	NSAIDS (Advil, Motrin, Naproxen), Celecoxib (Celebrex), Ketorolac (Toradol)
Anti-psychotics	Haloperidol (Haldol)[a], Quetiapine (Seroquel), Olanzapine (Zyprexa), Ziprasidone (Geodon)
Antidepressants	Mirtazapine (Remeron)[a], Citalopram (Celexa), Escitalopram (Lexapro), Sertraline (Zoloft)
Muscle relaxants	Cyclobenzaprine (Flexiril)[a], Methocarbamol (Robaxin)
Gastrointestinal drugs	Metoclopramide (Reglan), Anticholinergic agents (Glycopyrrolate, Bentyl), loperamide (Imodium)

[a] May have significant sedating effects compared to other medications in same class.

---

schedule and utilizing relaxation techniques can combat mood-related changes secondary to TBI.

Loss of smell/taste

After a brain injury, people may lose sense of smell due to injury to certain nerves that transmit information to the brain or injury to parts of the brain itself that process smell. It may also be due to infections, toxins, and medicines.[10,11] Damage to the cribriform plate (especially fractures along the roof of the nasal cavity) can disrupt bipolar olfactory receptor cells due to stretching or shearing injury. In addition, olfactory dysfunction can occur anywhere along the pathway from olfactory bulbs to the cortical processing centers of the frontal and temporal lobes. The primary olfactory cortex is located on the anteromedial portion of the uncus while olfactory tract is located along lateral surfaces of cerebral hemisphere.[11] As a result, loss of smell can lead to reduced appetite and lack of interest in food; this may result in a poor diet such as eating too little and unsafe weight loss or overeating with excess salt for flavor causing high blood pressure. Recovery can happen naturally in 30% of affected people. Other strategies to help deal with loss of smell or taste include cooking with flavorful food with different textures, setting reminders to eat, and taking vitamin supplements. It is also important to keep smoke alarms updated on every floor and natural gas detectors.

Balance

After TBI, people may develop dizziness, vertigo (room spinning), or loss of balance. Common causes of balance problems include severity/location of brain injury (brainstem/cerebellum), multiple orthopedic injuries, postural hypotension (blood pressure drop when standing), vision impairments, inner ear problems, and impaired sensation of extremities.[12] People who have balance impairment are unable to control the movement of their body and maintain a base of support leading to changes in posture and increased risk for falls. This can affect activities such as walking, self-care tasks like bathing, using the toilet, and dressing.[13,14] Balance can be improved through strength and flexibility, especially in ankle/hip muscles with physical/occupational therapies, developing strategies to increase base of support and addressing visual or inner ear impairments. In addition, it may be beneficial to practice in different conditions such as uneven ground or becoming accustomed to distracting environments.

ENVIRONMENTAL AND SOCIAL FACTORS IMPACTING COMMUNITY REINTEGRATION

Cognitive, emotional, and behavioral disturbances are common after TBI and can alter the trajectory of the life of the patient and their families.[15,16] While some patients are able to successfully return to their pre-injury lifestyle, those with moderate to severe TBI often require ongoing and extended care.[17,18] However, the transition to post-acute care is often poorly organized, leading to system breakdowns.[19] The process is further complicated by insufficient resources, lack of education, inadequate community facilities, financial limitations, and lengthy funding application procedures.[20–22] Consequently, many patients end up transitioning directly from acute or transitional services to their families' homes instead of appropriate post-acute outpatient or inpatient/residential programs. Families, despite the availability of community resources, are left to assume the role of caregivers without proper training. Unlike other types of long-term disabilities such as severe psychiatric disorders, neurodevelopmental disorders, and neurodegenerative diseases, families of individuals with TBI suddenly and without adequate preparation or time to plan, find themselves taking on the caregiver role.

Considerations for Caregivers

The intricate dynamics within and between individuals involved in the caregiver role, including pre-existing family dynamics, have a reciprocal impact on the well-being reported by both the caregiver and the patient. A breakdown of this framework can significantly hinder the adaptation process.[22] Everhart and colleagues define caregiver capacity as the degree to which caregivers possess the necessary knowledge and skills to provide care for the injured individual.[22] McIntyre and colleagues discovered that the ability of families to take on the caregiver role is influenced by various factors intrinsic to both the caregiver and the patient, as well as the level of support available and the dynamics within the family.[23]

It is crucial to prioritize the continuous support and well-being of both caregivers and patients in the long run.[19,24,25] Assessing the dynamics of the caregiver-patient relationship early on and on a regular basis is essential.[26,27] A study by Vangel and colleagues revealed a strong association between the life satisfaction of brain injury survivors and the level of perceived social support from their caregivers.[28] Additionally, the caregiver's own life satisfaction was identified as the most influential factor in predicting the emotional distress experienced by the patient. Importantly, a higher reported burden on the caregiver was linked to poorer neuropsychological functioning in the patient.[29] It should be noted that the manifestation of caregiver distress may vary among different caregivers.[30]

In order to achieve better and quicker outcomes in the long term, an overall proactive approach to intervention is necessary, with a focus on the caregiver, patient, and the caregiver-patient relationship. This approach should be comprehensive and involve early and regular clinical intervention, guidance, and education for the caregiver and the family. Critical elements for achieving these goals include addressing the evolving needs of the caregiver and patient, providing emotional and psychological support, offering anticipatory guidance, teaching problem-solving, stress management, and behavioral management strategies to the family, facilitating life planning, and promoting community integration.[31] Patients and their families still perceive shortcomings in the current service delivery system in these areas.

The process of community integration should be thorough and personalized, taking into account not only work-related aspects but also non-work related roles such as social relationships, leisure activities, and other environmental factors that can impact the effectiveness of intervention and outcomes.[32] This approach enables the identification of barriers and facilitators that affect community reintegration. It is important to recognize that community reintegration is a complex and dynamic process that reflects ongoing recovery, necessitating the review, and adjustment of goals as circumstances evolve over time.[33]

Individuals who experience a compromise in their community role and self-perception often express feelings of isolation and abandonment. The loss of social networks they once enjoyed before the injury, combined with a lack of skills to form new relationships, leads to dissatisfaction with their level of social integration. Social integration, on the other hand, plays a crucial role in fostering a sense of belonging, independence, and adjustment, and is linked to higher levels of life satisfaction for patients.[33–35] Loss of identity, purpose, independence, and social connections can exacerbate challenges in relationships with family and friends, leading to heightened feelings of loneliness, and resentment.

The patient's self-esteem is strongly connected to their sense of autonomy, which is nurtured through engagement in the community, including their work environment. This involvement allows the patient to experience a sense of purpose and agency as they contribute to society.[27,34] It is essential to address the long-term assistance required for community-based social integration and to implement more effective intervention strategies to help patients develop these skills. These efforts are necessary to enhance well-being and satisfaction.[34] Maximizing social integration is particularly crucial for patients with more significant impairments, as they are more likely to rely on ongoing support to improve their quality of life in the long term.

Specific Social Factors Impacting Community Reintegration

After TBI, questions arise about social and activity participation. Encouraging participation in various social activities is important to promote independence, however, the rehabilitation physician should ensure that activities are safe and appropriate for a patient's stage of recovery. Specific considerations are discussed later, including driving and community mobility, alcohol use, sexuality, and return to work/school.

Driving and Community Mobility

Return to driving is an important component of facilitating patients' independence after discharge, and is often limited for a period of time due to safety. Driving is a complex activity and many of the skills and senses used in driving are impacted after TBI, including vision, maintaining attention, short-term memory, dual-tasking, coordination, processing speed, reaction time, and safety awareness. Patients with post-traumatic epilepsy are restricted from driving for a period of time after their last seizure, as per state guidelines. Despite barriers, between 50% and 70% of people with moderate to severe TBI are able to return to driving after their injury.[36] A driving evaluation by a professional certified through the Association for Driver Rehabilitation Specialists (ADED) may be an important step toward returning to driving, and should be undertaken when the physician and patient agree that driving is an appropriate goal. The evaluation will include both a preliminary and on-the-road assessment of skills. If a patient is safe to return to driving, vehicle modifications to incorporate adaptive equipment may be required. If driving is not appropriate for a patient after community discharge, ensuring access to safe and reliable transportation to provide independence, and allow for participation in the community is crucial, either through family members, public transportation, or resources available specifically to people with disability.

Some patients with significant impairments after TBI may require a wheelchair or other assistive device for community mobility. Proper selection of an assistive device for community mobility is dictated by safety, comfort/positioning, and patient factors. The Americans with Disability Act dictates standards to improve community accessibility for patients with disabilities utilizing mobility devices.

Alcohol Use

Questions about alcohol consumption are common after TBI. Alcohol consumption after TBI can increase risk of re-injury, lower the seizure threshold, impair cognition, increase risk of depression, impact sexuality, and impede neurologic recovery.[37] Alcohol use disorder and TBI commonly co-occur, both before and after injury.[38] Alcohol consumption should be discouraged after TBI. If patients do consume alcohol after TBI, family members should be counseled on minimizing harm related to alcohol use to promote patient safety.

Sexuality

Sexual dysfunction may occur after TBI due to causes such as damage to the brain, hormonal changes, medication side effects, cognitive impairment, fatigue or physical impairment. Other factors that may impact sexual function include mood impairment or changes in relationships. This may lead to changes in sexual functioning such as increased/decreased desire, decreased arousal, difficulty/inability to reach orgasm/climax, or reproductive changes.[39] Physicians should screen for sexual dysfunction in the outpatient setting as patients may not feel comfortable asking questions about sexual function in the clinic setting. Depending on the patient's history and physical exam, more comprehensive testing including bloodwork to evaluate neuroendocrine dysfunction may be required. In addition, psychotherapy, counseling, open discussions with partners, and different environmental strategies may improve sexual function.

Return to Work/School

Returning to work and school can be difficult for patients after a brain injury. Symptoms may develop over time and manifest as physical changes, cognitive changes, emotional, or behavioral changes. For children returning to school, proper planning including early communication with family members and school personnel can help facilitate effective return.[40] For students with disabilities, working with trained educators in special programs can facilitate educational progress, however, not all students after a TBI require specialized programs. Specific laws such as Individuals with Disabilities Education Improvement ACT (IDEA), Section 5504 of the Rehabilitation Act and American with Disabilities Act (ADA) can provide accommodations for students with disabilities.[40] Neuropsychological testing can also help identify cognitive deficits and target them specifically prior to returning to class.

When returning back to work, secondary effects of TBI can present difficult challenges and may require simulation to prepare physically and mentally. Under the ADA, accommodations such as shorter hours, gradual return to work, breaks, and lighter/different roles can be discussed. In addition, modified desks or chairs, wheelchair accessibility, and computer programs can be discussed when returning to work. Working with vocational rehabilitation specialists to discuss different options and simulating work-related tasks with physical and occupational therapy can also facilitate employment. Other resources such as Social Security Disability Insurance (SSDI) or Supplemental Security Income (SSI) can provide benefits while a patient is incapacitated and recovering from a TBI.

COMMUNITY REINTEGRATION PROGRAM CHARACTERISTICS
Inpatient/Residential Program Characteristics

Community reintegration programs must be comprehensive, intensive, have credentialed staff, individualized, and well-coordinated. They must include a community-based multi-disciplinary approach to intervention and emphasize caregivers and families. To effectively reintegrate individuals into the community, inpatient/residential programs must possess specific characteristics. These programs should be suitable for patients and employ a multidisciplinary team approach to treatment development, coordination, implementation, and management.[41] Core areas of expertise that should be reflected in the multidisciplinary team are summarized in **Box 2**.

Unfortunately, many healthcare settings lack specialized personnel and personalized treatment options for individuals with TBI.[21] For instance, aged care facilities often fail to meet the unique needs of persons with TBI patients, and coordination of care is often deficient in other non-TBI settings as well. Comprehensive programs should include clinically trained staff those who specialize in treating individuals with TBI and their caregivers. It should also adopt an individualized approach to assessment, treatment, and patient monitoring.[42] This personalized approach enables therapists to leverage the strengths of patients, encourage prosocial behaviors, and address maladaptive behaviors, thereby maximizing long-term progress, particularly in older individuals.

In their review on the current state of TBI rehabilitation, Gordon and colleagues focused on research conducted between 1998 and 2004.[43] They noted that there was a greater understanding of various aspects of TBI and advancements in the development of reliable and valid measurement methods for post-TBI functions that were previously difficult to quantify. However, they found limited progress in evaluating the effectiveness of interventions and developing new treatments, primarily due to the heterogeneity of the TBI population and the complexity of brain injury.[43] It is evident that there is a need for methodological improvements to address the limitations in the existing literature. Despite these challenges, there is substantial evidence supporting the effectiveness of community reintegration programs, especially when they incorporate cognitive, psychosocial, and community components.[42,44–48]

Similarly, while there are documented benefits of community reintegration residential programs for individuals with TBI,[49] the variability across these settings makes it challenging to quantify their relative effectiveness.[50,51] The characteristics of home-

---

Box 2
Multidisciplinary rehabilitation team

- Neuropsychologists
- Speech/Language pathologists
- Occupational therapists
- Physical therapists
- Cognitive/Functional Life Skills Therapists

- Substance Use Therapists (Neuropsychologists and Doctoral Level Neuropsychology Externs)
- Vocational Therapists
- Residential Counselors
- Case Managers
- Physiatrist, ideally trained in Brain Injury Medicine
- Outside providers (eg, Neurology and Psychiatry)

based programs also vary, making them difficult to assess. However, an important finding by Eicher and colleagues was that intensive-based programs resulted in greater improvement compared to supported living programs, regardless of the living context (whether within the patient's home with associated outpatient and community-based services or within a programmatic residential setting).[52] In intensive-based programs, the staff consisted of licensed professionals such as neuropsychologists, occupational therapists, speech therapists, and physical therapists, while supported programs primarily relied on paraprofessionals. Malec & Kean also found that intensive-based programs were more effective than supported living settings.[53] Additionally, Cicerone and colleagues reported that intensive community-based treatment programs with a comprehensive integrated approach, particularly emphasizing psychosocial intervention, were more effective than programs that did not have such intensity.[54]

Outpatient Program Characteristics

Individuals with TBI may have the opportunity to participate in a day program at an outpatient facility, with flexible schedules tailored to their specific needs and other commitments, such as work, volunteering, and recreational activities. The level of independence granted to each patient is determined based on their individual requirements and functional abilities. Treatment within the program is typically overseen by neuropsychologists, who work alongside licensed therapists including speech pathologists, occupational therapists, and physical therapists. The team also may include certified cognitive/functional life skills and vocational therapists, who hold qualifications such as certification from the Academy of Certified Brain Injury Specialists (ACBIS), as well as consulting physiatrists. Having multilingual therapists and supporting staff is crucial not only for providing effective treatment to patients but also for establishing relationships and facilitating communication with their families and support systems.

An effective and well-coordinated multidisciplinary approach to patient treatment is crucial for various reasons. It enables the monitoring of medication side effects, facilitates prompt assessment of changes in medical condition, and helps identify psychosocial stressors and other indicators that may reflect changes in the patient's medical status. Patients with coexisting conditions such as psychiatric illness and neurologic disorders (such as seizure disorder) often require additional monitoring and coordination with medical disciplines beyond the community reintegration program. Treatment is tailored to address these specific disorders.[21] For instance, there is a significant presence of substance use disorders (SUD) within the population affected by TBI, and there is a noted increase in substance use following TBI.[37] This can have devastating consequences for both brain injury survivors and their families. Since general community support services often fail to adequately address the cognitive and behavioral effects of TBI,[55] it is important for a comprehensive program to provide an individualized approach to the assessment, treatment, and monitoring of individuals with coexisting TBI and SUD. This should be carried out by a team of professionals, including the neuropsychologist (Please refer to **Box 2** for details regarding the characteristics of the clinical team.).

Coordination of Care, Case Management, and Family Involvement

Regular clinical rounds, educational sessions, and case conferences involving families are common in both inpatient and outpatient healthcare settings. Typically, patients are assigned an internal case manager who maintains ongoing oversight of their clinical treatment. Case management can be described as a collaborative process that involves assessing, planning, coordinating, evaluating, and advocating for options and services to address the comprehensive health needs of individuals and their families. The goal is to promote quality outcomes in a cost-effective manner by utilizing effective communication and available resources.[56] Case managers who work with individuals with TBI often have backgrounds in clinical social work or other mental health professions. They possess education and training in psychology and clinical management and possess a solid knowledge base of TBI, substance misuse, and recovery. Many case managers in this field also hold ACBIS certifications, further enhancing their expertise.

Case managers play a crucial role in the care of patients, as they not only advocate for the patients but also ensure that the family is actively involved in the treatment process, fostering a collaborative, and individualized approach.[57,58] They establish effective communication channels among individuals with TBI, healthcare professionals, family members, and other support individuals. Additionally, case managers maintain connections with external community resources throughout the rehabilitation journey. They actively seek opportunities to enhance social engagement, leisure activities, and explore possibilities for employment or volunteer work. By developing and implementing monitoring protocols, they alleviate some of the burdensome responsibilities that caregivers and families may face across different care settings. Regular face-to-face contact between the case manager, patient, and family members is considered essential for maintaining the momentum of treatment, and this interaction occurs in various settings, including individual meetings, provider meetings, case conferences, and observational participation. The importance of well-coordinated interventions that involve multiple components integrated within the community-based service delivery system is supported, and case management is a critical component of such interventions.[59]

Continuous communication among all relevant parties, including prescribing doctors, therapists, families, supporting entities, and funding agents, is vital for optimizing the effectiveness and outcomes of treatment. Nevertheless, facilitating effective communication among multiple healthcare professionals can present challenges. In situations where individuals with TBI are at home or traveling outside of the rehabilitative program, families and friends often play a vital role in maintaining communication and providing support. However, case management is instrumental in establishing an efficient feedback loop among treating professionals, families, support persons, funding entities, and the individuals themselves. This ensures that the communication and support process is streamlined, particularly within a community re-entry setting.

SUMMARY

Community reintegration after TBI is multi-faceted: medical, environmental, and social factors should be considered to optimize success. Medical complications such as headaches, uncontrolled pain, seizures, visual/gustatory dysfunction, mood issues, and balance impairment can present significant barriers for patients. In addition, environmental challenges such as inadequate post-acute care and difficulty obtaining community resources can pose a significant caregiver burden. Inpatient/residential care programs (intensive-based programs vs supported-living settings) and outpatient day programs can provide an effective and well-coordinated multidisciplinary approach with trained professionals that can establish targeted rehabilitation while assessing for changes in medical status. Case management is also crucial to coordination of care and collaboration with families for resource management. Overall, identifying and addressing barriers for TBI patients reintegrating into the community is essential for a successful transition.

CLINICS CARE POINTS

- Community reintegration is an important component of recovery for patients with TBI
- Management of common medical complications related to TBI can facilitate community reintegration
- Asking patients about social factors including work or school, alcohol and drug use, as well as sexuality is important in the outpatient setting
- Inpatient/residential and outpatient programs may facilitate community reintegration for patients with TBI and should be staffed with a multidisciplinary rehabilitation team

DISCLOSURE

There are no disclosures or conflicts of interest reported by the authors. No funding was received by the authors for this work.

REFERENCES

1. Stacey A, Lucas S, Dikmen S, et al. Natural History of Headache Five Years after Traumatic Brain Injury. J Neurotrauma 2017;34(8):1558–64.
2. Brown AW, Watanabe TK, Hoffman JM, et al. Headache after traumatic brain injury: a national survey of clinical practices and treatment approaches. Pm r 2015;7(1):3–8.
3. Lee MJ, Zhou Y, Greenwald BD. Update on non-pharmacological interventions for treatment of post-traumatic headache. Brain Sci 2022;12(10).
4. Ritter AC, Wagner AK, Fabio A, et al. Incidence and risk factors of posttraumatic seizures following traumatic brain injury: A Traumatic Brain Injury Model Systems Study. Epilepsia 2016;57(12):1968–77.
5. Englander J, Bushnik T, Duong TT, et al. Analyzing risk factors for late posttraumatic seizures: a prospective, multicenter investigation. Arch Phys Med Rehabil 2003;84(3):365–73.
6. Thaxton L, Myers MA. Sleep disturbances and their management in patients with brain injury. J Head Trauma Rehabil 2002;17(4):335–48.
7. Barshikar S, Bell KR. Sleep Disturbance After TBI. Curr Neurol Neurosci Rep 2017;17(11):87.
8. Ripley DL, Politzer T. Vision disturbance after TBI. NeuroRehabilitation 2010; 27(3):215–6.
9. Bell KR. Fatigue and traumatic brain injury. Arch Phys Med Rehabil 2015;96(3): 567–8.
10. Hummel T, Whitcroft KL, Andrews P, et al. Position paper on olfactory dysfunction. Rhinol Suppl 2017;54(26):1–30.
11. Drummond M, Douglas J, Olver J. "I really hope it comes back" - Olfactory impairment following traumatic brain injury: A longitudinal study. NeuroRehabilitation 2017;41(1):241–8.
12. Patla AE, Shumway-Cook A. Dimensions of mobility: defining the complexity and difficulty associated with community mobility. J Aging Phys Act 1999;7(1):7–19.
13. Maskell F, Chiarelli P, Isles R. Dizziness after traumatic brain injury: overview and measurement in the clinical setting. Brain Inj 2006;20(3):293–305.
14. Katz DI, White DK, Alexander MP, et al. Recovery of ambulation after traumatic brain injury. Arch Phys Med Rehabil 2004;85(6):865–9.

15. Morton MV, Wehman P. Psychosocial and emotional sequelae of individuals with traumatic brain injury: a literature review and recommendations. Brain Inj 1995; 9(1):81–92.
16. Hoofien D, Gilboa A, Vakil E, et al. Traumatic brain injury (TBI) 10-20 years later: a comprehensive outcome study of psychiatric symptomatology, cognitive abilities and psychosocial functioning. Brain Inj 2001;15(3):189–209.
17. Lannoo E, Brusselmans W, Van Eynde L, et al. Epidemiology of acquired brain injury (ABI) in adults: prevalence of long-term disabilities and the resulting needs for ongoing care in the region of Flanders, Belgium. Brain Inj 2004;18(2):203–11.
18. Qadeer A, Khalid U, Amin M, et al. Caregiver's Burden of the Patients With Traumatic Brain Injury. Cureus 2017;9(8):e1590.
19. Gan C, Gargaro J, Brandys C, et al. Family caregivers' support needs after brain injury: a synthesis of perspectives from caregivers, programs, and researchers. NeuroRehabilitation 2010;27(1):5–18.
20. Turner B, Fleming J, Cornwell P, et al. A qualitative study of the transition from hospital to home for individuals with acquired brain injury and their family caregivers. Brain Inj 2007;21(11):1119–30.
21. Colantonio A, Howse D, Kirsh B, et al. Living environments for people with moderate to severe acquired brain injury. Healthc Policy 2010;5(4):e120–38.
22. Everhart DE, Nicoletta AJ, Zurlinden TM, Gencarelli AM. Caregiver issues and concerns following TBI: A review of the literature and future directions. Psychol Inj Law 2020;13(1):33–43.
23. McIntyre M, Ehrlich C, Kendall E. Informal care management after traumatic brain injury: perspectives on informal carer workload and capacity. Disabil Rehabil 2020;42(6):754–62.
24. Kreutzer JS, Rapport LJ, Marwitz JH, et al. Caregivers' well-being after traumatic brain injury: a multicenter prospective investigation. Arch Phys Med Rehabil 2009;90(6):939–46.
25. Ponsford J, Olver J, Ponsford M, et al. Long-term adjustment of families following traumatic brain injury where comprehensive rehabilitation has been provided. Brain Inj 2003;17(6):453–68.
26. Ergh TC, Rapport LJ, Coleman RD, et al. Predictors of caregiver and family functioning following traumatic brain injury: social support moderates caregiver distress. J Head Trauma Rehabil 2002;17(2):155–74.
27. Lefebvre H, Pelchat D, Swaine B, et al. The experiences of individuals with a traumatic brain injury, families, physicians and health professionals regarding care provided throughout the continuum. Brain Inj 2005;19(8):585–97.
28. Vangel SJ Jr, Rapport LJ, Hanks RA. Effects of family and caregiver psychosocial functioning on outcomes in persons with traumatic brain injury. J Head Trauma Rehabil 2011;26(1):20–9.
29. Lehan T, Arango-Lasprilla JC, de los Reyes CJ, et al. The ties that bind: the relationship between caregiver burden and the neuropsychological functioning of TBI survivors. NeuroRehabilitation 2012;30(1):87–95.
30. Perlesz A, Kinsella G, Crowe S. Psychological distress and family satisfaction following traumatic brain injury: injured individuals and their primary, secondary, and tertiary carers. J Head Trauma Rehabil 2000;15(3):909–29.
31. Rotondi AJ, Sinkule J, Balzer K, et al. A qualitative needs assessment of persons who have experienced traumatic brain injury and their primary family caregivers. J Head Trauma Rehabil 2007;22(1):14–25.

32. Sander AM, Clark A, Pappadis MR. What is community integration anyway?: defining meaning following traumatic brain injury. J Head Trauma Rehabil 2010; 25(2):121–7.
33. Shaikh NM, Kersten P, Siegert RJ, et al. Developing a comprehensive framework of community integration for people with acquired brain injury: a conceptual analysis. Disabil Rehabil 2019;41(14):1615–31.
34. Burleigh SA, Farber RS, Gillard M. Community integration and life satisfaction after traumatic brain injury: long-term findings. Am J Occup Ther 1998;52(1):45–52.
35. Gerber GJ, Gargaro J. Participation in a social and recreational day programme increases community integration and reduces family burden of persons with acquired brain injury. Brain Inj 2015;29(6):722–9.
36. Schultheis MT, Whipple E. Driving after traumatic brain injury: evaluation and rehabilitation interventions. Curr Phys Med Rehabil Rep 2014;2(3):176–83.
37. Zasler ND, Katz DI, Zafonte RD. Brain injury medicine : principles and practice. New York, NY: Springer Publishing Company; 2022.
38. Jorge RE, Starkstein SE, Arndt S, et al. Alcohol misuse and mood disorders following traumatic brain injury. Arch Gen Psychiatr 2005;62(7):742–9.
39. Sander AM, Maestas KL, Pappadis MR, et al. Sexual functioning 1 year after traumatic brain injury: findings from a prospective traumatic brain injury model systems collaborative study. Arch Phys Med Rehabil 2012;93(8):1331–7.
40. Keyser-Marcus L, Briel L, Sherron-Targett P, et al. Enhancing the schooling of students with traumatic brain injury. Teach Except Child 2002;34(4):62–7.
41. Gordon DJ, Persaud UD, Beitscher I, et al. Comprehensive community reintegration programming for persons with acquired brain injury 2021;52(4):343–51.
42. Hashimoto K, Okamoto T, Watanabe S, et al. Effectiveness of a comprehensive day treatment program for rehabilitation of patients with acquired brain injury in Japan. J Rehabil Med 2006;38(1):20–5.
43. Gordon WA, Zafonte R, Cicerone K, et al. Traumatic brain injury rehabilitation: state of the science. Am J Phys Med Rehabil 2006;85(4):343–82.
44. Cullen N, Chundamala J, Bayley M, et al. The efficacy of acquired brain injury rehabilitation. Brain Inj 2007;21(2):113–32.
45. Geurtsen GJ, van Heugten CM, Martina JD, et al. Comprehensive rehabilitation programmes in the chronic phase after severe brain injury: a systematic review. J Rehabil Med 2010;42(2):97–110.
46. Wade SD, Freed JA, Kyttaris VC, et al. Implementing a Virtual Flipped Classroom in a Rheumatology Fellowship Program. Arthritis Care Res 2021;75(3):634–9.
47. High WM Jr, Roebuck-Spencer T, Sander AM, et al. Early versus later admission to postacute rehabilitation: impact on functional outcome after traumatic brain injury. Arch Phys Med Rehabil 2006;87(3):334–42.
48. Braunling-McMorrow D, Dollinger SJ, Gould M, et al. Outcomes of post-acute rehabilitation for persons with brain injury. Brain Inj 2010;24(7–8):928–38.
49. Willer B, Button J, Rempel R. Residential and home-based postacute rehabilitation of individuals with traumatic brain injury: a case control study. Arch Phys Med Rehabil 1999;80(4):399–406.
50. Glenn MB, Rotman M, Goldstein R, et al. Characteristics of residential community integration programs for adults with brain injury. J Head Trauma Rehabil 2005; 20(5):393–401.
51. Trudel TM, Nidiffer FD, Barth JT. Community-integrated brain injury rehabilitation: Treatment models and challenges for civilian, military, and veteran populations. J Rehabil Res Dev 2007;44(7):1007–16.

52. Eicher V, Murphy MP, Murphy TF, et al. Progress assessed with the Mayo-Portland Adaptability Inventory in 604 participants in 4 types of post-inpatient rehabilitation brain injury programs. Arch Phys Med Rehabil 2012;93(1):100–7.

53. Malec JF, Kean J. Post-Inpatient Brain Injury Rehabilitation Outcomes: Report from the National OutcomeInfo Database. J Neurotrauma 2016;33(14):1371–9.

54. Cicerone KD, Mott T, Azulay J, et al. Community integration and satisfaction with functioning after intensive cognitive rehabilitation for traumatic brain injury. Arch Phys Med Rehabil 2004;85(6):943–50.

55. Parry-Jones BL, Vaughan FL, Miles Cox W. Traumatic brain injury and substance misuse: a systematic review of prevalence and outcomes research (1994-2004). Neuropsychol Rehabil 2006;16(5):537–60.

56. Available at:What is a case manager? Case Management Society of America; 2017 https://www.cmsa.org/who-we-are/what-is-a-case-manager/.

57. Heinemann AW, Corrigan JD, Moore D. Case management for traumatic brain injury survivors with alcohol problems. Rehabil Psychol 2004;156–66.

58. Tahan HA, Sminkey PV. Motivational interviewing: building rapport with clients to encourage desirable behavioral and lifestyle changes. Prof Case Manag 2012; 17(4):164–72 [quiz 73-4].

59. Boschen K, Gargaro J, Gan C, et al. Family interventions after acquired brain injury and other chronic conditions: a critical appraisal of the quality of the evidence. NeuroRehabilitation 2007;22(1):19–41.

Complementary and Integrative Medicine in Treating Headaches, Cognitive Dysfunction, Mental Fatigue, Insomnia, and Mood Disorders Following Traumatic Brain Injury

A Comprehensive Review

Bruno Subbarao, DO[a],*, Zayd Hayani, MD[b], Zeke Clemmens, DO[b]

KEYWORDS

- Complementary integrative medicine • Traumatic brain injury • Mindfulness
- Acupuncture • Yoga • Tai chi • Biofeedback • Supplements

KEY POINTS

- Complementary and integrative medicine shows promise in treating the spectrum of secondary complications following traumatic brain injury (TBI).
- For patients presenting with multiple complications of TBI, providers could consider mindfulness interventions and biofeedback as an adjuvant intervention. The evidence supports multiple benefits with a high safety profile.
- For patients with a mild TBI, a small randomized-controlled trial demonstrated statistically significant improvement in cognition that extended at least 6 months after intervention.

INTRODUCTION

Traumatic brain injury (TBI) is a significant global health concern, with an estimated 69 million individuals (about twice the population of California) sustaining TBI each year worldwide.[1] It is often accompanied by a range of persistent symptoms, including headaches, cognitive dysfunction, mental fatigue, insomnia, and mood disorders such as anxiety and depression. Conventional treatments for these TBI-related symptoms can sometimes be insufficient, but complementary approaches may provide

[a] Wellness and Administrative Medicine, Phoenix Veterans Healthcare System, 650 East Indian School Road, Phoenix, AZ 85012, USA; [b] HonorHealth, 8850 East Pima Center Parkway, Scottsdale, AZ 85258, USA
* Corresponding author. Whole Health, Phoenix Veterans Healthcare System, 650 E Indian School Road, Phoenix, AZ 85012.
E-mail address: bruno.subbarao@va.gov

Phys Med Rehabil Clin N Am 35 (2024) 651–664
https://doi.org/10.1016/j.pmr.2024.02.013
1047-9651/24/Published by Elsevier Inc.
pmr.theclinics.com

viable options to fill the void in helping to address these complex conditions. Complementary and integrative medicine (CIM) modalities offer a holistic and patient-centered approach in caring for individuals with TBI and consist of a wide array of therapeutic modalities. This article aims to provide a comprehensive overview of the current literature on CIM modalities in managing headaches, cognitive dysfunction, mental fatigue, insomnia, and mood disorders following TBI.

GENERALIZED TRAUMATIC BRAIN INJURY TREATMENTS
Herbal Supplements

Herbal supplementation and other natural dietary supplements may have a complementary role with more traditional medical interventions, but due to the vast range of available supplements, navigating the literature on what may be helpful for a particular patient may be daunting to providers. In this section, we aim to focus on supplementation with higher quality evidence of therapeutic effect in patients with TBI and its related conditions.

For generalized neurorecovery after TBI, there is some limited evidence to suggest at least theoretical benefit with certain supplements. Antioxidants, such as Zinc, Docosahexaenoic acid (DHA), and curcumin (a component of the spice turmeric) are being studied as a potential option to improve cognition following TBI. For example, curcumin has been shown in rat models to significantly improve spatial memory in a water maze test and decrease neuroinflammation when given for 28 days following TBI.[2] Unfortunately, these studies primarily utilize in vitro or non-human models, making it a challenge to comment on specific dosages or side effects at present.[2–4]

Looking at supplementation research with human studies, there is evidence that branched chain amino acid supplementation (BCAAs) may improve cognition following TBI.[5] Two randomized control trials (RCTs) in 2005 by Aquilani and colleagues and follow-up study in 2008 (total of n = 101) evaluated BCAAs in patients who were approximately 2 to 4 months post injury and recently admitted to rehabilitation service. [6,7] These studies found improvement in disability rating scale (DRS) scores in patients with severe TBI after supplementation with leucine (7500 mg/d), isoleucine (3010 mg/d), and valine (9100 mg/d). [6,7] BCAAs are generally well tolerated, with 1 systematic review finding no adverse effects reported after BCAA supplementation following TBI.[5] Notably, most research has been performed on patients after severe brain injury and it is still unclear the utility BCAAs may have in improving symptoms in patients with mild-moderate TBI.[5]

Acupuncture/Acupressure

Acupuncture is a practice commonly used as a part of traditional Chinese medicine whereby a thin needle is inserted into specific parts of the body.[8] In traditional Chinese medicine, it is believed that life energy, or Qi, is circulated throughout the body via meridians or energy channels. Restoring the flow of Qi through acupuncture is believed to return the body to a healthy state.[9] Acupuncture has been touted as a treatment for many conditions, several of which co-occur with TBI, and has a large evidence base to support its practice. Management of chronic pain is a common need following TBI, with an estimated 51% of TBI patients suffering from chronic pain of some kind.[10] The Veteran Administration's Evidence Synthesis Program (ESP) compiled an evidence map which showed at least moderate evidence of benefit of acupuncture in treating both chronic musculoskeletal pain and non-musculoskeletal pain, including migraine and tension headache.[11]

Mindfulness

Mind-body interventions, including relaxation techniques and meditation, have seen renewed popularity in the general population, especially in today's fast-paced world. Self-guided or more structured meditation and mindfulness programs have a low barrier to entry, especially with the implementation of mobile applications or online videos that can assist in guiding patients through mindfulness exercises. With increasing amounts of digital stimuli, turning inward and gaining more control over one's thoughts and feelings through meditation may be particularly helpful in the TBI patient population. Unfortunately, due to the heterogeneity and subjective nature of such interventions, developing high-quality standardized studies in this area has been challenging. However, one formal program that has been studied extensively is Mindfulness-based stress reduction (MBSR). MBSR is a 10-week course developed by Professor Kabat-Zinn in the 1980s whereby patients are guided to enhance their mind-body awareness and self-regulation. Preliminary studies have shown benefit in treating certain complications of TBI with MBSR as discussed later in this chapter.[9]

HEADACHES

Headaches are a very common symptom following TBI and can significantly impact quality of life, with an estimated 27% of patients experiencing post traumatic headache 6 months after head trauma.[12] Post traumatic headache is defined as headache with onset within 7 days following head or neck trauma, with the most common subtypes being migraine-like and tension-like headaches,[13] though post-traumatic headaches can resemble any headache phenotype.[14] Given that there is a lack of high-quality randomized controlled trials of pharmacotherapy specifically for post-traumatic headache,[13] it is reasonable to turn to studies on migraine and tension-type headaches for guidance.

Acupuncture/Acupressure

Although there have not been high quality randomized trials examining acupuncture in post-traumatic headache, one exploratory study of 45 service members with TBI found improved headache-related quality of life after either auricular or traditional Chinese acupuncture compared to usual care.[15] There is also evidence of its efficacy of acupuncture for other types of headaches. One meta-analysis examined five trials comparing acupuncture to sham acupuncture, which revealed a statistically significant decrease in tension-type headaches (51% compared with 43%).[16] However, study quality is limited given the difficulty in truly blinding participants given the nature of the procedure. Although rare, there are known risks of infection, pneumothorax, syncope, and hematoma, and it is important to refer to reputable and experienced practitioners.[17] Overall, evidence suggests acupuncture can and should be considered as an adjunct treatment given its potential benefits and low rate of adverse events.[8,18]

Herbal Supplements

There is much discussion regarding efficacy of herbal remedies in improving post-TBI headache, however there is limited evidence to directly support the use of any specific supplement. In examining literature on nutritional supplements for migraine prevention, the American Headache Society gives riboflavin a level B recommendation for migraine prevention,[19] and clinicians can consider trialing 400 mg daily. Of note, riboflavin can cause increased yellow-orange pigment of urine at higher doses but otherwise appears generally safe at the recommended dosage. Some headache societies recommend Coenzyme Q10 (100 mg TID) and magnesium citrate (600 mg daily) for migraine prevention as they appear to have minimal risk of adverse effects, though the conclusions are based on low-quality studies and not directly studied in TBI patients.[19] Butterbur root extract has demonstrated some efficacy in prevention of adult and childhood migraine episodes.[19,20] Unfortunately, there is a significant risk of hepatotoxicity, which has led to controversy and potential retractions of previous recommendations by some organizations.[19,21]

Mindfulness

Mindfulness and meditation programs have shown promise as an adjunct treatment for headache in the general population. One randomized controlled trial of 40 patients with chronic headache found that an 8-week course of MBSR significantly decreased perceived headache pain intensity reported by patients as compared to pharmacotherapy alone.[22] A meta-analysis of 10 studies found cognitive-behavioral therapy (CBT) to be significantly more effective in headache outcomes compared to individuals on the waiting list, however, there were 3 studies that found no significant difference.[23] Meditation and CBT have been employed in several multidisciplinary headache treatment programs and may also offer benefits in headache management.[24]

Biofeedback

Biofeedback is a process whereby a patient's physiologic measurement is used with the goal of training that individual to have increased voluntary control of their bodily state and furthermore their emotional and cognitive response. Biofeedback may have the potential to help individuals with post traumatic headaches. In one study of 221 military personnel at Naval Okinawa Neurology clinic, patients with post traumatic headache were taught lifestyle modification tips that included guided meditation, coupled with CBT and biofeedback exercises. The results were impressive as participants had a 36% decrease in headache frequency, a 56% decrease in headache severity, with 60% of patients reporting improved quality of life as compared to the 2 years prior, and 24% were able to reduce polypharmacy. Finally, the number of visits these participants had for migraine headaches was reduced from an average of 6.8% to 2.6% per year.[25] Though biofeedback played a role here, this study perhaps demonstrated better the utility and efficacy of a multidisciplinary approach in treating post-traumatic headaches.[25]

Though not specific to post-traumatic headaches or TBI, it should be noted that in 2019, a systematic review by Kondo and colleagues produced an evidence map in regard to the benefits of biofeedback across a number of conditions. At that time, the research team concluded that there was "clear, consistent evidence across a large number of trials that biofeedback can reduce headache pain." [26]

COGNITIVE DYSFUNCTION

TBI survivors frequently suffer from a variety of cognitive symptoms. The majority of these are seen in individuals who suffered moderate to severe TBI and can persist long after the injury.[27–29] These include executive functioning, memory, language, visuoperceptual functioning, psychomotor function, and attention.[27,30] These symptoms can and do significantly impair an individual's ability to integrate back into their community.[31] They can disrupt employment, social interactions and relationships, self-care, recreation, and a variety of other areas.

Cognitive rehabilitation following TBI is a multidisciplinary approach. Complimentary and Integrative medicine can work well in such models to serve as adjunctive therapy to ongoing care whether behavioral, pharmacologic or otherwise. Below are discussed a few options to consider in the treatment of cognitive dysfunction following TBI.

Mindfulness

Mediation comes in many forms. In a recent meta-analysis by Kim and colleagues, 10 recent studies focused on meditation in treatment of memory, attention, anxiety, and depression following TBI.[32] Of the 10 studies, 5 were quasi-experimental, 3 RCTs, one a mixed-method, and one a case report.[32] Seven of these studies used a meditation modality termed MBSR or a slightly modified version.[32] MBSR, in these studies, was defined as an evidence based 8-week program that combines meditation, yoga, and other mind body practices.[31] Other meditation interventions within their MBSR program included compassion-focused imagery, progressive muscle relaxation, and breathing-based attentional-control training.[31] Eight of the 10 studies showed positive benefits and improvement in the symptoms mentioned based on several difference scales including: perceived quality of life scale, perceived self-efficacy scale, neurobehavioral symptom inventory, continuous performance test of attention, and paced auditory serial addition test.[32] Of note, attention-control training and compassion-focused imagery did not show benefit, perhaps due to their shorter duration; one day for attention-control and four weeks for compassion-focused.[32] In conclusion, due its low risk profile and potential for improvement in quality of life, MBSR can be a great consideration to complement conventional treatments in TBI.

Yoga/Tai Chi

One RCT evaluated 96 adults aged 55 and older with mild TBI conducted in 50-minute weekly session of tai chi over 6 months.[32] It showed statistically significant improvement in cognition and sit-to-stand when compared with a computerized cognitive program and usual care.[32] These results were noted to be extended at least 6 months after the intervention was completed.32,33

Acupuncture/Acupressure

One RCT by McFadden and colleagues evaluated cognitive dysfunction following eight acupressure treatments performed over four weeks.[34] The study compared pre and post treatment self-report questionnaires, neuropsychological testing, and event-related potentials.[34] The result indicated clinically significant improvements in working memory and attention compared with the placebo group.[34] It was concluded from the results that acupressure likely improves cognition, psychologic, and neurophysiologic function by reducing stress and anxiety.[34] Unfortunately, a later systematic review was unable to confirm these results and concluded that there is very limited evidence that acupressure can improve working memory and attention following mild-to-moderate TBI. While there is an obvious need for further research, because of a high safety profile for acupressure, this modality can still be considered in TBI patients that are open to alternative treatment options that may potentially benefit their cognition.[32]

Biofeedback

Heart rate variability (HRV) can be used as a specific physiologic response to focus on during biofeedback. HRV is defined as the variation of heart rate and RR intervals (ie, the time between heartbeats) measured between consecutive R waves (ie, the peak ventricular polarization of an electrocardiography wave). HRV gives insight into the balance of sympathetic and parasympathetic activity on the sinus node of the heart more directly, and indirectly insight on baroreceptor function, hormone levels, and circadian rhythms. Parasympathetic activity overall increases HRV and sympathetic activity decreases it.[35–39] Heart rate variability biofeedback aims to reduce breathing rate by providing individuals with a technique to gain control over autonomic regulation and physiologic processes of the heartbeat teaching individuals to breathe at resonance frequency. More precisely, the goal is to achieve synchrony of respiration and heart rate, while blood pressure and heart rate oscillate with each other at 180°, thus producing increases in HRV.[40,41] High HRV has been associated with improved cognitive and physical functioning, as well as executive skills, working memory, sustained attention, and recovery of TBI symptoms.[42–44] In patients with moderate to severe TBI, HRV has been shown to be decreased.

In a systematic review performed by Talbert and colleagues, it was noted that biofeedback was associated with improved HRV following TBI.[41] There was a positive relationship between increased HRV and TBI recovery.[41] The studies reviewed all measured emotional functioning and five studies used neuropsychologic measures.[41] Participants completed eleven sessions of HRV biofeedback on average (range = 1–40). Though there was limited evidence overall, there did seem to be improvements in cognitive and emotional functioning, as well as sleep, headaches, and dizziness leading to a conclusion that HRV biofeedback has potential to complement conventional TBI care.[41]

Music Therapy

Mishra and colleagues evaluated 3 observational studies evaluating music therapy and its effects on executive functioning and memory.[45] Tests used to evaluate executive functioning included Wisconsin Card sorting, Paced Auditory Serial Addition Task, and Trial Making test.[45] There were 46 total participants who attended between 4 to 48 sessions, with the higher number of patients having 4 to 5 sessions total with pre and post testing.[45] Interestingly, the studies found significant improvement in executive function in patients with TBI following intervention, although no significant effect on memory was found.[45]

MENTAL FATIGUE

Mental fatigue is a pervasive symptom in a number of neurologic conditions, such as myasthenia gravis, stroke, multiple sclerosis (MS), TBI, and Parkinson's.[46–50] It can have significant negative impacts on rehabilitation, daily functioning, quality of life, rate of hospitalization, and mortality.[51] Fatigue is rated as a symptom with the highest impact on quality of life in 50% of individual with TBI.[52] It can manifest as lack of energy or initiative or increased tiredness.[53,54] CIM modalities, including mind-body interventions and acupuncture, have been explored for managing mental fatigue.

Mindfulness

Mind-body interventions, such as MBSR and relaxation techniques, have shown promise in reducing mental fatigue and improving psychological well-being in TBI patients.[55] This was demonstrated in a meta-analysis evaluating mindfulness practices in treatment of fatigue in neurologic conditions.[55] The four studies reviewed were RCTs and had a combined total of 257 participants with neurologic conditions such as TBI, stroke, and MS. Twenty-six participants had TBI.[55] Three of the studies used MBSR and the fourth used mindfulness-based cognitive therapy (MBCT).[55] The analysis of the data showed that mindfulness intervention did have a statistically significant positive effect on fatigue across the four studies, though it was of relatively low statistical power.[55]

Acupressure

A recent RCT by Chen and colleagues on the effects of acupressure to treat fatigue in individuals with TBI included 81 participants randomized into 3 groups: 1 group receiving 2-point acupressure (TPA), one receiving 5-point acupressure (FPA), and one control group with usual care.[56] The acupressure was self-administered and was conducted over a 3-minute duration, 3 times per week for 4 weeks at home.[56] Measurements included a multidimensional fatigue index (MFI), HRV, sleep quality index, and depression outcome scale.[56] The results showed significant improvement in all the measures noted over the study period with both the TPA and FPA groups compared to control.[56]

INSOMNIA

Insomnia is defined as the inability to sleep due to problems falling asleep or maintaining sleep. It is a common and distressing sleep disorder following TBI. It is estimated that 50% to 70% of individuals with TBI in the chronic phase of recovery suffer from sleep disturbances, which is much higher than the incidence in the general population.[57] Insomnia following TBI can have a negative impact on other injury-related symptoms prolonging recovery.[58] CIM modalities, including mind-body interventions and herbal remedies, have been investigated for managing insomnia in TBI patients.

Mindfulness

In recent years, there has been evidence that mindfulness has a significant effect on insomnia.[59] Tsai-Ling and colleagues performed a meta-analysis of seven RCTs evaluating MBSR with a total of 497 participants.[59] Treatment duration was 6-8 weeks and included a combination of in-person and at home practices.[59] The data revealed that even with variable numbers of session hours and weeks, MBSR did show significant improvement in sleep quality based on the Pittsburgh sleep quality index (PSQI).[59] This scale covers multiple facets of sleep, including sleep efficacy, duration, latency, and daytime dysfunction.[59] For most of the studies, follow-up after the completion of the intervention was not performed.[59] One study however did have follow-up and noted sustain effect of PSQI for approximately 5 months post intervention.[59] Similar to these studies an RCT that randomized 10 patients with TBI into an MBSR group found a significant difference in the Insomnia Severity Index after an 8 week program.[59] Because of the importance of improving sleep to help with general recovery after TBI, integrating mindfulness-based interventions into comprehensive treatment approaches for insomnia to improve sleep quality and enhance the overall well-being of individuals living with TBI should be strongly considered.

Herbal Remedies

Leach and colleagues conducted a meta-analysis of four commonly used herbal remedies for insomnia: valerian, chamomile, kava, and wuling.[60,61] The analysis included 1602 participants who met criteria for insomnia across 14 RCTs.[60] Twelve studies tested valerian, the majority using V. officinalis. The mean daily dose was 912 mg (ranging from 300 mg to 3645 mg daily) (13 studies).[60] Wuling had a dose of 0.33 g 3 times daily (1 study), Kava dose 100 mg 3 times daily (3 studies), and chamomile 270 mg twice daily(1 study).[60] The studies ranged in duration from 1 day to 6 weeks, with a mean study duration of 3 weeks.[60] The data showed no statistically significant difference between placebo and any of the 4 herbal remedies when assessing 13 measures of clinical efficacy.[60] No increased adverse events were noted with kava, chamomile, or wuling when compared with placebo[60] By contrast, a greater number of events per person were reported with valerian.[60] Based on this analysis there is insufficient evidence to support these 4 remedies for treatment of insomnia.

Suanzaoren is another remedy recently investigated for use in the treatment of insomnia. Yang and colleagues conducted a meta-analysis of 9 studies evaluating the use of suanzaoren for insomnia.[62] The studies included 785 patients with insomnia disorder and another 120 with sleep disturbances.[60] Doses and products were variable but were all taken by mouth several times a day for a mean of 4.5 weeks (range from 2-12 weeks).[62] Each study used either the Insomnia Severity Index (ISI) or the PSQI.[62] Though there was heterogeneity in the studies, subgroup analysis did show that suanzaoren had a significant improvement in the respective indexes compared to placebo.[62] Even compared with benzodiazepines or CBT, suanzaoren was associated with a significant decrease in insomnia severity at 4 weeks.[62] Long-term effects of suanzaoren are unknown but no major adverse effects were observed.[62] Though this meta-analysis is not specific to TBI, it does demonstrate promise for a potential treatment option in the future.

MOOD DISORDERS (ANXIETY/DEPRESSION)

Mood disorders, particularly anxiety and depression, are exceedingly prevalent following TBI and can significantly impact an individual's emotional well-being and overall recovery. The incidence of depression in patients with TBI is estimated to be 34.60 per 1000 person-years, compared to 21.42 in the general population.[63] One year following TBI, patients are at 11 times increased risk for development of depression.[63] Post Traumatic Stress Disorder (PTSD) is also a very common and debilitating comorbid psychiatric condition in patients with TBI. CIM modalities including mind-body interventions and herbal remedies have been explored for managing anxiety and depression in TBI patients.

Mindfulness

Mind-body interventions, such as mindfulness-based programs and meditation, have demonstrated benefits in managing symptoms of anxiety and depression among patients with a history of TBI.[64] More generally, several studies have shown that MBSR programs can significantly reduce depression and anxiety in patients with chronic illness.[65,66] One study of 200 patients who completed an 8-week MBSR program showed a 24% decrease in depression scores as measured by the Hospital Anxiety and Depression Scale- Depression subscale (HADS-D).[67] One small pilot study of nine veterans with PTSD and a history of mild TBI found improvement of attention and overall PTSD symptom scoring after a course of MBSR.[68]

Acupuncture

One meta-analysis conducted by Grant and colleagues including a total of 706 participants found very low quality of evidence in support of acupuncture as a treatment for PTSD symptoms or depressive symptoms in patients with PTSD. Additionally, across 7 RCTs reviewed, they found minimal risk for serious adverse events for patients utilizing this modality.[69]

Biofeedback

Biofeedback has the potential to help patients with mood disorders in addition to some of the aforementioned TBI sequelae. One systematic review showed evidence of HRV, temperature, and electromyography(EMG) biofeedback efficacy in decreasing anxiety and mood dysfunction following TBI.[32] One study of 32 survivors of intimate partner violence found a statistically significant decrease in depression, anxiety, and PTSD symptom scores after a neurofeedback program consisting of 42 30-min-long sessions using EEG feedback.[70] However, this study is limited in its lack of a control group.[70]

Herbal Supplements

Herbal remedies have been used for centuries to treat all ranges of ailments, and some have also shown potential in reducing anxiety and depression symptoms. One systematic review of five randomized controlled trials found a statistically significant decrease in depression symptoms in adults with major depressive disorder after taking Saffron 30 mg daily.[71] It is worth noting, however, there is some concern for financial conflict of interest involving the authors.[71] A more robust meta-analysis from Dai and colleagues of twelve studies showed improvement of mild-moderate depression in patients taking Saffron compared with placebo, without significant adverse effects attributed to the supplement.[72] Unfortunately, there have yet to be high quality studies on saffron on human subjects following TBI.

St John's wort is a dietary supplement extracted from the flowering plant, *Hypericum perforatum*.[73] Multiple meta-analyses of St. John's wort compared with placebo in the treatment of adults with depression showed improvement in depression scales.[74] These studies also showed no significant difference in depression scores between patients taking St. John's wort and traditional pharmacologic antidepressants (selective serotonin reuptake inhibitors or tricyclic antidepressants).[74] Overall, it appears St. John's wort is well tolerated, with only 2.6% of users reporting adverse effects, most commonly nausea and allergic rash.[73] However, clinicians should be aware that St. John's wort is a known inducer of the cytochrome P450 system, as well as case reports of it inducing supraventricular tachycardia.[75]

For individuals struggling with anxiety, dietary supplementation with Kava extract may be helpful. One systematic review of RCTs, with a total of n = 645 participants with generalized anxiety, found the Kava extract supplementation to be significantly more anxiolytic than placebo, with few, mild adverse events.[76]

SUMMARY

Complementary and integrative medicine approaches, including acupuncture, herbal remedies, nutritional supplements, and mind-body interventions, hold promise as adjunctive therapies for managing headaches, cognitive dysfunction, mental fatigue, insomnia, and mood disorders following TBI. Integrating CIM modalities into comprehensive TBI rehabilitation programs may offer a holistic approach to address these multifaceted symptoms and improve the overall well-being and quality of life of individuals with TBI. Further well-designed research studies will help establish their efficacy, safety, and optimal implementation in this specific population.

CLINICS CARE POINTS

- Patients can suffer from a wide spectrum of sequelae following traumatic brain injury, including insomnia, cognitive changes, mood disturbances, headache, and mental fatigue.
- There is evidence to suggest that acupuncture and acupressure may be helpful in common post

- TBI symptoms such as musculoskeletal pain and headache, however it is difficult to perform truly blinded and controlled studies.
- Biofeedback techniques have shown promising results in treatment of several different post
- TBI symptoms including cognitive function, mood, sleep, and headaches, however further development is needed to make this modality more standardized.
- Mindfulness is an inexpensive, therapeutic modality that has a low barrier of entry and has shown to be helpful in the treatment of post
- TBI related cognitive dysfunction, fatigue, insomnia, and mood dysfunction.

Pitfalls:
- There is limited high-quality evidence to suggest that specific herbal supplements are helpful in treatment of common post
- TBI related symptoms.-Research of the various CIM approaches have largely been conducted outside of the TBI population, and very few studies involve cohorts with severe TBI. More research is needed to understand the benefits and risks across the spectrum of TBI.

DISCLOSURE

There are no commercial or financial conflicts of interest from any of the authors.

REFERENCES

1. Dewan MC, Rattani A, Gupta S, et al. Estimating the global incidence of traumatic brain injury. J Neurosurg 2018;130(4):1080–97.
2. Sun G, Miao Z, Ye Y, et al. Curcumin alleviates neuroinflammation, enhances hippocampal neurogenesis, and improves spatial memory after traumatic brain injury. Brain Res Bull 2020;162:84–93.
3. Royes LFF, Gomez-Pinilla F. Making sense of gut feelings in the traumatic brain injury pathogenesis. Neurosci Biobehav Rev 2019;102:345–61.
4. Lucke-Wold BP, Logsdon AF, Nguyen L, et al. Supplements, nutrition, and alternative therapies for the treatment of traumatic brain injury. Nutr Neurosci 2018; 21(2):79–91.
5. Sharma B, Lawrence DW, Hutchison MG. Branched Chain Amino Acids (BCAAs) and Traumatic Brain Injury: A Systematic Review. J Head Trauma Rehabil 2018; 33(1):33–45.
6. Aquilani R, Iadarola P, Contardi A, et al. Branched-chain aminoacids enhance the cognitive recovery of patients with severe trau-matic brain injury. Arch Phys Med Rehabil 2005;86(9):1729–35.
7. Aquilani R, Boselli M, Boschi F, et al. Branched-chain aminoacids may improve recovery from a vegetative or minimally con-scious state in patients with trau-matic brain injury: a pilot study. Arch Phys Med Rehabil 2008;89(9):1642–7.
8. Linde K, Mulrow CD, Berner M, et al. St John's wort for depression. Cochrane Database Syst Rev 2005;(2):CD000448.
9. Drake DF, Hudak AM, Robbins W. Integrative Medicine in Traumatic Brain Injury. Phys Med Rehabil Clin N Am 2017;28(2):363–78. https://doi.org/10.1016/j.pmr.2016.12.011.
10. Nampiaparampil DE. Prevalence of Chronic Pain After Traumatic Brain Injury: A Systematic Review. JAMA 2008;300(6):711–9. https://doi.org/10.1001/jama.300.6.711.

11. Shekelle P, Allen J, Mak S, et al. Evidence map of acupuncture as treatment for adult health conditions: update from 2013–2021. Washington, DC: Evidence Synthesis Program, Health Services Research and Development Ser; 2022.

12. Baandrup L, Jensen R. Chronic post-traumatic headache—a clinical analysis in relation to the International Headache Classification 2nd Edition (published correction appears in Cephalalgia. 2005 Mar;25(3):240). Cephalalgia. 2005;25(2):132-138.

13. Larsen EL, Ashina H, Iljazi A, et al. Acute and preventive pharmacological treatment of post-traumatic headache: a systematic review. J Headache Pain 2019; 20(1):98.

14. Headache Classification Committee of the International Headache Society (I) The International Classification of headache disorders, 3rd edition. Cephalalgia. 2018;38(1):1-211.

15. Jonas WB, Bellanti DM, Paat CF, et al. A Randomized Exploratory Study to Evaluate Two Acupuncture Methods for the Treatment of Headaches Associated with Traumatic Brain Injury. Med Acupunct 2016;28(3):113–30.

16. Linde K, Allais G, Brinkhaus B, et al. Acupuncture for the prevention of tension-type headache. Cochrane Database Syst Rev 2016;4(4):CD007587.

17. He W, Zhao X, Li Y, et al. Adverse events following acupuncture: a systematic review of the Chinese literature for the years 1956-2010. J Altern Complement Med 2012;18(10):892–901.

18. Wong V, Cheuk DK, Lee S, et al. Acupuncture for acute management and rehabilitation of traumatic brain injury. Cochrane Database Syst Rev 2013;3: CD007700.

19. Rajapakse T, Pringsheim T. Nutraceuticals in Migraine: A Summary of Existing Guidelines for Use. Headache 2016;56(4):808–16.

20. Oelkers-Ax R, Leins A, Parzer P, et al. Butterbur root extract and music therapy in the prevention of childhood migraine: an explorative study. Eur J Pain 2008;12(3): 301–13.

21. Malone M, Tsai G. The evidence for herbal and botanical remedies, Part 1. J Fam Pract 2018;67(1):10–6.

22. Bakhshani NM, Amirani A, Amirifard H, et al. The Effectiveness of Mindfulness-Based Stress Reduction on Perceived Pain Intensity and Quality of Life in Patients With Chronic Headache. Global J Health Sci 2015;8(4):142–51.

23. Harris P, Loveman E, Clegg A, et al. Systematic review of cognitive behavioural therapy for the management of headaches and migraines in adults. Br J Pain 2015;9(4):213–24.

24. Andrasik F, et al. Behavioral treatment approaches to chronic headache. Neurol Sci 2016;37(Suppl 1):79–83.

25. Baker VB, Eliasen KM, Hack NK. Lifestyle modifications as therapy for medication refractory post-traumatic headache (PTHA) in the military population of Okinawa. J Headache Pain 2018;19(1):113.

26. Kondo K, Noonan KM, Freeman M, et al. Efficacy of Biofeedback for Medical Conditions: an Evidence Map. J Gen Intern Med 2019;34(12):2883–93.

27. Schretlen DJ, Shapiro AM. A quantitative review of the effects of traumatic brain injury on cognitive functioning. Int Rev Psychiatr 2003;15(4):341–9.

28. Lee B, Leem J, Kim H, et al. Herbal Medicine for Traumatic Brain Injury: A Systematic Review and Meta-Analysis of Randomized Controlled Trials and Limitations. Front Neurol 2020;11:772.

29. Goh M.S.L., Looi D.S.H., Goh J.L., et al., The Impact of Traumatic Brain Injury on Neurocognitive Outcomes in Children: a Systematic Review and Meta-Analysis. *J Neurol Neurosurg Psychiatry.* 2021:jnnp-2020-325066.

30. Sharbafshaaer M. Impacts of cognitive impairment for different levels and causes of traumatic brain injury, and education status in TBI patients. Dement Neuropsychol 2018;12(4):415–20.

31. Barman A, Chatterjee A, Bhide R. Cognitive Impairment and Rehabilitation Strategies After Traumatic Brain Injury. Indian J Psychol Med 2016;38(3):172–81.

32. Kim S, Mortera MH, Wen PS, et al. The Impact of Complementary and Integrative Medicine Following Traumatic Brain Injury: A Scoping Review. J Head Trauma Rehabil 2023;38(1):E33–43.

33. Hwang HF, Chen CY, Wei L, et al. Effects of Computerized Cognitive Training and Tai Chi on Cognitive Performance in Older Adults With Traumatic Brain Injury. J Head Trauma Rehabil 2020;35(3):187–97.

34. McFadden KL, Healy KM, Dettmann ML, et al. Acupressure as a non-pharmacological intervention for traumatic brain injury (TBI). J Neurotrauma 2011;28(1):21–34.

35. Cygankiewicz I, Zareba W. Heart rate variability. Handb Clin Neurol 2013;117: 379–93.

36. Esterov D, Greenwald BD. Autonomic Dysfunction after Mild Traumatic Brain Injury. Brain Sci 2017;7(8):100.

37. Heart rate variability: standards of measurement, physiological interpretation and clinical use. Task Force of the European Society of Cardiology and the North American Society of Pacing and Electrophysiology. Circulation 1996;93(5): 1043–106.

38. Blake TA, McKay CD, Meeuwisse WH, et al. The impact of concussion on cardiac autonomic function: A systematic review. Brain Inj 2016;30(2):132–45.

39. Bishop S, Dech R, Baker T, et al. Parasympathetic baroreflexes and heart rate variability during acute stage of sport concussion recovery. Brain Inj 2017; 31(2):247–59.

40. Conder RL, Conder AA. Heart rate variability interventions for concussion and rehabilitation. Front Psychol 2014;5:890.

41. Talbert LD, Kaelberer Z, Gleave E, et al. A systematic review of heart rate variability (HRV) biofeedback treatment following traumatic brain injury (TBI). Brain Inj 2023;37(7):635–42.

42. Abaji JP, Curnier D, Moore RD, et al. Persisting Effects of Concussion on Heart Rate Variability during Physical Exertion. J Neurotrauma 2016;33(9):811–7.

43. Hansen AL, Johnsen BH, Thayer JF. Vagal influence on working memory and attention. Int J Psychophysiol 2003;48(3):263–74.

44. Murray NP, Russoniello C. Acute physical activity on cognitive function: a heart rate variability examination. Appl Psychophysiol Biofeedback 2012;37(4):219–27.

45. Mishra R, Florez-Perdomo WA, Shrivatava A, et al. Role of Music Therapy in Traumatic Brain Injury: A Systematic Review and Meta-analysis. World Neurosurg 2021;146:197–204.

46. Chaudhuri A, Behan PO. Fatigue in neurological disorders. Lancet 2004; 363(9413):978–88.

47. DeLuca J, Genova HM, Hillary FG, et al. Neural correlates of cognitive fatigue in multiple sclerosis using functional MRI. J Neurol Sci 2008;270(1–2):28–39.

48. Cantor JB, Ashman T, Bushnik T, et al. Systematic review of interventions for fatigue after traumatic brain injury: a NIDRR traumatic brain injury model systems study. J Head Trauma Rehabil 2014;29(6):490–7.

49. Friedman JH, Abrantes A, Sweet LH. Fatigue in Parkin'on's disease. Expet Opin Pharmacother 2011;12(13):1999–2007.
50. Kluger BM, Krupp LB, Enoka RM. Fatigue and fatigability in neurologic illnesses: proposal for a unified taxonomy. Neurology 2013;80(4):409–16.
51. Juengst S, Skidmore E, Arenth PM, et al. Unique contribution of fatigue to disability in community-dwelling adults with traumatic brain injury. Arch Phys Med Rehabil 2013;94(1):74–9.
52. LaChapelle DL, Finlayson MA. An evaluation of subjective and objective measures of fatigue in patients with brain injury and healthy controls. Brain Inj 1998;12(8):649–59.
53. Glader EL, Stegmayr B, Asplund K. Poststroke fatigue: a 2-year follow-up study of stroke patients in Sweden. Stroke 2002;33(5):1327–33.
54. Choi-Kwon S, Kim JS. Poststroke fatigue: an emerging, critical issue in stroke medicine. Int J Stroke 2011;6(4):328–36.
55. Ulrichsen KM, Kaufmann T, Dørum ES, et al. Clinical Utility of Mindfulness Training in the Treatment of Fatigue After Stroke, Traumatic Brain Injury and Multiple Sclerosis: A Systematic Literature Review and Meta-analysis. Front Psychol 2016; 7:912.
56. Chen SM, Chen WL, Tai CJ, et al. Effects of Self-Administered Acupressure on Fatigue Following Traumatic Brain Injury: A Randomized Controlled Trial [published online ahead of print, 2023 Mar 23]. J Head Trauma Rehabil 2023. https://doi.org/10.1097/HTR.0000000000000.
57. Mathias JL, Alvaro PK. Prevalence of sleep disturbances, disorders, and problems following traumatic brain injury: a meta-analysis. Sleep Med 2012;13(7): 898–905.
58. Sandsmark DK, Elliott JE, Lim MM. Sleep-Wake Disturbances After Traumatic Brain Injury: Synthesis of Human and Animal Studies. Sleep 2017;40(5):zsx044.
59. Chen TL, Chang SC, Hsieh HF, et al. Effects of mindfulness-based stress reduction on sleep quality and mental health for insomnia patients: A meta-analysis. J Psychosom Res 2020;135:110144.
60. Werner JK Jr, Collen JF. 0391 Mindfulness Based Stress Reduction as a Treatment for Chronic Insomnia in Traumatic Brain Injury Patients. Sleep 2019;42: A158–9.
61. Leach MJ, Page AT. Herbal medicine for insomnia: A systematic review and meta-analysis. Sleep Med Rev 2015;24:1–12.
62. Yang M, Wang H, Zhang YL, et al. The Herbal Medicine Suanzaoren (Ziziphi Spinosae Semen) for Sleep Quality Improvements: A Systematic Review and Meta-analysis. Integr Cancer Ther 2023;22. 15347354231162080.
63. Choi Y, Kim EY, Sun J, et al. Incidence of Depression after Traumatic Brain Injury: A Nationwide Longitudinal Study of 2.2 Million Adults. J Neurotrauma 2022; 39(5–6):390–7.
64. Randolph C, et al. Mindfulness-based stress reduction for veterans with traumatic brain injury: Results from a pilot study. Mil Med 2017;182(9):e1798–805.
65. Bakhshani NM, Amirani A, Amirifard H, et al. The Effectiveness of Mindfulness-Based stress Reduction on Perceived Pain Intensity and Quality of Life in Patients With Chronic Headache. Global J Health Sci 2015;8(4):142–51.
66. Grossman P, Niemann L, Schmidt S, et al. Mindfulness-based stress reduction and health benefits: A meta-analysis. J Psychosom Res 2010;57(1):35–44.
67. Greeson JM, Smoski MJ, Suarez EC, et al. Decreased symptoms of depression after mindfulness-based stress reduction: potential moderating effects of

religiosity, spirituality, trait mindfulness, sex, and age. J Alter Complement Med 2015;21(3):166–74.

68. Cole MA, Muir JJ, Gans JJ, et al. Simultaneous treatment of neurocognitive and psychiatric symptoms in veterans with post-traumatic stress disorder and history of mild traumatic brain injury: a pilot study of mindfulness-based stress reduction. Mil Med 2015;180(9):956–63.

69. Grant S, Colaiaco B, Motala A, et al. Acupuncture for the Treatment of Adults with Posttraumatic Stress Disorder: A Systematic Review and Meta-Analysis. J Trauma & Dissociation 2018;19(1):39–58.

70. Brown L, Karmakar C, Gray R, et al. Heart rate variability alterations in late life depression: A meta-analysis. J Affect Disord 2018;235:456–66.

71. Hausenblas HA, Saha D, Dubyak PJ, et al. Saffron (Crocus sativus L.) and major depressive disorder: A meta-analysis of randomized clinical trials. J Integr Med 2013;11(6):377–83.

72. Dai L, Chen L, Wang W. Safety and Efficacy of Saffron (Crocus sativus L.) for Treating Mild to Moderate Depression: A Systematic Review and Meta-analysis. J Nerv Ment Dis 2020;208(4):269–76.

73. Gaster B, Holroyd J. St John's Wort for Depression: A Systematic Review. Arch Intern Med 2000;160(2):152–6.

74. Linde K, Mulrow CD, Berner M, et al. St John's wort for depression. Cochrane Database Syst Rev 2005;2:CD000448.

75. Fisher KA, Patel P, Abualula S, et al. St Johns Wort-induced Supraventricular Tachycardia. Cureus 2021;13(4):e14356.

76. Pittler MH, Ernst E. Kava extract for treating anxiety. Cochrane Database Syst Rev 2003;1:CD003383.

Medical-Legal Issues in Traumatic Brain Injury

Stuart J. Glassman, MD, MBA[a,b,]*

KEYWORDS

- Traumatic brain injury • Medical legal • Concussion • Ethics • Expert witness
- Medical evidence • Credibility • Damages

KEY POINTS

- Traumatic Brain Injury (TBI) cases often involve both medical and legal issues, litigation and prolonged recovery timelines.
- As TBI cases are often complex, and can have a significant impact on the lives of the patients and their families/caregivers, having a comprehensive understanding of the causes, diagnoses, treatments and long term outcomes will be valuable in understanding the medical and legal aspects of this type of injury.
- Patients, families, and health care professionals will all benefit from a deeper understanding of the medical and legal aspects of TBI, which should help improve rehabilitation and recovery outcomes.

INTRODUCTION

Understanding traumatic brain injury (TBI) is essential for medical professionals, legal professionals, and individuals/families affected by these injuries. TBI is a complex and potentially life-altering condition, and a deeper awareness of its causes, classifications, initial assessment, diagnosis, treatment, and long-term outcomes is crucial to a more comprehensive awareness of the medical and legal issues involved. Understanding the medical and legal aspects of TBI is crucial for health care professionals to provide appropriate care for their patients, and for individuals and their families to navigate the challenges and uncertainties that may arise during TBI recovery and rehabilitation. It is also vital for legal professionals involved in TBI cases to be aware of, and accurately represent, the medical aspects when advocating for the rights and compensation of TBI survivors. This interplay of medical and legal issues often occurs for many years after the initial injury, and can evolve through a patient's recovery and legal case progression. Patients with TBI are frequently involved in a litigation with

[a] Department of Physical Medicine & Rehabilitation, VA Northern California Healthcare System; 10535 Hospital Way, Mather, CA 95655, USA; [b] Department of Medicine, David Geffen School of Medicine at UCLA, 10833 Le Conte Avenue, Los Angeles, CA 90095, USA
* Corresponding author. VA Northern California Healthcare System, 10535 Hospital Way, Mather, CA 95655.
E-mail address: Stuart.Glassman@va.gov

Phys Med Rehabil Clin N Am 35 (2024) 665–678
https://doi.org/10.1016/j.pmr.2024.02.014
1047-9651/24/Published by Elsevier Inc.
pmr.theclinics.com

claim compensation proceedings because another person was partly or wholly at fault for causing the injury, in particular in the context of road traffic accidents.[1]

Understanding Traumatic Brain Injury

Definition of traumatic brain injury

Traumatic brain injury (TBI) is a medical condition that often results from an external force or trauma to the head. TBI can be caused by a forceful bump, blow, or jolt to the head or body, or from an object that pierces the skull and enters the brain.[2] This trauma can cause damage to the brain's structure or function, leading to a wide range of physical, cognitive, emotional, and behavioral impairments. TBI can vary widely in terms of presentation severity, from mild to severe. A TBI can lead to short- or long-term problems that may affect all aspects of a person's life, including the ability to work, or build relationships with others, and it can change how a person thinks, acts, feels, and learns.[3] TBI can result from various traumatic incidents,[4] including but not limited to.

- Falls: Especially common in young children and the elderly.
- Motor Vehicle Accidents: A leading cause of TBI, whereby head injuries often result from collisions or sudden deceleration.
- Sports-Related Injuries: Contact and/or collision sports, such as football or hockey, pose a risk of TBI due to head impacts.
- Assaults or Violent Encounters: Physical altercations can lead to head injuries, due to a blow/strike to the head.
- Explosions and Blasts: Military personnel, in particular, are at risk due to exposure to blasts, flying debris, pressure waves, and so forth.
- Penetrating Injuries: Gunshot wounds, shrapnel, or sharp objects can cause TBI.

Classification and Severity Levels of Traumatic Brain Injury

TBIs can be classified into 3 main categories based on severity.[5]

- Mild TBI (Concussion): most cases typically are not characterized by any loss of consciousness. Symptoms may include confusion, memory problems, and mild headaches. While most mild TBI cases resolve relatively quickly (days to weeks), some cases can persist for months or years.
- Moderate TBI: usually involves more pronounced cognitive and physical impairments, often with a loss of consciousness, and recovery may be more extended compared with a mild TBI.
- Severe TBI: Severe TBI cases often persist for months or years, and can result in significant and long-lasting cognitive, physical, and emotional impairments. Individuals with severe TBI may require extensive medical intervention and rehabilitation.

Medical Aspects of Traumatic Brain Injury

Initial assessment and diagnosis

Early and accurate diagnosis of TBI is crucial.[6] The process typically involves the following steps.

1. Clinical Assessment: Medical professionals, such as emergency physicians, trauma/neurosurgeons, neurologists, and physiatrists, assess the individual's condition, noting symptoms and signs of TBI, including loss of consciousness, amnesia, and neurologic deficits.

2. Neuroimaging: Diagnostic imaging techniques, such as CT scans and MRI scans, are often used to visualize the brain's structure and identify any abnormalities or damage.
3. Cognitive Testing: Neuropsychological testing may be used to assess cognitive functions, memory, and problem-solving abilities.
4. Physical Examination: This includes a comprehensive examination of the patient's physical condition, neurologic assessment, and balance, to identify any other associated injuries or complications.
5. Patient History: Gathering information from the patient or witnesses about the event leading to the injury can aid in diagnosis, including a self-reporting of symptoms such as the Graded Symptom Scale/Checklist
6. Glasgow Coma Scale (GCS): The GCS is a common tool used to assess a patient's level of consciousness, with lower scores indicating more severe injury.
7. Other Assessments: Depending on the circumstances and the severity of the injury, additional tests and assessments may be performed to rule out other conditions or injuries (PET scan, DTI scans, and so forth).

Clinical presentation and symptoms

The symptoms and clinical presentation of TBI can vary widely based on the severity and location of the brain injury.[7] Common symptoms include.

1. Headaches: Frequent or severe headaches are a common symptom of TBI.
2. Dizziness and Balance Problems: Individuals may experience difficulty maintaining balance or coordination.
3. Cognitive Impairments: This includes memory problems, difficulty concentrating, and decreased problem-solving abilities.
4. Sensory Disturbances: Changes in vision, hearing, or sensitivity to light and sound can occur.
5. Mood and Behavioral Changes: TBI can lead to mood swings, irritability, and behavioral issues.
6. Loss of Consciousness: Individuals may experience varying degrees of loss of consciousness.
7. Nausea and Vomiting: These symptoms can occur in the immediate aftermath of a head injury.
8. Motor Skill Impairment: Difficulty with motor functions, including weakness or co-ordination problems, can occur.
9. Seizures: Some individuals may experience seizures as a result of a TBI.
10. Coma: Severe TBIs can lead to a coma or a persistent vegetative state.

Diagnostic procedures

Diagnosing a traumatic brain injury can involve various testing/diagnostic procedures to assess the injury's extent and location.[8] Some of these include.

1. Computed Tomography (CT) Scan: CT scans are often used in the emergency room to visualize structural brain damage, hemorrhaging, and skull fractures.
2. Magnetic Resonance Imaging (MRI): MRIs provide more detailed images of the brain, making them valuable for assessing soft tissue damage and long-term effects, usually after the first 24 hours immediately following a traumatic brain injury.
3. Neuropsychological Testing: These assessments help evaluate cognitive functions, memory, and behavior.
4. Electroencephalogram (EEG): An EEG measures brain activity and is used to detect abnormalities, such as seizures.

5. Intracranial Pressure Monitoring: In severe cases, monitoring the pressure inside the skull can be necessary to prevent further damage.
6. Blood tests: The Banyan Brain Trauma Indicator (BTI) is a relatively new blood test that looks for proteins in a patients blood to indicate a mild TBI

Treatment options and rehabilitation

Treatment strategies for TBI can often depend on the severity of the injury.[9] Some treatment options include.

1. Mild TBI (Concussion):
   • Treatment primarily involves initial rest, symptom management, and close monitoring for complications. Physical and cognitive activity can gradually be increased as recovery progresses.
2. Moderate to Severe TBI:
   • Immediate medical intervention may be required to stabilize the patient. Surgical procedures may be necessary to remove blood clots, repair skull fractures, or relieve intracranial pressure. Rehabilitation programs aim to restore lost functions, including physical, cognitive, vision, and psychosocial aspects.
3. Medications
   Medications may be prescribed to manage symptoms such as headaches, seizures, balance problems, nausea or mood disorders.
4. Long-Term Rehabilitation
   Depending on the severity, individuals with TBI may require ongoing rehabilitation, including physical therapy, speech therapy, cognitive therapy, and vision therapy to regain functional independence.

Long-Term Effects and Prognosis of Traumatic Brain Injury

The prognosis for TBI varies widely based on the severity of the injury, the quality of medical care, and individual factors.[10] Long-term effects may include.

1. Cognitive Impairment: Memory problems, difficulties with attention and problem-solving, and changes in executive functioning.
2. Emotional and Behavioral Changes: Mood disorders, such as depression and anxiety, and personality changes are common.
3. Physical Impairments: Weakness, muscle spasticity, and coordination problems may persist.
4. Sensory Disturbances: Permanent changes in vision, hearing, or sensory perception can occur.
5. Seizures: Some individuals may develop epilepsy after a TBI.
6. Chronic Pain: Headaches or other chronic pain issues may persist.

Legal Framework for Traumatic Brain Injury Cases

TBI cases involve complex medical conditions and legal implications that require careful consideration due to their profound impact on the lives of affected individuals and their families.[11] The significance of medical-legal issues in TBI cases cannot be overstated. This significance arises from the complex medical nature of the injury, the need to establish causation and damages, the reliance on expert witnesses, issues of legal liability, insurance claims, statutes of limitations, and ethical considerations. Navigating these complexities requires a collaborative effort between legal and medical professionals to ensure just outcomes for TBI survivors and their families. Here are some key reasons why medical-legal issues in TBI cases are significant.

1. Complexity of TBI Diagnosis and Assessment:

- TBI cases often require in-depth medical expertise to properly diagnose and assess the extent of the injury. Accurate diagnosis is essential to determine the appropriate medical treatment and rehabilitation.
2. Establishing Causation:
    - In legal cases, it is crucial to establish a clear link between the traumatic event and the brain injury. Medical experts play a vital role in proving causation, helping the court understand how the injury occurred and its impact on the individual.
3. Determining Damages:
    - The severity of a TBI can vary significantly, and the extent of damages, including medical expenses, lost wages, and future care costs, must be accurately calculated. Medical experts can provide critical input on the long-term consequences of the injury, through consultative evaluations such as life care planning assessments.
4. Role of Expert Witnesses:
    - TBI case litigation, relative to the medical complexities, often relies on expert witnesses, including neurologists, neuropsychologists, and rehabilitation specialists. These experts provide essential testimony to help the court understand the medical aspects of the case.
5. Legal Liability and Negligence:
    - TBI cases may involve issues of liability and negligence, such as determining if a person or entity (eg, a driver, an employer, or a product manufacturer) was responsible for the injury. Legal professionals need to work closely with medical experts to establish negligence or liability.
6. Insurance Claims and Coverage:
    - TBI cases often intersect with insurance issues, including health insurance, auto insurance, and workers' compensation coverage. The involvement of medical-legal professionals is critical to navigate these complex insurance matters.
7. Statutes of Limitations:
    - Legal time limits, known as statutes of limitations, are applicable to TBI cases. Understanding these timeframes and ensuring timely legal actions is crucial.
8. Ethical Considerations:
    - Balancing the interests of the injured individual with the responsibilities of the legal and medical professionals requires ethical considerations. Ensuring fair compensation and access to necessary medical care is an ethical concern in TBI cases.
9. Settlement Negotiations and Trial Preparation:
    - Medical-legal experts play a significant role in settlement negotiations and trial preparations, often assisting lawyers to review the complex medical issues often seen in TBI cases.
10. Evolution of Legal Standards:
    - The legal landscape for TBI cases is continually evolving with changes in laws, regulations, and legal standards. Legal and medical professionals must stay informed about these developments and update their understanding of the medical-legal issues accordingly.

The legal framework in viewing traumatic brain injury (TBI) cases is a complex and essential aspect of addressing the legal rights and compensation for individuals who have suffered TBIs due to the negligence or fault of others. This framework encompasses personal injury claims, liability and negligence, statutes of limitations, and the role of insurance companies. Understanding this legal framework is crucial for legal professionals, TBI survivors, and their families.[12]

- Personal injury claims and TBI: TBI cases often fall under the broader category of personal injury law. Personal injury claims are legal actions pursued by individuals (plaintiffs) who have been harmed as a result of someone else's negligence, recklessness, or intentional actions.
- Liability and negligence in TBI cases: Establishing liability and negligence is a fundamental aspect of TBI cases. Plaintiffs must demonstrate that the defendant (the party responsible for the injury) owed a duty of care to the plaintiff, breached that duty, and that the breach directly caused the TBI. Negligence can occur in various situations, such as car accidents, premises liability (slip and fall cases), and medical malpractice. Comparative negligence laws in some jurisdictions assess the degree of fault on the part of both the plaintiff and the defendant, impacting the amount of compensation awarded.
- Statutes of limitations and filing deadlines: Statutes of limitations are legal time limits that dictate how long a plaintiff has to file a lawsuit after the injury occurs. These time limits vary by jurisdiction and the type of case but are typically between one to 6 years. In TBI cases, it is crucial to understand the relevant statute of limitations to ensure timely legal action. Certain circumstances, such as discovery rules (which start the clock when the injury is discovered), can affect the applicable deadline.
- Role of insurance companies: Insurance companies play a significant role in TBI cases, particularly in cases involving motor vehicle accidents, premises liability, and workers' compensation. Auto insurance, homeowner's insurance, and workers' compensation insurance may provide coverage for TBI-related claims. Negotiating with insurance companies and ensuring that victims receive fair compensation often involves legal professionals. Racial/ethnic minorities appear to be at increased risk for TBI and poor health outcomes after TBI, as racial/ethnic minorities are overrepresented among low-income populations and less likely to have medical insurance, which may contribute to their poor health status.[13]
- Workers' Compensation and TBI: In cases whereby TBI occurs in the workplace, individuals may be eligible for workers' compensation benefits. Workers' compensation is a system that provides medical treatment, wage replacement, and disability benefits to employees who suffer work-related injuries, including TBI.[14] Legal professionals may help individuals navigate the workers' compensation process and ensure they receive the appropriate benefits.
- Civil Court vs. Workers' Compensation: Determining whether to pursue a TBI case in civil court or through workers' compensation depends on the specific circumstances of the injury. Civil court cases often result in higher potential compensation but require establishing fault. Workers' compensation claims are generally less adversarial but may not cover noneconomic damages.

Medical Evidence Legal Issues in Traumatic Brain Injury Cases

Medical evidence plays a crucial role in traumatic brain injury (TBI) cases. Medical evidence is the backbone of evaluating TBI cases, and serves to help establish the reasonable medical probability of the diagnosis, causation, damages, and long-term effects of the injury. It is crucial for both plaintiffs and defendants to understand and effectively use medical evidence to advocate for their legal positions and ensure that TBI survivors receive fair compensation and appropriate medical care.[15] Gathering, presenting, and interpreting medical evidence is essential for both plaintiffs and defendants in TBI litigation, and often relies on a knowledgeable treating physician, and possibly an expert medical witness. Here is an overview of the significance of medical evidence in TBI cases.

- Establishing Diagnosis: Medical evidence, such as diagnostic imaging (CT scans, MRIs) and medical treatment records, is fundamental in confirming the diagnosis of TBI. It often provides objective and clinical proof that a brain injury occurred.
- Documenting Symptoms: Medical records and the testimony of health care professionals help document the symptoms experienced by the TBI survivor. This is critical for understanding the individual's pain and suffering, as well as the extent of their cognitive and physical impairments.
- Demonstrating Causation: Medical evidence is used to establish a clear link between the traumatic event (eg, a car accident, a fall, an assault) and the TBI. It helps demonstrate that the injury was a direct result of the defendant's actions or negligence.
- Assessing Damages: Medical evidence assists in calculating economic damages, such as medical expenses, lost wages, and future health care costs. It provides a basis for determining the financial impact of the TBI on the survivor and their family.

Types of Medical Evidence: there are various types of medical information that can be considered as crucial for the assessment of traumatic brain injuries. These include.

1. Medical Records: These include hospital records, physician notes, radiology reports, and therapy reports, which provide a detailed account of the medical care received.
2. Diagnostic Imaging: CT scans and MRIs offer visual evidence of the brain's structural changes or abnormalities caused by the TBI.
3. Neuropsychological Testing: Cognitive assessments, such as memory tests and psychological evaluations, can provide objective evidence of cognitive impairments resulting from the TBI.
4. Physical and Occupational Therapy Reports: These documents detail the patient's progress and limitations in regaining physical and cognitive function.
5. Vocational Assessments: For severe TBI cases, vocational assessments, usually done by vocational rehabilitation professionals, may be used to evaluate the individual's ability to work and earn a living postinjury.

Challenges in Gathering and Presenting Medical Evidence: as a medical-legal case comes together, there may be some pitfalls noted while reviewing the medical information. These can include.

1. Credibility and Bias: The credibility of medical professionals and the potential for bias can be issues raised during litigation, especially concerning the interpretation of medical treatment by those involved in the case.
2. Interpretation of Test Results: Complex medical tests and reports may require expert interpretation to explain their significance to the court.
3. Confidentiality and Privacy: Adhering to privacy and confidentiality regulations while disclosing medical records is essential.
4. Insurance Company Involvement: Insurance companies may dispute the medical evidence to limit their liability.
5. Pre-existing Conditions: Medical evidence must differentiate between pre-existing conditions and injuries resulting from the traumatic event, and whether there was any permanent worsening of the pre-existing condition.

Expert Witnesses in Traumatic Brain Injury Litigation

Expert witnesses, often medical professionals with specialized knowledge in TBI, provide critical testimony in court about the medical aspects of the case. Medical clinicians, including physiatrists, neurologists, neuropsychologists, and vocational rehabilitation specialists, are often called as expert witnesses.[16] They provide professional opinions on the TBI's causation, prognosis, and the required medical care and rehabilitation. These expert witnesses may or may not have performed an independent medical examination of the patient in question, but will often review the medical records and any legal testimony of the case. There is usually significant preparation time by the expert witness prior to any court deposition or testimony. Expert witnesses may also review and/or create life-care plans, which are used to determine the total cost of future care for an injured patient.[17] Medical experts should consider any potential ethical concerns with their involvement in a particular case.[18]

Traumatic Brain Injury Compensation and Damages

Compensation and damages in traumatic brain injury (TBI) cases are a critical aspects of legal proceedings. TBI survivors and their families often seek compensation to cover the costs of medical treatment, rehabilitation, lost income, and other losses resulting from the injury. Understanding the types of compensation and how damages are calculated is essential. Compensation and damages in TBI cases encompass economic, noneconomic, and, in rare cases, punitive damages.[19] Calculating these damages involves a combination of objective evidence (such as medical bills and lost wages) and subjective assessments (such as pain and suffering). Legal professionals and expert witnesses play a crucial role in presenting a comprehensive case for the fair compensation of TBI survivors and their families.

- Economic Damages
  - Medical Expenses: This includes the cost of emergency care, hospitalization, surgeries, medications, therapy, and assistive devices. Calculating medical expenses typically involves gathering evidence of past medical bills and obtaining expert opinions on future costs. Lost wages can be calculated based on the individual's pre-injury income, the time missed from work, and the estimated impact on future earning capacity.
  - Future Medical Costs: Damages may cover the estimated costs of ongoing medical care, rehabilitation, therapy, and necessary accommodations.
  - Lost Wages: Economic damages account for the income lost due to the TBI, including time off work, reduced earning capacity, or the inability to return to work.
- Non-Economic Damages
  - Pain and Suffering: These damages compensate TBI survivors for the physical pain, emotional distress, and loss of enjoyment of life resulting from the injury.
  - Loss of Consortium: Spouses or family members may be eligible for compensation if they have lost the companionship, care, or intimacy of the TBI survivor.
  - Loss of Quality of Life: Non-economic damages can address the impact of the TBI on the individual's overall quality of life, including mental and emotional well-being.
  - Determining non-economic damages such as pain and suffering can be challenging. These damages are often subjective and may involve expert testimony, psychological evaluations, and a review of the individual's mental and emotional state before and after the TBI. Loss of consortium and quality of life are typically assessed based on the specific impact of the TBI on the individual's relationships and daily life.

- Punitive Damages
  - In extreme cases of misconduct or recklessness, punitive damages may be awarded to punish the defendant and deter similar behavior in the future. Punitive damages are not common in TBI cases but may be considered in cases of gross negligence or intentional harm. The awarding of punitive damages is less common in TBI cases. To justify punitive damages, plaintiffs need to demonstrate that the defendant's actions were malicious, intentional, or exhibited a reckless disregard for safety. Courts consider the defendant's financial situation and the degree of misconduct when determining punitive damages.

Challenges in calculating damages

1. Proving Noneconomic Damages: Calculating noneconomic damages such as pain and suffering is challenging as they involve intangible losses. Expert witnesses and psychological evaluations may be required.
2. Long-Term Prognosis: Determining the future costs of medical care and lost earning capacity can be challenging, especially in severe TBI cases whereby the prognosis is uncertain.
3. Comparative Negligence: If the plaintiff contributed to the accident in any way, this can impact the final damages awarded. Some jurisdictions follow comparative negligence laws, which reduce damages in proportion to the plaintiff's level of fault.
4. Insurance Coverage Limits: In cases involving insurance companies, there may be limits on the amount of compensation available, and the defendant's financial resources may affect the final award.

Recent Legal Trends and Case Studies

Recent legal trends and case studies in traumatic brain injury (TBI) litigation reflect evolving standards and the application of the law to address the complex issues surrounding TBI. These trends and cases offer insights into legal developments and highlight the significance of medical-legal issues in TBI cases. Here are some recent legal trends and notable case studies.

LEGAL TRENDS

1. Focus on Concussions in Youth Sports, Collegiate, and Professional Sports
   - Recent legal trends have seen an increased focus on sports-related concussions, particularly in professional, collegiate, and amateur sports. High-profile lawsuits have been filed against sports organizations, towns and coaches, alleging negligence in managing and preventing concussions, leading to more stringent concussion protocols and greater awareness of TBI risks in sports.[20] Legal trends reflect a growing awareness of TBI risks among young athletes and students. All states have implemented laws requiring concussion protocols in schools and youth sports, as noted in the 'Heads Up' campaign from the Centers for Disease Control, with potential legal repercussions for institutions failing to comply.[21] Lawsuits have been filed against youth soccer organizations, claiming that they failed to adequately address concussions and protect young players. These cases highlight the increasing scrutiny of concussion protocols in youth sports and the focus on improving safety measures for young athletes.
   - The National Collegiate Athletic Association has also improved its focus on athlete concussion awareness and safety practices at all Divisions within the NCAA, with the creation of the Concussion Safety Protocol Checklist. Policies

and procedures for concussion and TBI assessment, management, and prevention have been updated in the last decade to improve player safety.[22]
- Several high-profile lawsuits in professional sports have focused on the long-term consequences of concussions. Settlements and legal actions in these cases have raised awareness about the need for improved player safety measures. The National Football League (NFL) faced a class-action lawsuit brought by former players who alleged that the league failed to protect them from the long-term consequences of concussions. The case resulted in a landmark settlement in 2013 of approximately $1 Billion, requiring the NFL to compensate affected players and fund medical research into brain injuries.[23]

2. Military and Traumatic Brain Injury
   - Lawsuits and legal actions involving TBI in military personnel have gained attention, particularly in cases related to blast injuries and post-traumatic stress disorder (PTSD). Recent studies have shown a high prevalence of TBI cases in military personnel, including those with multiple head injuries.[24] These cases have prompted discussions about military responsibility and the long-term consequences of TBI on veterans. Legal actions related to blast injuries and TBI in military personnel have resulted in compensation for affected veterans, included a recent settlement of a class-action lawsuit by the United States Army, concerning Other Than Honorable ('OTH') discharges for thousands of soldiers who suffered various conditions, including traumatic brain injuries, during military operations in Iraq and Afghanistan.[25] These cases raise awareness about the unique challenges and consequences of TBI in military settings.

3. Workers' Compensation and Occupational TBI:
   - Cases involving TBI in the workplace have prompted discussions about workers' compensation claims and employer responsibility for safety. Legal trends may involve a focus on improving workplace safety measures to prevent TBI. Cases involving mild TBI in the workplace have underscored the importance of recognizing and addressing less severe TBIs. Legal actions have prompted discussions about workers' compensation and employer liability.[26]

These legal trends and case studies emphasize the evolving legal landscape in TBI litigation, including a growing awareness of the long-term consequences of TBI, an increased focus on prevention and safety, and the need for compensation and support for TBI survivors. As legal standards and public understanding of TBI continue to evolve, medical and legal professionals and advocacy groups play a crucial role in driving these changes.

Ethical Considerations in Traumatic Brain Injury Cases

Ethical considerations play a crucial role in traumatic brain injury (TBI) cases, especially those with severe TBI, affecting the behavior and decisions of all parties involved, including health care professionals, legal professionals, and TBI survivors and their families. These ethical considerations are integral to ensuring that the rights, well-being, and dignity of TBI survivors are respected throughout the legal and medical processes.[27] Here are some key ethical considerations in TBI cases.

Informed consent
In the medical context, obtaining informed consent from TBI survivors is essential. Individuals and/or their guardians must understand the proposed treatments, potential risks, and available alternatives before making decisions about their care. Ensuring that patients with cognitive impairments due to TBI can provide informed consent is

an ethical challenge. In such cases, proxy decision-makers may be involved, and their decisions should align with the patient's best interests.

Truthfulness and honesty
Medical professionals and legal representatives have an ethical obligation to provide truthful and honest information to TBI survivors and their families. This includes providing accurate information about the diagnosis, prognosis, treatment options, and the potential long-term consequences of TBI.

Confidentiality
Protecting the privacy and confidentiality of TBI survivors' medical and legal information is paramount. Health care providers and legal professionals should ensure that sensitive medical and legal records are safeguarded and only disclosed with proper consent or in compliance with relevant laws.

Competence and diligence
Health care professionals must provide competent care for TBI survivors, adhering to established medical standards. Legal professionals must diligently represent their clients, advocating for their best interests and legal rights.

Advocacy for the vulnerable
TBI survivors may be particularly vulnerable, especially if they have severe cognitive impairments or communication difficulties. Ethical considerations require that health care professionals, legal representatives, and family members advocate for the best interests of the survivor when they cannot advocate for themselves.

Balancing legal and medical concerns
Ethical dilemmas can arise when legal and medical concerns conflict. For example, a TBI survivor's desire to participate in a lawsuit might conflict with their medical best interests. Recent studies have shown that traumatic brain injury may be a potential risk factor for criminal activity.[28] Achieving a balance between legal rights and medical well-being requires open communication, ethical reflection, and shared decision-making. Some medical professionals may have a better understanding of the legal system, and some legal professionals develop a better understanding of the medical system through their career path and client representation. Traumatic brain injury has been shown to be a potential risk factor in violent crime activity.

Quality of life and dignity
Maintaining a focus on the TBI survivor's quality of life and preserving their dignity is a paramount ethical consideration. Decision-making should take into account the individual's values, goals, and preferences, even if they have cognitive impairments.

End-of-life and palliative care
In severe TBI cases, discussions about end-of-life care, including do-not-resuscitate orders and palliative care, are ethically complex. Health care professionals and legal representatives must engage in sensitive conversations and respect the values and wishes of the TBI survivor and their family. Encouraging TBI survivors to create advance directives or living wills that outline their preferences for medical care in case they become unable to make decisions is an ethical consideration. Respecting these directives is essential, even if they limit the scope of medical interventions.

Cultural competence and diversity
Recognizing and respecting the cultural, religious, and personal beliefs of TBI survivors and their families is an ethical imperative. Health care and legal professionals

should provide culturally competent care and consider diverse perspectives in decision-making.

Guardianship and legal capacity

When TBI survivors lack legal capacity, ethical questions arise about guardianship and decision-making on their behalf. Legal professionals and courts must act in the best interests of the survivor and ensure that their rights are protected, while medical professionals must respect the decisions of the guardians of their patients with TBI in cases where the patient no longer has the decision-making capacity for medical issues. These ethical considerations involve navigating complex medical and legal decisions, respecting individual autonomy and dignity, and advocating for the best interests of the TBI survivor.[29] Ethical conduct by health care and legal professionals is essential in upholding the principles of beneficence, autonomy, and justice in the care and representation of individuals affected by TBI.

SUMMARY

In conclusion, there are many issues to consider in the medical-legal context of traumatic brain injuries. A proper understanding of the medical definitions, complications, and ethical issues in the TBI population is crucial for any health professional that will be treating these patients. Since many TBI cases will at some point likely have some type of legal involvement, knowledge of the legal aspects of TBI cases will assist the medical professional in being able to advocate for their patients who may have to be involved with this medical-legal process. Recent events in the sports-related concussion legal arena have shown that ongoing expertise in dealing with medical-legal parameters will be of value in future TBI litigation cases.

CLINICS CARE POINTS

- Understand the classification and severity of traumatic brain injury (TBI).
- Be familiar with the medical aspects of TBI care, including assessment, diagnosis, treatment, rehabilitation, and long term recovery issues.
- Recognize the legal aspects of traumatic brain injury cases, including economic damages and compensation, medical-legal expert testimony, recent case law decisions, and ethical considerations.

DISCLOSURE

The author has nothing to disclose.

REFERENCES

1. Bayen E, Ruet A, Jourdan C, et al. Lawsuit and Traumatic Brain Injury: The Relationship Between Long-Lasting Sequelae and Financial Compensation in Litigants. Results From the PariS-TBI Study. Front Neurol 2019;10:320. Available at: https://www.ncbi.nlm.nih.gov/pmc/articles/PMC6473085/.
2. Available at: https://www.ninds.nih.gov/health-information/disorders/traumatic-brain-injury-tbi. Accessed November 28, 2023.
3. Available at: https://www.cdc.gov/traumaticbraininjury/health-disparities-tbi.html. Accessed October 19, 2023.

4. Available at: https://www.mayoclinic.org/diseases-conditions/traumatic-brain-injury/symptoms-causes/syc-20378557. Accessed February 4, 2021.

5. Available at: https://bestpractice.bmj.com/topics/en-us/515. Accessed July 11, 2023.

6. Scorza KA, Cole W. Current Concepts in Concussion: Initial Evaluation and Management. Am Fam Physician 2019;99(7):426–34. Available at: https://www.aafp.org/pubs/afp/issues/2019/0401/p426.html.

7. Available at: https://www.nichd.nih.gov/health/topics/tbi/conditioninfo/symptoms. Accessed November 24, 2020.

8. Available at: https://my.clevelandclinic.org/health/diseases/8874-traumatic-brain-injury. Accessed January 25, 2024.

9. Jha S, Ghewade P. Management and Treatment of Traumatic Brain Injuries. Cureus 2022;14(10):e30617. Available at: https://www.ncbi.nlm.nih.gov/pmc/articles/PMC9681696/.

10. Bramlett H, Dietrich WD. Long-Term Consequences of Traumatic Brain Injury: Current Status of Potential Mechanisms of Injury and Neurological Outcomes. J Neurotrauma 2015;32(23):1834–48. Available at: https://www.ncbi.nlm.nih.gov/pmc/articles/PMC4677116/.

11. Herbert DL. Medical-Legal Issues of Mild Traumatic Brain Injury. Curr Sports Med Rep 2007;6(1):20–4. Available at: https://journals.lww.com/acsm-csmr/fulltext/2007/02000/medical_legal_issues_of_mild_traumatic_brain.7.aspx.

12. Hawley L, Hammond FM, Cogan AM, et al. Ethical Considerations in Chronic Brain Injury. J Head Trauma Rehabil 2019;34(6):433–6. Available at: https://www.ncbi.nlm.nih.gov/pmc/articles/PMC6986275/.

13. Gao S, Kumar RG, Wisniewski SR, et al. Disparities in health care utilization of adults with traumatic brain injuries are related to insurance, race and ethnicity: A systematic review. J Head Trauma Rehabil 2018;33(3):E40–50. Available at: https://www.ncbi.nlm.nih.gov/pmc/articles/PMC5857393/.

14. Konda S, Al-Tarawneh IS, Reichard AA, et al. Workers' compensation claims for traumatic brain injuries among private employers– Ohio, 2001–2011. Am J Ind Med 2020;63(2):156–69. Available at: https://www.ncbi.nlm.nih.gov/pmc/articles/PMC10088096/.

15. Kaufman N, Bush SS, Aguilar MR. What Attorneys and Factfinders Need to Know About Mild Traumatic Brain Injuries. Psychological Injury and Law 2019;ume 12: 91–112. Available at: https://link.springer.com/article/10.1007/s12207-019-09355-9.

16. Zasler ND, Bigler E. Medicolegal Issues in Traumatic Brain Injury. Phys Med Rehabil Clin 2017 May;28(2):379–91. Available at: https://pubmed.ncbi.nlm.nih.gov/28390520/.

17. Zasler ND, Ameis A, Riddick-Grisham SN. Life care planning after traumatic brain injury. Phys Med Rehabil Clin 2013;24(3):445–65. Available at: https://pubmed.ncbi.nlm.nih.gov/23910485/.

18. Kass JS, Rose RV. Ethical challenges for the medical expert witness. AMA Journal of Ethics; 2016. Available at: https://journalofethics.ama-assn.org/article/ethical-challenges-medical-expert-witness/2016-03.

19. Available at: https://www.biausa.org/public-affairs/media/should-i-accept-a-traumatic-brain-injury-settlement. Accessed January 1, 2024.

20. Bell JM, Master CL, Lionbarger MR. The Clinical Implications of Youth Sports Concussion Laws: A Review. Am J Lifestyle Med 2019;13(2):172–81. Available at: https://www.ncbi.nlm.nih.gov/pmc/articles/PMC6378501/.

21. Available at: https://www.cdc.gov/headsup/policy/index.html. Accessed February 25, 2022.

22. Available at: https://www.ncaa.org/sports/2016/7/20/concussion-safety-protocol-management.aspx. Accessed January 15, 2024.

23. Available at: https://www.nfl.com/news/nfl-ex-players-agree-to-765m-settlement-in-concussions-suit-0ap1000000235494. Accessed August 29, 2013.

24. Lindquist LK, Love HC, Elbogen EB. Traumatic Brain Injury in Iraq and Afghanistan Veterans: New Results from a National Random Sample Study. J Neuropsychiatry Clin Neurosci 2017;29(3):254–9. Available at: https://www.ncbi.nlm.nih.gov/pmc/articles/PMC5501743/.

25. Available at: https://www.kennedysettlement.com/. Accessed January 1, 2024.

26. Chang VC, Guerriero EN, Colantonio A. Epidemiology of work-related traumatic brain injury: A systematic review. Am J Ind Med 2015;58:353–77. Available at: https://onlinelibrary.wiley.com/doi/abs/10.1002/ajim.22418.

27. Ezer T, Wright MS, Fins JJ. The Neglect of Persons with Severe Brain Injury in the United States: An International Human Rights Analysis. Health Hum Rights 2020; 22(1):265–78.

28. Williams WH, Chitsabesan P, Fazel S, et al. Traumatic brain injury: a potential cause of violent crime? Lancet Psychiatr 2018 Oct;5(10):836–44. Available at: https://www.ncbi.nlm.nih.gov/pmc/articles/PMC6171742/.

29. Anderson TP, Fearey MS. Legal guardianship in traumatic brain injury rehabilitation: Ethical implications. J Head Trauma Rehabil 1989;4(1):57–64. Available at: https://psycnet.apa.org/record/1989-27251-001.

Printed and bound by CPI Group (UK) Ltd, Croydon, CR0 4YY

14/10/2024

01774104-0001